T0202401

The Mismatch negativity (MMN)

The Mismatch negativity (MMN)
A window to the brain

Risto Näätänen
Professor Em. of Psychology
University of Helsinki, Finland
Professor of Cognitive Neurosciences,
Department of Psychology, University of Tartu, Estonia

Teija Kujala
Professor of Psychology,
Cognitive Brain Research Unit, Department of Psychology and
Logopedics, Faculty of Medicine, University of Helsinki, Finland

Gregory Light
Professor of Psychiatry,
University of California, San Diego, USA

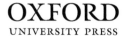

OXFORD
UNIVERSITY PRESS

OXFORD
UNIVERSITY PRESS

Great Clarendon Street, Oxford, OX2 6DP,
United Kingdom

Oxford University Press is a department of the University of Oxford.
It furthers the University's objective of excellence in research, scholarship,
and education by publishing worldwide. Oxford is a registered trade mark of
Oxford University Press in the UK and in certain other countries

Published in the United States of America by Oxford University Press
198 Madison Avenue, New York, NY 10016, United States of America

British Library Cataloguing in Publication Data
Data available

Library of Congress Control Number: Data available

ISBN 978-0-19-870507-9

Printed and bound by
CPI Group (UK) Ltd, Croydon, CR0 4YY

This book is dedicated to Professor Donald B. Lindsley, UCLA,
and to the MMN community.

Preface

In the 1960s, information processing theories were beginning to be applied to the study of cognition, with an emphasis on the conditions by which unattended information could reach consciousness and be acted on or stored for later processing. At the time, the brain was increasingly compared to a computer with subsystems in place for receiving external sensory stimuli, storing them in a buffer that would then undergo additional analysis in transient storage (e.g. RAM) for relevance and meaning, followed by intermediate steps that ultimately resulted in the transfer of information into longer-term storage (i.e. hard drive). The role of attention on sensory inputs was an area of particularly intensive debate with clever behavioural studies designed to parse the extent to which attended and unattended inputs become accessible to conscious, effortful processing. Behavioural studies alone, however, could not fully disentangle the rapid time course or neurophysiological substrates of the complex orchestration of the earliest stages of human information processing. It is in this context that a Finnish graduate student, Risto Näätänen, embarked upon a journey to the laboratory of Professor Donald Lindsley at the University of California at Los Angeles (UCLA) 1965–1966 to learn and conduct cognitive event-related potential studies. These early studies contributed to the genesis of a new field of study centered around the EEG measure, Mismatch Negativity (MMN), the topic of this book.

After completing his EEG studies at UCLA on an analog amplifier, Risto packed up his large bundle of recently collected paper-based EEG-recording plots and boarded a bus from Los Angeles to New York that was followed by a boat ride to Helsinki via London. On this trip, Näätänen prepared his doctoral-thesis work 'Selective Attention and Evoked Potentials', which he defended in the University of Helsinki in 1967. Näätänen's findings, published in the *Annales Academiae Scientiarum Fennicae*, identified critical experimental design limitations of previous ERP studies of the role of attention and perception. One such commonly used, but suboptimal design feature of the time, was the reliance on a fixed, predictable sequence of stimuli that fundamentally confounded the interpretation of results.

Inspired by Näätänen's 1967 thesis work, a separate thread of investigation was taking place in the laboratory of Steven Hillyard at the University of California, San Diego. Hillyard attempted to overcome the previous limitations noted in other studies by using unpredictable stimulus sequences in an active auditory oddball task. Armed with the improved methodology, Hillyard's early studies assessed the extent to which attention could modulate early sensory evoked potentials (i.e. N100), resulting in his seminal 1975 *Science* publication. Concurrently in 1975, at the age of 36 and with a career total of 13 academic publications, Näätänen continued his ERP studies at the Institute for Perception in the Netherlands where he, together with Anthony Gaillard and Sirkka Mäntysalo, conducted the experimental studies that that aimed to determine whether there is evidence of 'preattentive' or preconscious processing of unattended sounds in the brain potentials. This published work called for a reinterpretation of Hillyard's early selective attention effect and served as the basis for the discovery of Mismatch Negativity (MMN; Näätänen, Gaillard & Mäntysalo, *Acta Psychologica.*, 1978). Näätänen and colleagues observed 'a negative shift superimposed on the EP waveform, herein called "mismatch negativity," [that] can be observed when a deviating stimulus is delivered among much more numerous "standard" stimuli.' They went on the note that this 'reflects specific auditory stimulus-discrimination processes ... suggested to be largely automatic, beyond the control of will, instructions, etc ... '

Hillyard and Näätänen continued their collegial scientific debate over the role of preattentive vs attention-dependent processing on early evoked potential components. Ultimately, thousands of studies convincingly demonstrated that both were correct—there are both selective attention effects on early evoked potentials as well as evidence of preattentive processing that occurs in the brain outside of conscious awareness.

From these modest, and somewhat contentious beginnings, the study of MMN extended beyond their relatively circumscribed laboratories in Scandinavia and Southern California. On the 40th anniversary celebration of the discovery of MMN at the University of Helsinki, it was pointed out that there have been approximately 5000 scientific reports with mismatch negativity as a key topic with studies conducted in nearly 70 countries and published in at least 11 different languages. Cumulatively, these MMN papers have been cited over 145,000 times in more than 44,000 citing articles. On average, each MMN paper is cited ~30 times and there are now more than 150 MMN papers that have each been cited at least 150 times. These papers are primarily within the fields of neuroscience, psychology, and psychiatry, but also extend to seemingly distant fields such as electrical engineering, artificial intelligence, and veterinary science.

It is important to note that the rise of MMN was neither immediate nor possible without the tireless efforts of many early adopters of the work. In the early years of this work, only basic science research questions of cognitive neuroscience such as the nature of sound discrimination and role of sensory memory in normal cognition were addressed. It was eventually determined that this tool could also be used for the understanding of normal as well as impaired neural systems that underlie, for example, neurodevelopmental and neuropsychiatric disorders. In fact, from Näätänen's own humble discovery of mismatch negativity now 40 years ago, he has amassed over 400 publications, including 125 articles that have each been cited at least 125 times and obviously stimulated the work of countless scientists as evidenced by the 20th year anniversary of the formation of the International Congress on MMN—a rare international conference dedicated to the many applications of a measure as opposed to a disorder or a discipline.

There has been a remarkable growth of research in the use of MMN that spans a wide range of basic and clinical science applications. MMN has already profoundly contributed to theories of hearing, language acquisition, and cognitive development. In the 5-year period from 2012 to 2017 while this book was being written, an average of over 300 new MMN articles were added to the scientific literature *each year*. While this book attempts to cover some of the trends in MMN research over the past 40 years, it is admittedly not a comprehensive review of the many applications of this fundamental tool of neuroscience. Instead, a heavier emphasis is provided on how MMN can contribute to our understanding of neurodevelopmental, psychiatric, and neurodegenerative disorders. As a translational tool that can be used in contexts ranging from preclinical animal studies to human studies conducted in non-specialty clinical treatment centres, MMN shows tremendous promise for accelerating the pace of development of new therapeutics for disorders of the central nervous system. In this context, MMN is viewed as a 'breakthrough biomarker,' but it has not yet graduated from the confines of specialized academic laboratories to widespread use in real world clinical settings.

The authors of this book humbly thank those pioneering researchers over the past four decades as well as the early career trainees/investigators who are just now beginning to embark upon their own journeys with the study of MMN. From the careful visual inspection of paper plots on cross-country greyhound buses and transatlantic boats that started this new field of study, cloud computing, video conferencing, and big data analytics are bringing together investigators from around the world and revealing the clues hidden in neurophysiological datasets at an unparalleled rate of discovery. We eagerly anticipate what new discoveries and applications will develop over the next 40 years of study.

Risto Näätänen
Teija Kujala
Gregory Light
July 2018

Acknowledgements

Risto Näätänen wishes to acknowledge the support of Professor Leif Östergaard, the Head of the Center of Cognitive Neuroscience of the University of Århus, where the book project was initiated, and that of Professor Juri Allik, Department of Psychology, the University of Tartu, Tartu, Estonia, where the book project continued. Also, he and Teija Kujala wish to acknowledge their original home institute, the Cognitive Brain Research Unit (CBRU), which is currently at the Department of Psychology and Logopedics, Faculty of Medicine of the University of Helsinki, Helsinki, Finland for continued support throughout this book project and before. Gregory Light wishes to acknowledge his colleagues Professors David Braff and Neal Swerdlow for their mentorship and pioneering neurophysiological studies of neuropsychiatric patient populations. The authors are grateful for the financial support of the Academy of Finland, Jane and Aatos Erkko foundation, the National Institute of Mental Health, the Brain and Behavior Research Foundation, and the Sidney R. Baer, Jr. Foundation. They also warmly thank Nella Moisseinen, Peter Palo-oja, Sanna Talola, Heidi Juntunen, Anastasia Gallen, Joyce Sprock, Melissa Tarasenko, and Aria Nisco for their help in editing the book.

Contents

List of abbreviations

AD	Alzheimer's disease	ERP	Event-related potential
aMCI	Amnestic MCI	EP	Evoked potential
ALS	Amyotrophic lateral sclerosis	eLORETA	Exact Low Resolution Electromagnetic Tomography
AS	Asperger syndrome	FM	Fibromyalgia
ARMS	At-Risk Mental States criteria	fMMN	Frequency-MMN
ADHD	Attention deficit and hyperactivity disorder	fMRI	Functional magnetic resonance imaging
ACT	Auditory consonant trigrams	GCS	Glasgow Coma Scale
ASD	Autism spectrum disorders	HA	Harm-avoidance
ANS	Autonomic nervous system	HSE	Herpes simplex encephalitis
BIS	Behavioral inhibition system	HD	Huntington's disease
BECTS	Benign Epilepsy with Centro-Temporal Spikes	IQ	Intelligence quotient
BD	Bipolar Disorder	ISI	Inter-stimulus interval
BAC	Blood alcohol content	ITI	Inter-train interval
BPRS	Brief Psychiatric Rating Scale	LKS	Landau-Kleffner syndrome
CNS	Central nervous system	LDN	Late differentiating negativity
CSF	Cerebrospinal fluid	LC	Locus coeruleus
CL/A	Cleft lip with or without a defect in the alveolar arch	LTM	Long-term memory
		LTP	Long-term potentiation
CP	Cleft of palate	MMNm	Magnetic equivalent of MMN
CLP	Cleft of the lip and palate	mGFP	Magnetic local field power
CPO	Clefts of the soft palates only	MRI	Magnetic resonance imaging
CHR	Clinical high-risk	MEG	Magnetoencephalography
CHI	Closed-head Injury	MDD	Major Depressive Disorder
CI	Cochlear implants	MTLE	Mesial temporal-lobe epilepsy
CSWS	Continuous spikes and waves during slow-wave sleep	MLR	Middle-latency responses
		MCI	Mild Cognitive Impairment
COPS	Criteria of Prodromal Syndromes	MCS	Minimally conscious state
DBS	Deep brain stimulation	MMSE	Mini-Mental State Examination
DLB	Dementia with Lewy bodies	MMN	Mismatch negativity
DAI	Diffuse axonal injury	MMR	Mismatch response
DA	Dopamine	MMNi	Integrated MMN
dMMN	Duration-MMN	MS	Multiple sclerosis
DUP	Durations of untreated psychosis	NAC	N-acetyl-cysteine
DCM	Dynamic Causal Modeling	NMDAR	N-methyl-D-aspartate glutamate receptors
EDN	Early discriminative negativity		
ERAN	Early right anterior negativity	NES	Non-epileptic seizures
ECD	Equivalent current dipole	NE	Norepinephrine

NH	Normal hearing	sMMN	Somatosensory MMN
oMMN	Olfactory MMN	SPL	Sound pressure level
OI	Optical imaging	SLI	Specific language impairment
PD	Parkinson's disease	STWI	Spectro-temporal window of integration
PDD	Parkinson's disease dementia		
PIQ	Performance IQ	SOA	Stimulus onset asynchrony
PVS	Persistent vegetative state	STN	Subthalamic nuclei
PACT	Pharmacologic augmentation of cognitive training	TCT	Targeted Cognitive Training
		TWI	Temporal Window of Integration
PET	Positron-emission tomography		
PTSD	Post-traumatic Stress Disorder	TLE	Temporal-lobe epilepsy
A1	Primary auditory cortex	HCS	The Halifax Consciousness Scanner
PN	Processing negativity		
PWD	Pure Word Deafness	MMP	Mismatch positivity
REM	Rapid eye movement	TCI	Temperament and character inventory
RT	Reaction time		
rCBF	Regional cerebral blood flow	TPD	Two-point discrimination
RON	Re-orienting negativity	VNS	Vagal nerve stimulation
BSE-R	Revised Behavior Summarized Evaluation Scale	VS	Vegetative state
		VIQ	Verbal IQ
SCD	Scalp current density analysis	vMMN	Visual MMN
SZ	Schizophrenia	WMS	Wechsler Memory Scale

Chapter 1

The mismatch negativity (MMN): An introduction

1.1 Introduction

This book introduces the electrophysiological change detection response called the mismatch negativity (MMN) and its magnetoencephalographic (MEG) equivalent MMNm, together with their different clinical applications. MMN/MMNm is elicited by any discriminable change in auditory stimulation occurring within the time span of sensory memory, even in the absence of attention and task performance. An analogous response can be recorded in the other sensory modalities: visual MMN (vMMN), somatosensory MMN (sMMN), and olfactory MMN (oMMN). MMN has opened an unprecedented window to central auditory processing and the underlying neurophysiology affected in different cognitive brain disorders. MMN in audition enables one to reach a new level of understanding of the brain processes forming the biological substrate of central auditory processing and the different forms of auditory memory, as well as the attentional processes controlling the access of sensory input to conscious perception and higher forms of memory. Most importantly, MMN provides an index of general brain plasticity (e.g. Näätänen & Kreegipuu, 2010), accounting for its very wide clinical perspective. Consistent with the wide range of clinical applications, MMN deficiency indexes cognitive and functional status in different neuropsychiatric, neurological, and neurodevelopmental brain disorders, irrespective of their specific aetiologies and the symptoms of the disorder (Baldeweg & Hirsch, 2015; Light et al., 2015; Näätänen, et al., 2011; 2012, 2014; Thomas et al., 2017).

1.2 What is MMN?

MMN (in audition) is a response of the brain to any discriminable change in the stream of auditory stimulation. Fig. 1.1 illustrates MMN to a minor frequency change in a simple repetitive 1000 Hz tone stimulus of 50 ms in duration ('standards') in subjects instructed to ignore all auditory stimulation and to read a book. Standards, delivered at a constant inter-stimulus interval (ISI) of 1 s, were occasionally and randomly interspersed with deviant stimuli (the proportion being 20% of the stimuli), of a slightly higher frequency (from 1004 to 1032 Hz, in separate stimulus blocks) but otherwise identical to the standards. The standards elicited a simple P1-N1-P2 waveform (Näätänen & Picton, 1987), whereas the deviants also elicited an additional, separate negative component at

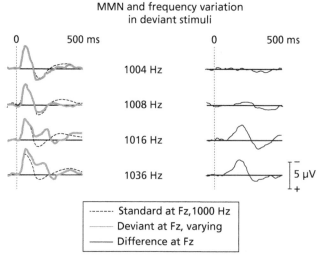

Fig. 1.1 MMN to tone-frequency changes (standards 1000 Hz, deviants 1004-1032 Hz in separate stimulus blocks). Left: Frontal event-related potentials to standard and deviant stimuli. Right: Difference waves, where the standard-stimulus ERP has been subtracted from the deviant-stimulus ERP. Difference wave highlights the MMN.

Data from Sams, M., Hämäläinen, M., Antervo, A., Kaukoranta, E., Reinikainen, K. & Hari, R., *Cerebral neuromagnetic responses evoked by short auditory stimuli*, Electroencephalography and clinical neurophysiology, 61 (4), 254–266, https://doi.org/10.1016/0168-5597(85)90054-1, 1985.

a latency range of 100–200 ms from stimulus onset visible in difference waves formed by subtracting the event-related potential (ERP) to the standards from that to the deviants. These difference waves display the quite surprising sensitivity of MMN, considering the fact that subjects were reading a book: MMN was in fact elicited at the same sensitivity as that shown by subjects behaviourally when they tried to discriminate deviants among standards in a corresponding behavioural discrimination task (Sams et al., 1985; Sculthorpe et al., 2008).

The change used to elicit MMN can also be abstract, such as a violation of regularity or a 'rule' obeyed by auditory stimulation (Carral et al., 2005a, 2005b). This more cognitive aspect of MMN, showing the presence of genuine cognitive processes of an automatic nature at the level of the sensory cortex, gave rise to the concept of 'Primitive Sensory Intelligence' (Näätänen et al., 2001; for reviews, see Bendixen et al., 2007, 2012; Näätänen et al., 2010). Currently, primitive sensory intelligence constitutes an intense focus in cognitive and neuropsychiatric research. Since MMN can be evoked by perceptual deviance as well as more abstract pattern violations, MMN is now commonly characterized as a regularity-violation response rather than just as a sound-change response.

To place MMN into a wider context, let us consider the main functions of the sensory systems. First, sensory systems develop representations of the environment, i.e. memory traces corresponding to the stimuli and their regularities, with perception occurring at the transient phase of the emergence of a memory trace. Secondly, the brain must continuously keep updating these representations to maintain their correspondence with the environment. It is here that MMN enters the picture: MMN generated by the auditory sensory-specific cortices is elicited by this updating process. Furthermore, this sensory change-detection signal has high priority access to the frontal mechanisms of attention control, explaining an involuntary attention switch to sensory change. Thirdly, the sensory systems also have a predictive, anticipatory function, based on the automatic detection of sequential and combinatory stimulus rules obeyed by the stimulus stream. Even this function, an expression of primitive sensory intelligence, is reflected by MMN generation.

1.3 **MMN: The original description**

MMN (Fig. 1.2) was discovered as late as the end of the 1970s (Näätänen et al., 1978) but nevertheless has emerged as one of the most intense research foci across multiple scientific fields, now with more than 4500 published journal articles published in at least 11 different languages. Articles listing 'mismatch negativity' as a keyword have amassed more than 125,000 citations. Moreover, eight major international congresses have already been dedicated to MMN and its different clinical and other applications. In the early years of MMN, however, the response was not so favourable. A neurophysiological measure presumed to reflect an automatic discrimination process between two very similar sounds occurring in the full absence of directed attention, and hence outside of our conscious mind, appeared neither plausible nor interesting. It was rather thought that

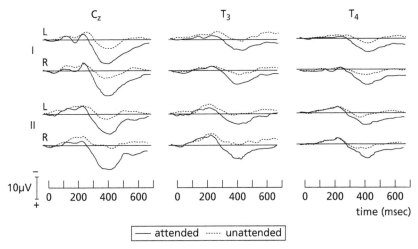

Fig. 1.2 The difference between ERPs to deviants and standards separately for the left (L) and right (R) ears when attended and when unattended. I refers to Experiment 1, where deviants were slightly louder than standards. II refers to Experiment 2, where deviants had a slightly higher pitch. Stimuli were presented randomly at either ear and subjects attended to one ear at a time. Reprinted from Acta Psychologica, 42(4), Näätänen, R., Gaillard, A.W. & Mäntysalo, S., *Early selective-attention effect on evoked potential reinterpreted*, 131–329, Copyright 1978, with permission from Elsevier.

such fine-grained discrimination could only occur when supported by attention and active voluntary effort. Therefore the main lecture hall of the 1983 Congress of Cognitive Event-Related Potentials in Florence was almost empty when MMN was introduced in one of the keynote addresses.

Secondly, in particular in active oddball paradigms, there is an overlap of a multitude of parallel ERP components, most remarkably so in the N2-P3 time zone. In fact, MMN was isolated from 'N2' and 'N2-P3a' wave complexes (Ford et al.1976a, 1976b; Simson et al., 1976, 1977; Snyder & Hillyard, 1976; Squires et al., 1975, 1976), typically elicited in oddball paradigms, by Näätänen et al. (1978; see also Näätänen 1975), through the analysis of deviant-standard difference waves. This resulted in division of N2 into an automatic MMN (N2a) and attention-dependent N2b (Näätänen & Gaillard, 1983; Näätänen & Michie 1979; Näätänen et al., 1978, 1982). N2b has a topography posterior to those of N1 and MMN and, together with the accompanying P3a, forms the N2-P3a or N2b-P3a complex. This complex is elicited by deviants when the stimulus sequence is attended or when there is an 'attention leak' to the to-be-ignored channel (Näätänen & Gaillard 1983). For an illustration of the different ERP components in ignore and attend conditions, see Fig. 1.3.

It is of utmost importance to make a clear distinction between deflections as measured in scalp ERPs (waves that can be directly seen in ERP waveforms) and their underlying components (contributions of separable brain processes, usually with different loci of origin and functional significances) to the total ERP waveform. According to Näätänen and Picton (1987), the evoked potential (EP) 'consists of a sequence of positive and negative waves or peaks'. Although these deflections in the waveform provide a convenient point for measurement, they are not necessarily generated by distinct cerebral events and generators. At any point in time, multiple cerebral processes may contribute to the EP waveform. In fact, scalp-recorded ERP waves represent a variable mixture of multiple brain and even non-brain (e.g. ocular or muscle artefacts) that summate to produce the peaks and valleys of the surface waveforms (Rissling et al., 2014). We thus define an EP 'component' as the contribution to the recorded waveform of a particular generator process, such as the activation of a localized area of cerebral cortex by a specific pattern of input. A component is therefore related to the 'source potential' defined by Scherg and von Cramon (1986) as 'the compound local activity of a circumscribed brain region'. Whereas the peaks or deflections of an EP can be directly measured from the averaged waveform, the components contributing to these peaks can usually be inferred only from the results of experimental manipulation or source decomposition using high-density recordings that are now more commonly used. Donchin et al. (1978) defined an ERP component as 'a source of controlled, observable variability'. Our definition is similar with respect to how the components are determined, but it limits the component by referring it back to a localized physiological activity (Näätänen and Picton (1987), p.376).

Interestingly, around the same time, an analogous division to automatic and controlled processing in visual search and other cognitive performance tasks was proposed by other researchers (Shiffrin & Schneider, 1977; Schneider & Shiffrin, 1977). Moreover,

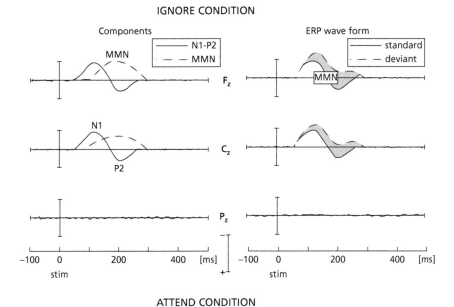

Fig. 1.3 A schematic illustration of ERP components elicited by standards and deviants in IGNORE (top) condition in which only obligatory ERP components are elicited by standard stimuli. In the ATTEND condition (bottom), the responses are overlapped by attention-dependent responses, such as N2b-P3a, P3, and a slow parietal positivity.

Reproduced from Näätänen, R., Kujala, T., and Winkler, I., *Auditory processing that leads to conscious perception: A unique window to central auditory processing opened by the mismatch negativity and related responses*, Psychophysiology, 48 (1), 4–22, Figure 1, DOI: 10.1111/j.1469-8986.2010.01114.x, Copyright © 2011, John Wiley and Sons.

even P3 was subjected to an analogous division when Squires et al. (1975) proposed that P3 is often composed of two separable components: the less attention-dependent P3a, with fronto-central scalp topography and shorter peak latency (220–250 ms), and the attention-dependent P3b, with a posterior topography and longer peak latency of around 300 ms.

1.4 **MMN as the first objective index of auditory discrimination**

Several early studies showed that from the sensitivity of MMN to small stimulus changes in passive recording conditions, with the subject attending, for instance, to a movie, one can predict his/her behavioural discrimination accuracy. Lang et al. (1990) found that the behavioural discrimination of a frequency difference between two successively presented tones strongly correlated with the MMN amplitude (recorded in a passive condition). Their subjects were high school pupils of 17 years of age. Three groups ('good', 'moderate', and 'poor') were formed based on their accuracy of behavioural pitch discrimination in a same–different task. In subsequent MMN recordings, the standard stimulus frequency was 698 Hz, whereas that of the deviant stimulus was different in different blocks. In the good behavioural discrimination group, MMN was elicited with a frequency deviation of 19 Hz or smaller. In contrast, with the poor performers, the frequency deviation had to be increased to 50–100 Hz until MMN was elicited. The mediocre performers took an intermediate position between the two extreme groups (Fig. 1.4). (For corroborating results, see Tiitinen et al. (1994)).

Consistent with these findings of relationships between active behavioural tasks of auditory discriminability and MMN, employing rhythmic stimulus patterns with an occasional order reversal of two tones belonging to such a pattern, Tervaniemi et al. (1997) found that subjects detecting these reversals in a behavioural discrimination task (a test of musical abilities) with a high accuracy had a considerably larger amplitude MMN elicited by order reversals in a passive condition than those with a poorer behavioural discrimination. Moreover, with MMN, one can monitor the progress of sound discrimination as a function of training/exposure. Näätänen et al. (1993), using a complex spectro-temporal stimulus pattern as their standard stimulus, found that subjects who were able to discriminate a slightly deviant pattern behaviourally showed MMN to this deviant stimulus pattern in a subsequent passive condition (Fig. 1.5). In contrast, no MMN was elicited in subjects who were not able to behaviourally discriminate stimuli in the preceding discrimination condition. However, after they learned to discriminate stimuli behaviourally, then MMN was elicited by the deviant patterns in the subsequent passive condition.

An equivalent training effect, but one with short (eight tone) melodies randomly occurring at 12 different frequency levels, with the deviant melodies having a slightly different contour than that of the standard melodies, was found by Tervaniemi et al. (2001), although in 'musical' subjects only. In 'non-musical' subjects, no MMN emerged at any phase of the experiment, and they never learned to discriminate deviants from standards.

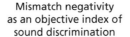

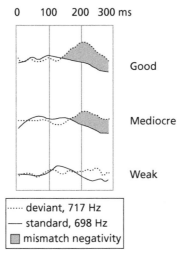

Data from Lang HA, Nyrke T, Ek M, Aaltonen O, Raimo I, Näätänen R., *Pitch discrimination performance and auditory event-related potentials*, Psychophysiological brain research, 1, 294–298, 1990.

Fig. 1.4 The mismatch negativity (MMN) serves as an objective index of sound discrimination accuracy. Some of the subjects were very good in behavioral tone discrimination and showed a large- amplitude MMN (blue in the figure) in a separate passive stimulus condition. Subjects with a less accurate pitch-discrimination ability showed a smaller-amplitude MMN, and subjects with weak behavioral discrimination ability showed no MMN in the passive condition (but started to disclose an MMN when frequency change was increased).

MMN and discrimination training

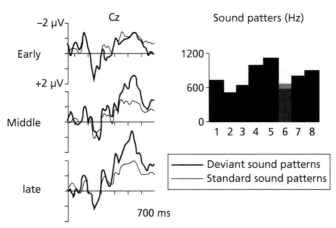

Fig. 1.5 Left: In subjects trying to learn to discriminate a minor change in a complex spectro-temporal stimulus pattern, no MMN is elicited in the early third of trials but an MMN is elicited in the middle third of trials, which is enhanced in amplitude in the late third of the trials. Consistently with this, the subjects' performance in a discrimination task, where they had to press button to each deviant stimulus, improved after each stage. Right: The standard and deviant sound patterns consisted of eight sinusoidal segments of different frequencies, their only difference being that in the deviant patterns, the frequency of the sixth segment (indicated by grey) was higher than that in the standard patterns.

Data from Näätänen, R., Schröger, E., Karakas S., Tervaniemi, M., & Paavilainen P., *Development of a memory trace for a complex sound in the human brain*, NeuroReport, 4, 503–506, http://dx.doi.org/10.1097/00001756-199305000-00010, 1993.

A discrimination-training effect with phonetic stimuli was found by Kraus et al. (1995a, 1995b) who used different variants of the /da/ syllable initially impossible for subjects to discriminate from one another. Importantly, the improved behavioural discrimination performance along with enhanced MMN amplitude was present even at one month after the end of the training.

Moreover, MMN also indexes the learning of the mother tongue speech sounds, being stronger in amplitude to native- than foreign-language phonemes (Fig. 1.6). MMN can also index memory representations of even larger linguistic units such as words (Pulvermüller et al., 2001). In addition, other aspects of language processing, besides phonetics and semantics, can be studied with MMN, for instance, syntactic processing (Pulvermüller & Shtyrov, 2006) and morphology (Leminen et al., 2013).

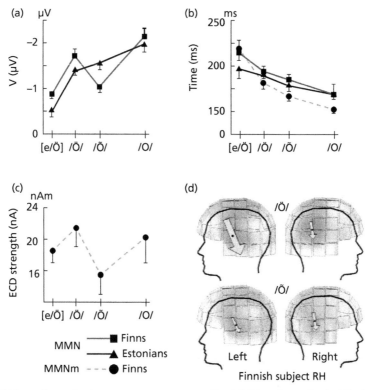

Fig. 1.6 Evidence for native-language memory traces. The MMN peak amplitude (**A**), the MMN and MMNm peak latencies (**B**), and equivalent current dipole (ECD) strengths (**C**) in Finns and Estonians for vowel changes. A drop in the magnitude of the MMN amplitude and MMNm ECD strength in Finns can be seen for vowel /õ/, which does not belong to the Finnish language. ECDs from a typical Finnish subject for deviants /ö/ (top) and /õ/ (bottom) (**D**), suggesting left-lateralized activation for the native /ö/ vowel.

Furthermore, learning a second language after childhood (Winkler et al., 1999; see also Tremblay et al., 1997, 1998) also caused an MMN-amplitude enhancement (for reviews, see Kraus & Cheour 2000; Näätänen, 2001). The standard stimulus was a vowel that is perceived as /e/ by both Finns and Hungarians, whereas the deviant stimulus was the Finnish /ä/ which in the Hungarian language (spoken in the Budapest region) belongs to the same phoneme category as /e/ used as the standard. It was found that Hungarians who knew no Finnish had no MMN to the deviant /ä/ in the ignore condition and were very poor in discriminating it behaviourally from /e/ (Fig. 1.7). In contrast, Hungarians who had lived in Finland for years and learned to speak fluent Finnish had a distinct MMN to /ä/, similar to that of native Finns, and were also able behaviourally to discriminate it from /e/. These results thus demonstrated the formation of new phoneme categories in Hungarian adults, with the original wide /e/ category (also incorporating /ä/) being divided into

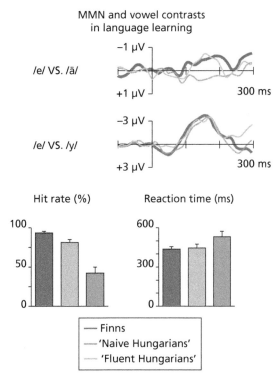

Fig. 1.7 MMN to vowel contrasts (top) and performance in a vowel identification task (bottom). No MMN was elicited in 'naïve' Hungarian subjects (no exposure to Finnish) by a deviant /ä/ when the standard was /e/ but in Hungarians who lived in Finland, a robust MMN was elicited by this contrast common in the Finnish but not in the Hungarian language. Hit rate and reaction-time data were consistent with these results. A sizable MMN was elicited in both subject groups by /y/ as a deviant, which is common in both languages.

Data from Winkler, I., Kujala, T., Tiitinen, H., Sivonen, P., Alku, P., Lehtokoski, A., Czigler, I., Csepe, V., Ilmoniemi, R.J. & Näätänen, R., *Brain responses reveal the learning of foreign language phonemes*, Psychophysiology, 36 (5), 638–642, 1999.

separate /e/ and /ä/ categories. Taken together, these results show that with MMN, one can monitor how the discrimination of foreign-language phonemes improves during learning new languages.

Importantly, Tremblay et al. (1998) found that MMN emerged before the improvement in the behavioural discrimination of the phoneme contrast used to train subjects could be detected. Moreover, Tremblay et al. (1997) found a transfer of a discrimination-training effect to an untrained discrimination. English-speaking adults were trained to discriminate and identify a voicing contrast not existing in English but being phonetically salient in Hindi. These subjects were trained to hear the distinction of voice onset time in a bilabial context, but were evaluated before and after training on their ability to discriminate and identify the voicing contrast, both in the bilabial (training condition) and alveolar context (transfer condition). After training, subjects could identify and discriminate both the training and transfer contrasts behaviourally. These effects were also manifested by increases in the MMN area and duration, which were more pronounced over the left than right frontal areas.

Most of the MMN studies with speech sounds used only one (acoustically constant) exemplar of each phonetic category included, even though when we hear speech in real life its acoustic properties are changing all the time, due to, for instance, prosodic variation. To address this issue, Shestakova et al. (2002) presented 150 different male voice exemplars of three different vowels (a, u, i) to adult Russian males in short sequences with continuously varying exemplars (standards), there being no break before the onset of a sequence of another vowel (e.g. five exemplars of /a/, followed by three exemplars of /u/, and these followed by four exemplars of /i/). Hence, the first stimulus of each sequence served as a deviant stimulus. An MMNm, lateralized to the left hemisphere, was elicited, suggesting that the central auditory system could extract the invariant phonetic features from the acoustically varying input (Fig. 1.8). This strong lateralization to the left hemisphere probably occurred because the acoustic MMNm component was omitted as there was no acoustically fixed standard (see also Jacobsen et al., 2004).

Obviously, this left-hemispheric phonetic MMNm depended on the presence of long-term memory traces for the mother tongue vowels which are able to recognize the invariant vowel-identity code amongst wide acoustic variation. This code must be identical, or roughly identical, in any sound perceived as, for instance, /e/ irrespective of whether it is uttered by a male, female, or child's voice. The core property of this phoneme-identity code hence must be its invariance in the midst of acoustical variation, suggesting that there must be neuronal populations which may detect such invariance. As this invariance cannot involve any level of an acoustical feature per se, it probably is of a relational nature, i.e. the phoneme identity would be based on certain fixed relations or ratios between the different levels of the acoustic features involved (Näätänen, 2001).

Neuronal populations which may underlie phoneme discrimination were found by Paavilainen et al. (1999). Their within-tone-pair frequency change was ascending both in

(a) Magnetic responses

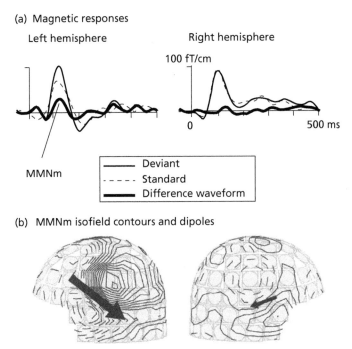

Fig. 1.8 Abstract phoneme representations in the left temporal cortex as shown by the MEG equivalent of the MMN in one, typical subject. The stimuli were each uttered by a different speaker and belonged to three different vowel categories. (a) MEG responses from one channel over the auditory cortex of each hemisphere. (b) MMNm isofield contour maps over each hemisphere. The arrows indicate the locations and orientations of the MMN equivalent current dipoles (ECD). The dashed lines represent the magnetic flux entering and solid lines exiting the head. The MMNm is markedly stronger in the left than in the right hemisphere.

Reproduced from Anna Shestakova, Elvira Brattico, Minna Huotilainen, Valery Galunov, Alexei Soloviev, Mikko Sams, Risto J. Ilmoniemi, and Risto Näätänen, *Abstract phoneme representations in the left temporal cortex: magnetic mismatch negativity study*, NeuroReport, 13 (14), p. 1814, Figure 2, http://journals.lww.com/neuroreport/Abstract/2002/10070/Abstract_phoneme_representations_in_the_left.25.aspx © 2002 Lippincott Williams.

the standard and deviant pairs. The standard pairs had a constant within-pair frequency ratio of five musical steps between the two tones, whereas the deviant pairs either had a larger (seven or eight steps) or smaller (two or three steps) within-pair frequency ratio. In addition, the stimulus pairs randomly varied over a wide frequency range. Nevertheless, MMN was elicited by deviant pairs. Moreover, an analogous result was obtained even when the two tones were simultaneously presented as a complex tone consisting of two different frequency components (with the frequency level of the stimuli again varying across an extensive range).

Consequently, MMN provides an objective means for assessing auditory discrimination and its improvement by exposure or training. Previously, in the absence of an attention or behavioural task, ERPs could index detection only, i.e. whether the central auditory system detected the presence of stimulus energy, but could not index whether sounds were also discriminated. (For the objective ERP audiometry, see Rapin et al., 1966). Hence, a person could have a 'normal' ERP response to auditory input but nevertheless did not understand speech in his/her mother tongue.

In recent years, the sensitivity of MMN to auditory system experience or training has assumed a role of great importance in neuropsychiatry. There is growing recognition that the cognitive impairments (e.g. verbal learning and memory) observed in many disorders (e.g. schizophrenia) are not fixed but may be ameliorated with cognitive exercises that target low-level auditory sensory processing. When measured at the group level, large effect size gains are evident in schizophrenia patients after 40 h of auditory system training. Response is variable, however, with 40–45% of patients showing no response to such time- and resource-intensive interventions. Perez and colleagues (2017) showed that MMN is malleable to even a 'single-dose' of auditory discrimination training and that pre-exposure MMN amplitude correlates with the amount of perceptual 'learning' that takes place during the initial hour of training. These results encourage the use of MMN as a leading candidate biomarker of auditory system 'target engagement' in auditory training that may be used to predict and monitor response to time- and resource-intensive cognitive training interventions (Light & Näätänen, 2013; Light & Swerdlow, 2015). MMN may thus be used to assign patients who are acutely sensitive to auditory system training to receive longer-term (and presumably therapeutic doses) of the exercises.

1.5 Which neurons generate MMN?

Recent studies found that MMN may, in fact, be preceded by change-detection responses of a very small amplitude within the first 50 ms from sound onset, i.e. at the latency range of the middle-latency responses (MLR) (for a review, see Grimm & Escera, 2012). Previous studies showed that MMN may commence at as early as 50 ms from stimulus onset (change in the spatial locus of sound origin; Paavilainen et al., 1989). The more recently described even earlier change-detection responses appeared either as enhancements of the MLRs (Sonnadara et al., 2006) or as an addition to a slower early shift of a short duration (Althen et al., 2011).

The type of neurons automatically responding to sound change by generating a change-detection signal reflected by MMN was hotly debated. The original interpretation (Näätänen & Michie, 1979; Näätänen et al., 1978) stressed the fact that MMN is generated by a genuine change-detection process using the memory trace representing the preceding stimuli (standards) as a reference. Standards automatically form (short-lived) neural sensory-memory representations for all the features of these stimuli, strengthened by subsequent stimulus repetitions, whereas deviant stimuli elicit a 'neuronal mismatch' response (cf. Sokolov 1963) generating the scalp-recorded MMN. On this view, MMN itself is not generated by afferent neurons but rather by a separate, memory-based, change-detection process, implicating the participation of memory neurons beyond the central afferent system (Bellis et al., 2000; Näätänen et al., 2011). According to an alternative interpretation, MMN is just due to the different degrees of refractoriness of N1 neurons (see Butler, 1968) responding to standards and deviants, for the neurons responding to deviants are stimulated at much longer time intervals than those responding to standards (May & Tiitinen, 2010). The currently predominant view maintains that whereas the early part of the deviant–standard difference wave may, depending on the type of stimulus change, include a contribution from the N1 neurons, the later part of the difference wave is solely due to the 'genuine', memory-based, MMN. This is nicely illustrated by the deviant–standard difference wave as a function of frequency change in a 1000 Hz standard tone by Tiitinen et al. (1994). For very small frequency changes, two separate peaks (N1 and MMN) can be observed in the difference waves, which gradually merge when the magnitude of frequency change is increased and eventually become inseparable.

The separate N1 and MMN contributions to the ERP wave form are also illustrated in Fig. 1.9 of Näätänen et al. (1989). The standard stimulus was of an intensity of 80 dB sound-pressure level (SPL) and, in different blocks, the deviant stimulus was an intensity decrement or increment. The subject was instructed to read a book and to ignore auditory

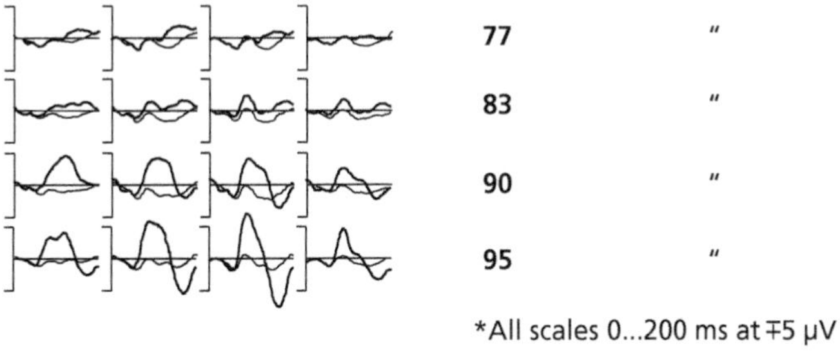

**MMN and intensity variation
of the deviant stimulus**

Fpz	Fz	Cz	Pz	Deviant	Standard
				57 dB SPL	80 dB
				70	"
				77	"
				83	"
				90	"
				95	"

*All scales 0...200 ms at ∓5 µV

Fig. 1.9 With a standard-tone intensity of 80 dB sound pressure level (SPL), in separate stimulus blocks, an MMN is elicited both by intensity increments and decrements, and the amplitude is increased with an increasing difference from the standard. N1 peak amplitude, on the other hand, only increases when the deviant-tone intensity increases, which can be seen in the three bottom rows of the figure.

Data from Näätänen, R., Paavilainen, P., Alho, K., Reinikainen, K., & Sams, M., *Do event-related potentials reveal the mechanism of the auditory sensory memory in the human brain?*, Neuroscience Letters, 98 (2), 217–221, doi:10.1016/0304-3940(89)90513-2, 1989.

stimuli. The response to the 77 dB deviant stimulus shows two consecutive negative waves of which the earlier may be mainly interpreted in terms of the N1 component (that of the three 'genuine' N1 components generated on the supra-temporal plane; see Näätänen & Picton 1987) and the later in terms of the MMN component. When the intensity of the deviant stimulus is further reduced then MMN becomes larger in peak amplitude and earlier in peak latency, overlapping N1 (Fig. 1.9).

The increase of the response amplitude with a decrease of stimulus energy can only be understood in terms of an increase of the difference between the deviants and standards. That is, MMN is a response to the *difference* between the present stimulus and the previous stimuli rather than that to the present stimulus per se. This means that a stimulus change is necessary for MMN elicitation: If we omit the intervening standards, then no MMN is elicited (Cowan et al. 1993; for a review, see Näätänen et al., 2007). Consistent with this, when intensity increments are used as deviant stimuli, then MMN becomes larger and earlier for larger stimulus changes. In contrast, the N1 component, getting larger in amplitude with increased intensity but smaller with softer intensity, reflects the intensity of the eliciting stimulus rather than the relation between the intensity of this stimulus to that of the preceding stimuli (Näätänen & Picton, 1987) (Fig. 1.9).

MMN is also elicited by other forms of discriminable acoustic changes such as sound-duration decrement or increment (Näätänen et al., 1989; Kaukoranta et al., 1989; Grimm et al.,2004), change of the locus of sound origin (Paavilainen et al., 1989; Nager et al., 2003; Pakarinen et al., 2007; Tata & Ward, 2005; Vaitulevich & Shestopalova, 2010; Richter et al.,2009; Grimm et al., 2012; Bennemann et al., 2013; Sonnadara et al., 2006; Deouell et al., 2006), or even by sound omission (when stimuli are presented at a fast rate; Yabe et al.,1997, 1998; Salisbury, 2012). In the case of MMNs elicited in response to stimulus omissions, MMN cannot be accounted for by new afferent elements.

Moreover, even the MMN generation locus can be separated from that of N1. In humans, MMN/MMNm to frequency change is generated in the supra-temporal cortex 3–10 mm anteriorly to the N1m source (Scherg et al., 1989; Sams et al., 1991; Csepe et al. 1992; Hari et al., 1992; Huotilainen et al., 1993, 1998; Tiitinen et al., 1993; Levänen et al., 1993; Levänen et al., 1996; Liasis et al., 1999, 2000; Korzyukov et al., 1999; Rosburg, 2003; Rosburg et al., 2004; Sams & Hari 1991). Optical imaging (OI) also shows a clear separation between the N1 and MMN generators. The separate OI equivalents of stimulus detection and deviance detection were observed by Rinne et al. (1999) in a passive oddball paradigm with longer tones (75 ms) as standards and shorter (25 ms) ones as deviants. The stimulus-detection effect, peaking at about 100 ms from stimulus onset, was elicited by the 75 ms standards, whereas no significant signal at this latency could be found for the 25 ms deviants, which rather elicited a considerably later response, one peaking at 160–200 ms and corresponding in latency to MMN recorded in parallel with OI. These two OI signals, the earlier for detection and the later for discrimination, were recorded by different sensors, indicating different intra-cranial generators (which in turn corresponded to the dipole-modelled N1m and MMNm sources, respectively (Huotilainen et al., 1993, 1998; Levänen et al., 1996).

In addition, intracranial recordings in humans (Kropotov et al., 1995, 2000; Rosburg, 2003) indicate that MMN to deviant sounds among standard sounds and the enhanced N1 to infrequent sounds occurring with no intervening standards are generated by different neuronal populations. Intra-cranial animal data also support the separability of MMN from the afferent responses. On the basis of their cat recordings, Pincze et al. (2001, 2002) concluded that MMN was generated in the rostro-ventral part of the secondary auditory cortex, clearly separated from the P1 and N1 sources. Moreover, in monkey, it was found that an NMDA receptor antagonist MK-801 eliminated MMN to frequency and intensity deviants but left the afferent responses N1 and P2 intact (Javitt et al., 1996; see also Javitt et al., 1992, 1994), which strongly supports the separability of MMN from the afferent responses (see also Korzyukov et al., 1999).

1.6 **The memory dependence of the MMN**

It became clear that MMN elicitation is a strictly memory-dependent process. At the beginning of a stimulus block, two or three standard stimuli need to be presented before a deviant stimulus can elicit MMN (Cowan et al., 1993). In contrast, in the next block with identical stimuli as standards, a deviant stimulus in the second stimulus position elicited MMN but did not if the standard stimulus was different from that of the first stimulus block (called the roving-standard condition). This suggests that the memory trace for the standard of the preceding block was 'dormant' when the first stimulus of the next stimulus block was presented but was reactivated by this stimulus. The duration of this 'active' state (i.e. when deviants may elicit MMN) is about 10 s in young healthy subjects (Böttcher-Gandor & Ullsperger, 1992) but is considerably shortened by aging and different clinical conditions, in particular, in degenerative brain diseases, as will be reviewed later in this book (*Chapter 6*). So, MMN is based on sensory-memory traces closely resembling those assumed to underlie echoic memory (Cowan, 1984, 1988).

Furthermore, MMN can also reflect long-term traces such as those of the native language speech sounds located in left auditory cortex (Näätänen et al., 1997). Corroborating evidence was provided by Finnish–Hungarian (Winkler et al., 1999) and French–Hindi (Dehaene-Lambertz, 1997) cross-language studies. In sum, MMN enables one to probe all the different levels of auditory memory representations extending from the short-term memory traces developed in the beginning and during an experimental session, to long-term or permanent ones. Importantly, these traces also include temporal stimulus aspects (Warren & Obusek, 1972); consequently, these traces do not correspond just to static stimulus features and their combinations but rather to stimuli as events in time as auditory stimulus events are represented in our sensory memory (Näätänen & Winkler, 1999).

1.7 **MMN and the emergence of perception**

When a sound is presented, the auditory system encodes this stimulus information in a very short time. According to Näätänen and Winkler (1999), this stimulus code, containing precise sensory information, undergoes several transformations as it moves from the peripheral to the central auditory system. At the level of auditory cortex, the neuronal populations underlying the supra-temporal N1 retain information on individual static stimulus features for several seconds, not, however, representing the combination (integration) of these features or the (higher order) temporal aspects of stimulation (such as the order of the elements of complex auditory events) that are present in perception. Therefore, the stimulus information contained by the refractoriness patterns of the neurons generating the supra-temporal N1 still undergo some transformation (at least integration) and may be complemented with temporal stimulus information. Näätänen and Winkler (1999) proposed that the critical borderline to stimulus representations is crossed when stimulus effects, i.e. the outcomes of the previous processing stages, accumulate in the neural system accommodating the traces involved in MMN generation and underlying sensory memory. The neural traces then developed contain the highly stimulus-specific feature-integrated sensory information that is present in perception and sensory memory. Auditory stimuli are represented by these traces as auditory events in time rather than as only their static features (Warren & Obusek, 1972).

A parsimonious way to understand the emergence of the percept is to associate it with the fast initial emergence of the sensory-memory representation of a stimulus, as illustrated in Fig. 1.10 for a brief sound. In this trace-formation phase, the outcomes of the different feature analysers are integrated, so that the developing trace can represent a unitary auditory event. This integration process uses, presumably, a sliding temporal window of some 150–200 ms in duration (the temporal window of integration, TWI; Cowan, 1984; Näätänen & Winkler, 1999; Yabe et al., 1997, 1998, 1999, 2005, 2001a, 2001b; Zwislocki, 1960). This is followed by a latent period during which the sound representation is subjectively silent (sensory memory) but can be brought into conscious experience by involuntary or voluntary attention. Further, if a sound is not repeated within a few seconds, then its representation decays from sensory memory so that no MMN can be elicited by a deviant stimulus (Sabri & Campbell, 2001).

How fast, then, is the memory-trace formation process that, according to the present model, lasts until the emergence of a fully developed percept? Backward recognition masking studies (e.g. Massaro, 1975) provided an estimate of 200 ms. In these studies, a masker stimulus was presented very soon after a brief test sound to be identified by the subject. When mask onset followed the onset of a brief test stimulus with an interval shorter than 150–200 ms, then stimulus features were incompletely perceived, leading to an estimate that some 200 ms from stimulus onset are needed for the trace development. This might then be the time needed for a fully elaborated percept to emerge. The masking results can hence be explained with TWI: a sliding window of integration of about 200 ms in duration integrating acoustic information from the same source or channel (i.e. of

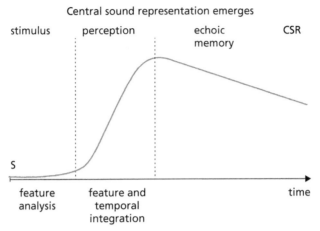

Central sound representation emerges

Fig. 1.10 The emergence and decay of central sound representation (CSR) elicited by a brief sound. After stimulus onset, its different sensory features are analyzed, which is followed by feature and temporal integration resulting in perception and the formation of CSR in sensory (echoic) memory. The abrupt emergence of the CSR provides the specific information contents for the sound percept. The subsequent slowly decaying phase represents the sensory-memory trace of the sound.
Based on Näätänen and Winkler (1999).

similar acoustic parameters and of approximately the same spatial origin) into a unitary auditory percept. As the more recent sound components weigh more in the temporal-integration process (Zwislocki, 1960, 1969), with 50–100 ms test-to-mask intervals, the integrated standard and mask and deviant and mask traces are dominated by the mask, preventing the recognition (discrimination) of the standard and deviant stimuli (Winkler et al., 1993). A TWI of about 200 ms in duration is also supported by loudness summation for brief sounds occurring up to durations of about 200 ms (Moore, 1989).

A TWI may also be of central importance for speech and music perception, which depend on the simultaneous perceptual presence of auditory stimulation from a time window of some (short) duration rather than that from any given instant. Thus, auditory perception does not correspond to the immediately present acoustic reality but rather to the outcome of temporal integration over the immediate 200 ms. Näätänen (1990; see also Wang et al., 2005, 2015) proposed that the continuously sliding TWI provides this temporally stretched perceptual presence. TWI may considerably expand 'the perceptual presence in audition relative to the timeless "cutting edge" of physical presence that continuously turns the future into the past' (p. 275).

Hence, the sensory-memory trace formation is a fast, automatic process that is complete by about 200 ms from stimulus onset and underlies (provides the specific sensory informational contents for) the transient percept of the sound. In this memory-trace formation process, both parallel (feature integration using the outputs from the different feature analysers) and sequential (temporal) integration of sensory information occurs.

The temporal integration process, however, sometimes results in loss of sensory infor-mation, as in detection and recognition masking (Massaro, 1975; Moore, 1989; Winkler et al., 1993; Zwislocki, 1972; Zwislocki et al., 1959). However, 'it is expected that a smooth [frequency] transition would prevent the backward masking of recognition of segments within the sound' (Cowan, 1984, p. 359). Such transitions form an essential element in natural sounds such as speech and music. Therefore, according to Näätänen (1995), ra-ther than condensing the time dimension, temporal integration binds together tempor-ally closely spaced events at the perceptual level (e.g. the integration of two closely spaced sounds as a single perceptual event; Csépe et al., 1997; Loveless et al., 1996; Tervaniemi et al., 1994; Winkler & Näätänen 1994). Hence, this integration usually is of constructive nature, structuring or segmenting the auditory perceptual world (see also Bregman et al., 1990). In conclusion, the representation of an auditory event (an auditory sensory-memory trace) emerges at a stage at which the outcomes of the different feature detectors are accommodated into the neuronal circuits of sensory memory. Here, the stimulus code carried by the stimulus-initiated process reaches the phase of elaboration at which it cor-responds to that read to perception and subjective experience. This means that the dif-ferent stimulus features are integrated into a unitary veridical sound percept projected onto the temporal coordinates: The sensory-memory system (probed with MMN) rep-resents an auditory event in time. Similarly as space is the medium of visual perception (Treisman, 1988), time is the medium of auditory perception.

1.8 Attention-independent elicitation of MMN

It is well established that MMN can be elicited even in the absence of attention. This was already implicated in the original description of MMN: Näätänen et al. (1978) pro-posed that 'it may well be that a physiological mismatch process caused by a sensory input deviating from the memory trace ("template") formed by a frequent "background" stimulus is such an automatic basic process that it takes place irrespective of the inten-tions of the experimenter and the S, perhaps even unmodified by the latter' (pp. 324–5). This is indicated by MMN elicitation in an irrelevant input stream even in the presence of a highly demanding primary task in the auditory or visual modality, with this task in the auditory modality then usually involving a separate input channel such as the opposite ear (for a review, see Näätänen et al., 2007). Moreover, MMN can be recorded even in sleep (Atienza & Cantero, 2001, Atienza et al., 1997, 2000, 2001, 2002, 2004, 2005; Nashida et al., 2000; Sallinen et al., 1994, 1996; Sculthorpe et al., 2009) and in patients in coma and persistent vegetative state (PVS), thus predicting the recovery of their consciousness in the near future (Fischer et al., 1999; Kane et al., 1993, 1996, 2000; Wijnen et al., 2007).

Even though MMN is elicited in the absence of attention, its amplitude may under some conditions be attenuated by strongly focusing attention elsewhere (Woldorff & Hillyard, 1991; Woldorff et al., 1998; for a review, see Näätänen et al., 2007). In contrast, when the stimulus stream is attended, then a sequence of attention-related ERP compo-nents also emerges, overlapping MMN (Fig. 1.3). The activation of the MMN generator leads to attention switch to the eliciting stimulus change, representing a biologically vital warning function that makes the organism immediately inspect the origin of auditory change (cf. passive attention; James, 1890; see also Sokolov, 1963; Näätänen et al., 2007). Hence, P3a, appearing as a sharp positive peak at about 220–250 ms from stimulus onset, reflects involuntary attention switch to the deviant stimulus initiated by MMN generation, resulting in the conscious perception of auditory change (Escera et al., 1998; see also Fig. 1.3).

1.9 **The MMN subcomponents**

The scalp-recorded MMN has its largest amplitude over the fronto-central scalp areas. The modelling of the generator sources of MMN with equivalent current dipoles (ECD) suggests that the fronto-centrally predominant scalp distribution of MMN is mainly explained by the sum of the activity bilaterally generated in the supra-temporal cortices (Giard et al., 1990, 1995; Jemel et al., 2002; Rinne et al., 2000; Scherg et al., 1989). This is supported by MMNm recordings (Alho et al., 1996; Csépe et al., 1992; Hari et al., 1984; Levänen et al., 1996; Sams et al., 1985, 1991) showing signal maxima bilaterally over the supra-temporal cortices. Moreover, intracranial MMN recordings also indicated MMN generation in the auditory cortex. These recordings were made in mouse (Umbricht et al., 2005), guinea pig (King et al., 1995; Kraus et al., 1994a), cat (Csépe, 1995; Csépe et al., 1987; Pincze et al., 2001, 2002), rat (Astikainen et al., 2006, 2011; Ruusuvirta et al., 1998, 2007, 2013), rabbit (Astikainen et al., 2000, 2005), dog (Howell et al., 2012), pigeon (Schall et al., 2015), monkey (Javitt et al., 1992, 1994, 1996), and humans (Baudena, 1995; Halgren et al., 1995, 1998; Kropotov et al., 1995, 2000; Liasis et al., 1999, 2000, 2001; Rosburg et al., 2005; see also Rosburg et al., 2007).

Importantly, at least partially different neural populations in the auditory cortex are activated by different types of auditory change, as proposed by Paavilainen et al. (1991) who found different polarity reversal ratios (mastoid/vertex) for the frequency, duration, and intensity MMNs in their mastoid recordings using a nose reference. Subsequently, studies using the dipole modelling of the MMN and MMNm sources reported differences in the range of a few mm in location and/or differences in orientation between the sources of the MMN/MMNm to intensity, frequency, ISI, or duration changes (Frodl-Bauch et al., 1997; Giard et al., 1995; Levänen et al., 1993, 1996; Rosburg, 2003; see also Deouell & Bentin, 1998; Deouell et al., 1998, 2003). Different, attribute-specific sources are also supported by results showing that MMN to the second of two consecutive deviants is not attenuated if the two deviants differ from the standard in different attributes (Nousak et al., 1996) but are attenuated if the two deviants differ from standards in the same attribute (Sams et al., 1983, 1984). Furthermore, a functional magnetic resonance imaging (fMRI) study by Molholm et al. (2005) also found that frequency and duration changes activate different areas both in the supra-temporal and frontal cortices. Moreover, unlike MMN/MMNm to changes in non-phonetic sounds, that to phoneme changes was predominantly elicited in the auditory cortex of the left hemisphere (Alho et al., 1996, 1998; Kuuluvainen et al.,

2014; Näätänen et al., 1997; Rinne et al., 1999; Shestakova et al., 2002; Tervaniemi et al., 1999; for supporting positron-emission tomography (PET) results, see Dittmann-Balçar et al., 2001; Müller et al., 2002; Tervaniemi et al., 2000). In addition, Alho et al. (1996) found that the MMNm sources for changes in simple and complex sounds differed from each other in the right-hemisphere temporal cortex.

Besides the bilateral supra-temporal cortices, other cortical areas are also involved. A frontal-lobe involvement in MMN generation was already proposed by Näätänen et al. (1978; see also Näätänen & Michie, 1979). This was supported by MMN scalp-potential distribution (scalp current density analysis, SCD), which indicated an additional MMN source in the frontal lobes (Deouell et al., 1998; Giard et al., 1990; Yago et al., 2001a, 2001b). Frontal MMN sources were also suggested by source-current modelling (Fig. 1.11; Rinne et al., 2000; Waberski et al., 2001) and multi-dipole modelling (Jemel et al., 2002) as well as by intracranial ERP (Baudena et al., 1995; Halgren et al., 1995; Kropotov et al., 1995, 2000; Liasis et al., 1999, 2000, 2001; Rosburg et al., 2005, 2007), PET (Dittmann-Balcar et al., 2001; Müller et al., 2002; Tervaniemi et al., 2000), fMRI (Celsis et al., 1999; Doeller et al., 2003; Molholm et al., 2005; Opitz et al., 2002; Restuccia et al., 2005; Rinne et al., 2005; Schall et al., 2003; Schönwiesner et al., 2007), OI recordings (Rinne et al., 1999; Sable et al., 2007; Tse & Penney, 2007, 2008; Tse et al., 2006, 2013). Consequently, MMN gets a contribution from at least two intracranial processes: (1) a bilateral supra-temporal process generating the supra-temporal MMN subcomponent (and the polarity reversed 'MMN' in nose-referenced mastoid recordings); (2) a predominantly right hemispheric frontal process, generating the frontal MMN subcomponent.

The supra-temporal component is, presumably, associated with pre-perceptual change detection, whereas the frontal component, triggered by the auditory-cortex change detection signal with a delay of some 20–30 ms (Rinne et al., 2000; Rissling et al., 2012), is related to involuntary attention switch to auditory change (Näätänen et al., 1978; Näätänen & Michie 1979; Giard et al., 1990; Alho et al., 1997; Escera et al., 1998, 2000a, 2000b, 2001, 2002; Schröger, 1994, 1995, 1996, 1997; Schröger et al., 2000; Schröger & Wolff, 1996, 1998a, 1998b; Wolff & Schröger, 2001a, 2001b; Berti 2008a, 2008b, 2012, 2013; Berti & Schröger, 2001, 2003, 2004, 2006; Berti et al., 2004; Jankowiak & Berti, 2007; Rinne et al., 2006; Roeber et al., 2003a, 2003b; Shestakova et al., 2002; Yago et al., 2001a, 2001b; Rissling et al., 2012). In addition, MMN receives a contribution from the parietal lobes (Kasai et al., 1999; Lavikainen et al. 1995, 1996; Molholm et al., 2005; Schall et al., 2003; Takahashi et al., 2013; Wang et al., 2005). This activation, however, occurs later than the temporal one, and might therefore be related to subsequent processes triggered by the MMN generator activation. In conclusion, the auditory cortex MMN/MMNm generators reflect the nature of stimulus change. For example, these responses usually are left-lateralized for language stimuli. Further, MMN/MMNms for changes in different auditory attributes are generated in different loci of auditory cortex which might enable one to map, by using MMN and its PET, fMRI, and OI analogues, the neuroanatomical and physiological basis of auditory sensory memory.

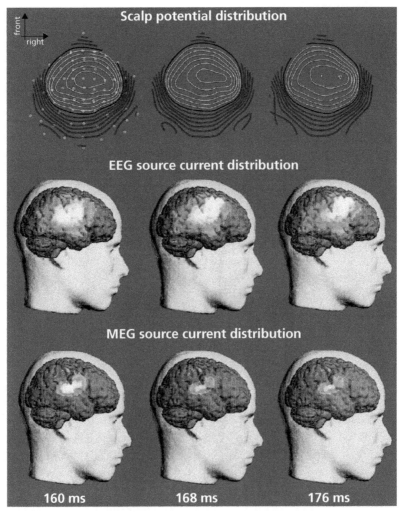

Fig. 1.11 EEG and MEG source current distributions at 160, 168, and 176 ms from change onset in a single subject. Top: Scalp distributions of the MMN, seen from above. Negativity is marked in yellow and the electrode locations are marked with grey circles. Middle: Minimum-norm estimation (MNE) map calculated from the scalp potential. Bottom: MNE map calculated from the magnetic field. From these figures, it looks like the auditory cortex generator of MMN is activated before the frontal MMN generator.

Reprinted from NeuroImage, 12(1), Rinne, T., Alho, K., Ilmoniemi, R.J., Virtanen, J. & Näätänen, R., *Separate Time Behaviors of the Temporal and Frontal Mismatch Negativity Sources*, 14–19, Copyright 2000, with permission from Elsevier.

1.10 **The MMN and involuntary attention**

As already noted, the activation of the auditory change-detection mechanism reflected by MMN also triggers the switching of attention to potentially important auditory events, supported by numerous studies reviewed. These results indicated that MMN-eliciting sound changes in irrelevant auditory background stimulation distract primary-task performance and elicit P3a associated with the actual orienting of attention to a change (see also Squires et al., 1975). This is also supported by the fact that MMN may also be followed by autonomic nervous system (ANS) responses associated with the involuntary orienting of attention such as heart-rate deceleration and the skin-conductance response (Lyytinen & Näätänen, 1987; Lyytinen et al., 1992; see also Sokolov et al., 2002).

Schröger (1994), using a selective dichotic-listening paradigm, found that the reaction time (RT) to an infrequent softer intensity stimulus in the right ear was increased and the hit rate decreased when this target stimulus was preceded (with a 200 ms lead time) by a frequency deviant rather than a standard in the opposite ear. When the frequency deviation was 50 Hz (standard 700 Hz), then the RT increased by 12 ms, and with a frequency deviation of 200 Hz, the RT prolongation amounted to 26 ms. Both frequency deviants elicited MMN while the wider frequency deviant also elicited N2b-P3a. According to Schröger (1994), this decrement in performance was probably triggered by deviants in the to the to-be-ignored channel, which captured attention, concluding that their data pattern supports the hypothesis that the neural processes generating MMN may be involved in passive attention switch.

Interestingly, MMN elicited by occasional intensity increments is followed by P3a, whereas that elicited by equivalent intensity decrements is not (Rinne et al., 2006). Intensity decrements do not catch attention in the same way that intensity increments do. This might be due to the fact that intensity increments also activate fresh afferent neurons (resulting in N1-component enhancement), whereas intensity decrements (resulting in N1 attenuation; Näätänen et al., 1989; Rinne et al., 2006) appear to activate no, or only a small number of, such neurons. In general, this attention-switching mechanism responds even to minor changes, with its sensitivity approaching that of the behavioural discrimination in attend conditions. For instance, Berti et al. (2004) found that subjects' performance in a tone-duration discrimination task deteriorated in almost half the trials even by an occasional 1% frequency change in this tone. In contrast to MMN, P3a and the reorienting negativity (RON; Schröger & Wolff 1998a) were only elicited in trials with an RT prolongation, i.e. when an involuntary attention switch to frequency change indeed occurred.

The prefrontal cortex has a central role in controlling the direction of attention (Knight et al., 1989; Näätänen, 1988, 1990, 1992), presumably to prevent irrelevant sensory inputs from bombarding consciousness and disrupting the ability to attend to task-relevant or salient information (e.g. Rissling et al., 2014). Therefore, the frontal MMN might signify a call for, or the initiation of, the involuntary orienting of attention to a change in the acoustic environment detected by the pre-attentive auditory-cortex MMN mechanism (Giard et al., 1990; Näätänen, 1985, 1988, 1990, 1992; Näätänen & Michie, 1979; Näätänen et al., 1978; Rinne et al., 2000). Consistent with this view, the time course of this frontal activation to auditory change (the frontal MMN subcomponent) is slightly (by ca. 20 ms) delayed relative to that of the auditory-cortex subcomponent (Kwon et al. 2002; Opitz et al. 2005; Rinne et al., 2000). More recently, the view maintaining that the

auditory-cortex change detection precedes the frontal-cortex activation has been qualified by results suggesting that MMN is, in fact, generated by a very rapid sequence of
interacting processes occurring between the auditory and frontal cortices (Choi et al.,
2013; Garrido et al., 2007, 2009; Hsiao et al. 2010; Tse et al., 2013). Tse et al. (2013) concluded that the prefrontal cortex is involved in both pre- and post-deviance detection,
depending on the magnitude of stimulus change, as previously proposed by Opitz et al.
(2002) and Rinne et al. (2006).

1.11 **MMN as an expression of sensory cortex 'primitive intelligence'**

Saarinen et al. (1992), in a pioneering study, presented tone pairs to their subjects instructed to ignore auditory stimuli. The tone pairs varied in frequency, there being no
identical, repetitive standard stimulus. Instead, the constant feature of the standard pairs
was an abstract, or second order one: the standard pairs were ascending ones (with the
second tone being higher in frequency than the first tone), whereas the deviant pairs were
descending ones. Thus, the abstract attribute defining the standards was the rule governing
the frequency relationship between the two tones forming a pair. Nevertheless, MMN was
elicited by deviant pairs, showing that the pre-attentively formed sensory representations
encoded the abstract attribute ('ascending pair'), i.e. derived the common invariant feature from a set of physically varying stimulus events (Fig. 1.12); for similar results in
children of 8–14 years of age, see Gumenyuk et al. (2003). In addition, Korzuykov et al.
(1999) located the source of the abstract-feature MMNm in the auditory cortex anterior
to that of N1m. Furthermore, Paavilainen et al. (1995) replicated the Saarinen et al. (1992)
results with a more strict control of attention and concluded that they indeed represented
pre-attentive processing rather than post-perceptual cognitive operations.

In addition, Tervaniemi et al. (1994) found that an occasional repetition in a sequence
of steadily ascending tones elicited MMN in reading subjects, concluding that their central auditory system, on the basis of the ascending trend automatically detected, had
extrapolated the next stimulus and used it as a reference in the automatic comparison
process. This suggests that the brain does not only model the immediate auditory past but
also forms extrapolatory traces on the basis of regularities automatically detected in the
ongoing stimulus sequence (predictive coding; Friston, 2005; for reviews, see Baldeweg,
2007; Summerfield & Egner, 2009; see also Grimm & Schröger 2007; Todd et al. 2010).
In these studies, MMN was elicited when a stimulus violated such a regularity or trend.
Consequently, traces representing anticipated auditory events, rather than those of the
auditory past, were used in the automatic comparison process: MMN was elicited by a
stimulus differing from that represented by the extrapolatory trace.

More recently, Paavilainen et al. (2007) presented their subjects with a sequence of four
tones: short-low, short-high, long-low, and long-high. This tone sequence was constructed
by obeying the rule that short tones are followed by low ones and long tones by high ones.
MMN was elicited, in subjects instructed to ignore stimuli, by violations of the sequential

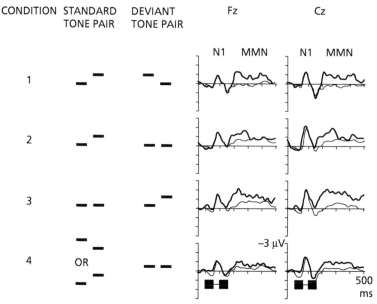

Fig. 1.12 N1 and MMN to standard and deviant tone pairs when the frequency level of stimulus pairs randomly varied across a wide frequency range (stimuli schematically illustrated on the left). ERPs to standard tone pairs are marked with thin lines and ERPs to deviant tone pairs are marked with thick lines. Timing of the stimuli is presented below the graphs. N1 waves were very similar in responses to both standard and deviant tone pairs, while MMN was only elicited by the deviant tone pairs.

Reproduced from Jukka Saarinen, Petri Paavilainen, Erich Schöger, Mari Tervaniemi, and Risto Näätänen, *Representation of abstract attributes of auditory stimuli in the human brain*, NeuroReport, 3 (12), p. 1150, Figure 1, http://journals.lww.com/neuroreport/Abstract/1992/12000/Representation_of_abstract_attributes_of_auditory.30.aspx © 1992, (C) Lippincott-Raven.

rules, e.g. when a high tone followed a short one. Interestingly, subjects were able, in a subsequent active detection condition, to detect correctly only about 15% of the rule-violating stimuli, and none of them could describe the rule verbally. Furthermore, using an even more complex sequential stimulus-contingency rule, Bendixen and Schröger (2008) found that when such a rule was unexpectedly changed during an ongoing stimulus block, then only two to four exemplars of stimuli, depending on the complexity of the new rule, sufficed for rule updating; MMN was soon elicited by a stimulus violating the new rule. Importantly, all this complex rule extraction, encoding, and monitoring for possible rule violation occurred in the absence of attention in subjects performing a difficult primary task (although being transiently distracted by instances of automatic detection of rule violation; Schröger et al. 2007) and who showed no sign of explicit knowledge of the rule when asked about it. Moreover, this rule extraction and modelling occurred equally rapidly irrespective of whether the subject attended to the stimulus sequence or not (Bendixen & Schröger, 2008). Such results suggest the automatic elicitation of this MMN, reflecting the automatic detection of violations of the stimulus-contingency rules automatically extracted during the stimulus block. Furthermore, recent evidence for the full automaticity of rule detection was obtained by Sculthorpe et al. (2009) who found MMN in subjects in rapid eye movement (REM) sleep to violations of a sequential auditory stimulus pattern. Interestingly, Wang et al. (2012) have recently shown, using MMN, that there is a kind of sensory intelligence in the perception of Chinese lexical tones, too, concluding that humans can automatically extract abstract auditory rules in speech at a pre-attentive stage to ensure speech communication in complex and noisy auditory environments without drawing on conscious resources.

On the basis of these and further related human and animal studies, Näätänen et al. (2001, 2010) proposed that there exists a category of complex higher-order automatic processes of perceptual–cognitive nature at the level of auditory cortex: these findings were surprisingly similar irrespective of the species, the ontological stage of development, or the state of consciousness, hence revealing a shared, relatively state-independent, perceptual-cognitive core of human and animal cognition.

1.12 Model of central auditory processing

Näätänen et al. (2011) subsequently presented a new model of automatic and attentive central auditory processing, aiming at defining the borderline between the automatic and attention-dependent processing in audition and at illustrating the emergence of conscious auditory percepts. As already reviewed, the outputs of the different feature detectors are automatically integrated in time (TWI, with a duration of approximately 200 ms; Atienza et al., 2003; Näätänen & Winkler, 1999; Nousak et al., 1996; Oceák et al., 2006; Tervaniemi et al., 1994; Yabe et al., 1997) and across the different features (Gomes et al., 1995, 1997; Ritter et al., 2000; Takegata & Morotomi, 1999; Takegata et al., 1999, 2005; Winkler et al., 2005). For instance, loudness integration continues for about 200 ms from stimulus onset, with the outcome of this process determining the loudness, the perceived intensity of a sound (Scharf & Houtsma, 1986), which provides an estimate of the duration of TWI. During TWI, masking may also occur, with a subsequent stimulus often preventing the accurate perception of the preceding stimulus (Bazana & Stelmack, 2002; Cowan, 1984; Hawkins & Presson, 1977; Massaro, 1970). Consistent with this, as already reviewed, MMN is abolished when a masking stimulus follows each stimulus of the oddball paradigm with a very short interval. Therefore MMN can also be used for determining the TWI duration (Winkler et al., 1993; Yabe et al., 1997, 1998; Yabe et al., 2001, 2005). Furthermore, the vMMN recordings of Czigler et al. (2006) suggest that the TWI duration is about 200 ms in the visual modality also.

The outputs from the TWI process then accumulate in the neural populations that underlie sensory memory (see Fig. 1.13). Further, the rapid accumulation of this stimulus-specific information underlies transient stimulus perception. This stimulus-specific information, in turn, becomes consciously perceived in the absence of attention if the N1 transient-detector system, activated by the same stimulus, generates a signal (attention call) that is strong enough to exceed some temporally varying threshold (Fig. 1.13). The

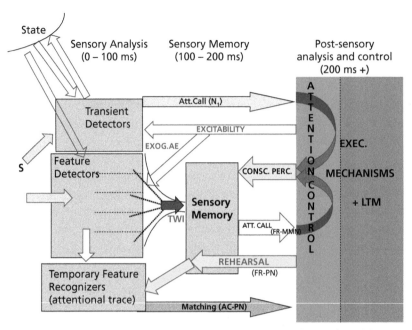

Fig. 1.13 The model of central auditory processing (Näätänen 2007, fig.4; adapted from Näätänen 1990). First the stimulus is analyzed by Permanent Feature-Detector and Transient-Detector Systems. This information from the Permanent Feature-Detector System is encoded in Sensory Memory. If this new information deviates from that represented by Sensory Memory, then an automatic change-detection signal eliciting an MMN is generated alerting Executive Mechanisms which may result in a Response of the organism. In case of selective attention, a Temporary Feature-Recognition System (Attentional Trace) is also activated, serving a rapid identification of task-relevant stimuli subjected to further analysis. The Transient-Detector System is particularly sensitive to abrupt changes in stimulus energy, serving an alerting function of the organism in its interaction with the environment.

N1 amplitude apparently reflects the magnitude of the sensory 'refreshment' of the feature traces involved (Näätänen, 1984). The biological significance of the long duration of these N1 refractoriness patterns might lie in 'optimizing' the strength and frequency of the attention-call signals elicited. This transient-detector system (Loveless, 1983; MacMillan, 1973; Walter, 1964) mainly consists of N1 neurons of non-specific or relatively nonspecific type. Consistent with this, Walter (1964) suggested that the 'vertex potential' notified the brain that something was happening while the specific sensory areas determined what it was (see also Davis & Zerlin, 1966; Näätänen 1975).

The second major cerebral route to attention switch/conscious perception is activated by violations of the automatic predictions (i.e. anticipatory memory traces) that are based on the regularities extracted from the preceding sequence. The MMN generator process then also causes attention switch to the eliciting auditory event. This is mediated by the auditory-cortex MMN process activating the frontal-cortex MMN. Furthermore, a deviant stimulus may, in addition to activating the MMN attention-call mechanisms, also activate the generator process of the N1 component (when new afferent elements are also activated). In either case, exceeding the threshold of attention switch results in the conscious perception of the parallel feature and temporally integrated sensory contents incorporated in the memory trace. (For a description of the parallel processing of features and the integrated stimulus representation, see Ritter et al., 1995). As already mentioned, attention switch to, and conscious perception of, auditory change is also accompanied by P3a (e.g. Escera et al., 1998, 2001; Friedman et al., 2001) or N2b-P3a responses (Näätänen et al., 1982; for a review, see Näätänen, 1992). In addition, P3 (Sutton et al., 1965) and slower parietal positivity are also elicited, at least when the stimulus is recognized as a target. Moreover, ANS responses may also be observed (Lyytinen & Näätänen, 1987; Lyytinen et al., 1992). This attention switch is also manifested by a transient deterioration in primary-task performance that accompanies MMN to a task-irrelevant change, as already reviewed (Escera et al., 1998).

The conscious perception of auditory stimulus representations (perception or rehearsal) is shown by yellow arrows in Fig. 1.13. Conscious perception/awareness of the contents of sensory memory occurs either when an attentional-call process is strong enough to exceed some momentarily varying threshold (Näätänen, 1982, 1992; Näätänen et al., 1978) or when the stimulus features of the to-be-attended stimulus are voluntarily maintained (rehearsed) in the form of the attentional trace (selective attention; Alho et al., 1992, 1994; Näätänen, 1982, 1990, 1992). The presence of the attentional trace continuously depends on its conscious, voluntary maintenance by the attentional control mechanisms reflected by the frontal processing negativity (PN) component (Hansen & Hillyard, 1980, 1983, 1984; Näätänen, 1982; Okita et al., 1983). During the lifetime of the attentional trace, each stimulus initiates a comparison with the stimulus represented by the attentional trace, with this comparison process being on-line reflected by the auditory-cortex PN. Further, the more discernible the current stimulus is from that represented by the attentional trace, the sooner the comparison terminates. Hence, this comparison process runs its full time course only when the input fully matches with the stimulus represented by the attentional trace (Alho, 1987a, 1987b) and is then subjected to further processing. This is illustrated by the arrow at the bottom of Fig. 1.13. Also illustrated is another type of attention effect (EXCITABILITY) which is channel rather than stimulus specific, supported by the very early Hillyard type of N1 effect found when the subject attends to stimuli presented to the designated ear at a very rapid rate (Hillyard et al., 1973), expressing 'a tonically maintained set rather than an active discrimination and recognition of each individual stimulus' (p. 179).

The present model closely corresponds to Näätänen and Winkler's (1999) distinction between the representational and pre-representational systems. According to these authors, the representational system contrasts with the pre-representational system in that the stimulus code: (a) is stable, even though it is subject to decay and interference;

(b) contains the outcome of complete sensory analysis, has temporal properties, and corresponds to the percept; (c) can be brought into conscious experience by a stimulus-triggered attentional-call process or subject-initiated voluntary attention, imagination, or rehearsal; hence these stimulus codes are accessible to top-down operations and may contact long-term memory (LTM), which results in the recognition of the stimulus and semantic activation (Pulvermüller & Assadollahi, 2007; Pulvermüller & Shtyrov, 2006). The present model is consistent with these suggestions, but it can also accommodate the very early attention effects on auditory processing. Even though these effects are manifested peripherally from the suggested borderline between the representational and pre-representational systems, their nature nevertheless is channel rather than stimulus specific, in agreement with the borderline proposed. Finally, the general vigilance state of the organism is also illustrated (Fig. 1.13). The excitability of the transient detectors depends on the subject's state (Eason et al., 1964; Fruhstorfer & Bergström, 1969; Hermanutz et al., 1981; Näätänen, 1975; Näätänen & Picton, 1987).

1.13 MMN as seen by different brain research technologies

As already reviewed, MMN can also be recorded with MEG (MMNm; Hari et al., 1984) which can detect MMN-related activity in the supra-temporal cortex but is blind to radially oriented brain activity (Hämäläinen et al., 1993). Consequently, MMNm is primarily generated by supra-temporal activation (Lütkenhöner & Steinsträter, 1998; Korzyukov et al., 1999; Kreitschmann-Andermahr et al., 2001; Sams & Hari, 1991). This is not simply a handicap, however: the component identification becomes easier because of less component overlap. Furthermore, the parallel use of MEG and EEG would be helpful in disentangling the different temporally overlapping components because of the differential sensitivity of these technologies to different brain events (Näätänen, 1992; Scherg, 1992).

fMRI, in turn, displays fMRI equivalents for both the temporal and frontal lobe MMN subcomponents (Celsis et al., 1999; Doeller et al., 2003; Molholm et al., 2005; Opitz et al., 2002, 2005; Schall et al., 2003). Moreover, the two MMN subcomponents can also be seen with PET (Dittmann-Balcar et al., 2001; Muller et al., 2002; Tervaniemi et al., 2000) and OI (Tse & Penney, 2007, 2008; Tse et al., 2006). Of particular interest are the MEG (Levänen et al., 1996; Rosburg, 2003) and fMRI (Molholm et al., 2005) results showing the feature-specific organization of the supra-temporal MMN generator, as previously suggested by Paavilainen et al. (1991) on the basis of their MMN recordings. For example, Molholm et al. (2005) demonstrated with fMRI that the supra-temporal MMN generators for frequency and duration changes are differently located in the auditory cortex. Moreover, as already reviewed, an OI equivalent of MMN (Rinne et al., 1999a; Sable et al., 2007; Tse et al., 2006; Tse & Penney, 2007, 2008) could be separated from the OI equivalent of N1 both in timing and locus of generation, consistent with EEG (Huotilainen et al., 1998) and MEG recordings (Levänen et al., 1996).

1.14 **MMN in animals**

MMN can also be recorded in different animals: in monkey (Javitt et al., 1992, 1994, 1996), cat (Csepe, 1995; Csépe et al., 1987a, 1987b; Pincze et al., 2001, 2002), rabbit (Astikainen et al., 2000, 2001, 2005; Ruusuvirta et al., 2010), rat (Ahmed et al., 2011; Astikainen et al., 2006, 2011; Ruusuvirta et al., 1998, 2007, 2013; Roger et al., 2009; Tikhonravov et al., 2008, 2010), guinea pig (Kraus et al., 1994a, 1994b; King et al., 1995; Okazaki et al., 2006, 2010), pigeon (Schall et al., 2015), dog (Howell et al., 2012), and mouse (Ehrlichman et al., 2008, 2009; Umbricht et al., 2005). The first animal recordings of MMN were conducted by Csepe et al. (1987a, 1987b, 1989) who demonstrated an animal analogue of the human MMN in cat. These recordings were made with epidural electrodes placed over the primary and secondary auditory cortices, auditory association cortex, and vertex area of freely moving cats. Frequency deviants elicited a negativity that closely resembled the human MMN, but occurred at a considerably shorter latency. As in humans (Sato et al., 2000), this negativity was larger in amplitude with smaller deviant-stimulus probabilities and was elicited even in slow-wave sleep.

MMN under pentobarbitol (Nembutal) anaesthesia in cat was found by Csépe et al. (1989). This MMN of a small size was confined to the primary auditory cortex only, there being no MMN in recordings over the association cortex. This MMN occurred only when the deviants differed from the standards at least by 10% in tone frequency. In wakefulness, too, the MMN amplitude was enhanced with an increasing frequency difference but reached a plateau with a difference of 15%. Interestingly, the smaller the stimulus change, the larger was the cortical area activated (determined with recordings through 20 closely spaced electrodes arranged in the form of a matrix), as if representing an automatic cortical contrast-enhancing mechanism of the brain.

Csépe et al. (1989) also found early MMN kinds of effects from electrodes placed both in the medial geniculate body and hippocampus. These MMNs corresponded in latency to those recorded over the nonspecific cortex, and were earlier than those recorded over the auditory-specific cortex. Both cortical and subcortical electrodes also showed MMN during the slow-wave sleep, but only at lower deviant-stimulus probabilities and with a longer peak latency than that recorded during wakefulness.

Subsequently, Pincze et al. (2001) recorded ERP responses to tone-frequency changes from awake, freely moving cats by using a permanently implanted epidural electrode matrix covering both the primary and secondary auditory fields. The P1 and N1 components both to standard and deviant tones appeared with the highest amplitudes in the middle ectosylvian gyrus, whereas the amplitude maximum of MMN was ventral and rostral to P1 and N1 in the AII area. The authors concluded that MMN is generated in the rostroventral part of the secondary auditory area, well separated from the sources of the afferent P1 and N1 components. Further strong evidence for this separability of MMN from these exogenous responses was provided by Pincze et al.'s result that both the peak latency and amplitude of MMN depended on the magnitude of stimulus deviation, whereas the N1 peak latency was not affected. Corroborating results showed that an increasing probability of deviant stimuli strongly attenuated the MMN amplitude, whereas it had no effect on the P1 and N1 amplitudes (Pincze et al., 2002). This data pattern further supports the separability of MMN from the afferent responses.

Epidural monkey recordings (Javitt et al., 1992; see also Javitt et al., 1994) also support the separability of MMN from the afferent P1 and N1 responses. The authors found that in the oddball paradigm, occasional softer tones elicited a long-duration fronto-central negativity (apparently MMN), peaking at approximately 85 ms, that was superimposed upon cortically generated obligatory (afferent) ERP components. Importantly, Javitt et al. (1996) found that this MMN in monkey to tone-intensity decrement was abolished by epidural MK-801 (an NMDA receptor antagonist) injection which left the afferent responses, P1 and N1, generated in layer four, intact, lending further strong support to the separability of MMN from the afferent responses. Moreover, Tikhonravov et al. (2008) found that MK-801 attenuated the MMN amplitude for a tone-frequency change in intracranial recordings in rat and Ehrlichman et al. (2008) observed similar ketamine (another NMDA-receptor antagonist) effects with a tone-frequency change MMN in mouse. Subsequently, Tikhonravov et al. (2010), using anaesthetized rats, found that a small dose of memantine, a low-affinity NMDA-receptor antagonist used to treat cognitive symptoms in Alzheimer's disease, prolonged the duration of MMN in response to tone frequency change, but blocked the MMN generation with a high dose.

More recently, several further rat-MMN studies of major interest were conducted. Astikainen et al. (2011), using epidural recordings above the primary auditory cortex of urethane-anesthetized rats, found that a mismatch response of positive polarity to tone-frequency change was asymmetric in that it was elicited by frequency increments of 5% and 12.5% but not by the corresponding frequency decrements from a standard of 4000 Hz. In addition, the mismatch response could be elicited at least with an ISI (offset to onset) of 375 ms and even with that of 600 ms for the larger one of the frequency changes used (12.5%). No mismatch types of responses were, however, observed when the ISI was prolonged to 1000 ms. The authors concluded that the memory trace for the standard had to be highly accurate to permit the discrimination of a frequency change of 5% in magnitude as this frequency difference is close to the behaviourally assessed Weber ratios for the frequency-difference limen in awake rats, varying from 3.7% to 7.3% (Syka et al., 1996). Consequently, these results provide an estimate for the sensory-memory duration in the rat which appears to be shorter than 1 s.

Moreover, Ahmed et al. (2011), recording local field potentials above the primary auditory cortex of urethane-anesthetized rats, found an MMN kind of response for the synthesized spoken speech sound syllable contrast /ba/ - /wa/ (but not for the /da/ - /ga/). These results resemble those of Kraus et al. (1994a, 1994b) who were the first to describe MMN for speech sounds in animals. Kraus and associates, recording from the thalamus (the caudo-medial portion of the medial geniculate nucleus) of anesthetized guinea pigs, found a mismatch response for the /ga/ - /wa/ but not for the /da/ - /ga/ speech-sound contrast. However, on the epidural midline surface (secondary albeit not primary auditory cortex), an MMN type of response was found for both speech-sound contrasts. In addition, importantly, it was found by Ruusuvirta et al. (2010) that the hippocampus reacts to auditory change in the rabbit, suggesting the involvement of hippocampus in auditory change detection.

1.15 MMN as an index of the functional condition of the NMDA-receptor system

The very wide applied perspectives of the MMN/MMNm, can mainly be accounted for by the fact that, besides serving as an objective index of central auditory processing, it provides a noninvasive index of the NMDA-receptor functioning. We already reviewed recent animal results showing that different NMDA-receptor antagonists selectively abolished MMN in monkey (Javitt et al., 1996), rat (Tikhonravov et al., 2008; see also 2010), and mouse (Ehrlichman et al., 2008). Moreover, analogous results were obtained in normal healthy humans in whom ketamine attenuated the MMN amplitude for tone frequency and duration changes (Umbricht et al., 2000), prolonged the MMNm peak latency for frequency, duration, and intensity changes, and also decreased the MMNm dipole moment, whereas it affected neither the peak latency nor dipole moment of N1m (Kreitschmann-Andermahr et al., 2001), lending further strong support to the separability of MMN from the afferent ERP responses.

Furthermore, quite surprisingly, Umbricht et al. (2002) found that normal healthy young subjects with a smaller amplitude MMN for tone-frequency change (before any drug intake) were more affected by a small dose of ketamine than were subjects with a larger amplitude MMN, as indexed by a larger number of 'psychotic' responses on the Brief Psychiatric Rating Scale (BPRS). In addition, an analogous data pattern was obtained for duration changes. Consequently, MMN/MMNm seems to index the width of the safety margin an individual has for conversion to psychosis, providing a measure of the intact functioning of the NMDA receptor system and brain plasticity. Moreover, Lavoie et al. (2007) found that a 6-week administration of N-acetyl-cysteine (NAC), a glutathione precursor that can potentiate the activity of the NMDA receptors, corrected the MMN-amplitude deficiency for tone-frequency change in patients with schizophrenia. Most recently, Swerdlow and colleagues (2016) found that a single dose of the non-competitive NMDA receptor antagonist memantine, a medication approved for the treatment of Alzheimer's disease, enhances MMN in both healthy subjects and schizophrenia patients. These results, collectively, support the use of MMN to select clinical subgroups of patients who are sensitive to the enhancing or disrupting effects of drugs that target the NMDA receptor.

1.16 MMN in other sensory modalities

For many years, it was believed that an MMN kind of response could be obtained in the auditory modality only (Näätänen, 1990; Nyman et al., 1990). However, more recently, a visual analogue (vMMN) of the auditory MMN for different kinds of changes in unattended visual stimulation was described. In these studies, a vMMN, a posterior negativity at around 100–150 ms from change onset (Kimura et al., 2006a, 2006b, 2009, 2011; Urakawa et al., 2010a, 2010b), was elicited by a change of colour (Czigler et al., 2002), shape (Alho et al., 1992; Stagg et al., 2004; Tales et al., 1999), motion direction (Pazo-Álvarez et al., 2004a, 2004b), orientation (Astikainen et al., 2008), spatial frequency (Kenemans et al., 2003), brightness (Stagg et al., 2004; Kimura, Katayama & Murohashi, 2008a), size (Kimura et al., 2008b), spatial location (Berti & Schröger, 2001, 2004, 2006), and facial emotional expression (Stefanics et al., 2012). Moreover, a vMMN was also reported for a sequential regularity violation (Stefanics et al., 2011).

As for the N1/MMN controversy familiar from the auditory MMN studies, a general conclusion from the vMMN studies using appropriate control conditions (Kimura et al., 2009; Grimm et al., 2009; Li et al., 2012) was that in the deviant-standard difference wave, the early part is due to the infrequent stimulation of the afferent elements specific to deviants (the N1 time zone) and the later part to a genuine memory-based vMMN. This is illustrated in Fig. 1.14 from Kimura et al. (2011; see also Maekawa et al., 2009; Urakawa et al., 2010). Further support for the separability of N1 and MMN in the visual modality was provided by results showing that vMMN emerges not only for a change in single stimulus features but also for that in the conjunction of stimulus features (Winkler et al., 2005), and deviation from a regular sequential pattern of stimulation (Czigler, 2006a, 2006b). Moreover, vMMN was also elicited by infrequent feature conjunctions between the colour and orientation of a grating pattern (Winkler et al., 2005) and by the omission of a visual stimulus within the window of integration (about 170 ms) in vision, closely corresponding to that in audition (Czigler et al., 2006a, 2006b, 2007; Czigler & Pato, 2009). In addition, infrequently breaking a repetitive visual stimulus pattern elicited vMMN relative to the ERP elicited by the same stimulus presented at the same low probability in a sequence of several different visual stimuli, each at the same low probability, i.e. when no repetitive standard was presented (Czigler et al., 2002; Pazo-Álvarez et al., 2004a, 2004b); see also Fig. 1.14.

Consequently, all these results point to the conclusion that sensory-memory processes are involved in vMMN generation (Czigler et al., 2007). Subsequent research has qualified this conclusion by indicating that the visual sensory system automatically encodes sequential stimulus regularities and, further, that the automatic stimulus- or event-comparison process does not use just a visual memory representation as a reference but rather one extrapolated into the future as a continuation of the sequential regularities automatically extracted from the stimulus sequence by the visual system (Czigler & Pato, 2009; Kimura et al., 2009, 2010b, 2012; Stefanics et al., 2011). According to Czigler et al. (2007), the existence of such a memory representation of the regularities of the immediate past seems to be reasonable because it would play a critical role in predicting events of the immediate future.

Furthermore, the fact that vMMN was observed regardless of the relevance of the sequential regularities to the current task supports the notion that not only sensory non-specific systems but also sensory-specific ones contribute to these automatic cognitive operations in vision (Kimura et al., 2009). These studies also showed that whereas the

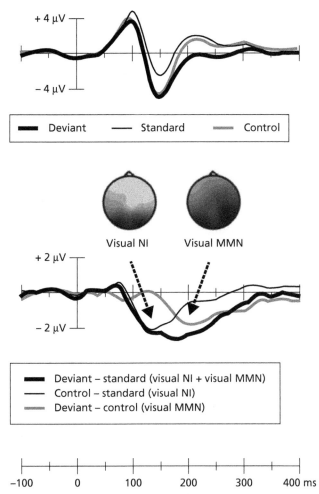

Fig. 1.14 Visual MMN elicited by orientation deviations in an oddball sequence. Due to the different probabilities of deviant and standard stimuli, a visual N1 response to deviant stimuli can be greater than that in response to standard stimuli. Consequently, visual N1 can also contribute to the negative waveform, in addition to visual MMN. Kimura et al. used an additional control sequence with equiprobable control stimuli in five different orientations, subtracting the ERPs elicited by these control stimuli from those elicited by the deviant stimuli to extract genuine visual MMN.

Reproduced from Motohiro Kimura, Erich Schröger, and István Czigler, *Visual mismatch negativity and its importance in visual cognitive sciences*, NeuroReport, 22 (14), p. 670, Figure 1c, doi: 10.1097/WNR.0b013e32834973ba © 2011 Lippincott Williams.

visual N1 is generated by large areas including the primary and non-primary visual cortical areas, vMMN emanates from a relatively small, non-primary visual area (Kimura et al., 2010a). In addition, prefrontal areas also contribute to vMMN. Recently, evidence for the human visual system automatically representing large-scale (long-duration pattern) regularities was also provided by Kimura, et al. (2010c). Such results extend the estimated duration of sensory memory in vision to several seconds, usually understood in terms of a very short-duration 'iconic' memory lasting for a few hundred ms only (Atkinson & Shiffrin, 1968). Kimura et al. (2011), in their recent review, proposed that a large number of vMMN findings can be regarded as suggestive of the existence of unintentional prediction about the next state of a visual object in the immediate future on the basis of its temporal context ('unintentional temporal context based prediction in vision') and, further, that such an automatic predictive process might be qualitatively similar to that underlying behavioural results involving perceptual sequence learning. According to the authors, such automatic predictive visual processes may provide advantages for the adaptation to our visual environment at the computational, neural, and behavioural levels, concluding that in concert with such behavioural phenomena, vMMN could provide 'a unique tool for tapping into the predictive power of the human visual system' (p. 669).

In the somatosensory modality, too, there exists an MMN kind of response, i.e. the somatosensory MMN, sMMN. Kekoni et al. (1997) found that an occasional short tactile pulse given to one skin location (the middle finger) but of the same frequency and amplitude as that of standards repetitively delivered to another location in the skin (the thumb), or vice versa, elicited an extra negativity at a latency of 100–200 ms from stimulus onset, interpreted in terms of a possible analogy of the auditory MMN. Subsequently, sMMNs were reported by several other groups (e.g. Shinozaki et al., 1998; Astikainen et al., 2001; Akatsuka et al., 2005, 2007a, 2007b; Restuccia et al., 2005, 2007, 2009; Wei et al., 2002; Spackman et al., 2007, 2010; Strömmer et al., 2014). Akatsuka et al. (2007a, 2007b) found that with sMMN, one could objectively determine the two-point discrimination (TPD) threshold. The TPD test is widely used in the clinic as an index of the patient's somatosensory perception but there are two serious problems when trying to determine the TPD threshold in the clinic: the examiner's skill and the patient's ability and willingness to give adequate responses. According to the authors, if patients do not understand the meaning of the test, due to, for example, dementia, or if they lie to make symptoms seem less or more serious, the examiner cannot determine whether there really is a disorder; therefore, a more objective approach is needed.

In stimulus blocks with a deviant stimulus at a distance from the standard stimulus approximating the behaviourally determined TPD threshold, sMMN was elicited when the two-point distance slightly exceeded the behavioural threshold but was not elicited for distances below this threshold. Therefore, the authors concluded that their newly developed, computer-assisted procedure enabled them, by using the magnetic equivalent of sMMN (sMMNm), to objectively determine the subject's TPD threshold in the ignore condition. There are three advantages of their method as follows. First, this objective method is not affected by the individual's judgment at all, since the mismatch responses are generated automatically. Second, it does not depend on the examiner's practical skills. Third, it can be applied to any part of the body surface and at any time on different days.

Finally, even though MEG was used to determine the TPD accuracy, EEG can be similarly used (Akatsuka et al., 2007b).

MMN was also described in the olfactory modality, i.e. the olfactory MMN, oMMN. Krauel et al. (1999) found, in subjects instructed to ignore odours and to perform an auditory task, that oMMN was elicited at a long peak latency of 500–600 ms from infrequent odour onset within a constant air flow to the subject's nostril. Dilutions of linalool (lavender) and eugenol (clove) were employed because the two odours can be well discriminated and are predominantly processed by the olfactory system. This parietally predominant response was elicited independently of the odour quality used. The authors concluded that this response resembled the auditory MMN, even though it occurred at a considerably longer latency (directly after the olfactory N1 at 400–500 ms from stimulus onset). For a review of the oMMN studies, see Pause and Krauel (2000).

1.17 MMN as an index of cognitive capacity

An MMN deficit indexes cognitive and functional decline in a variety of different neuropsychiatric, neurological, and neurodevelopmental disorders (Näätänen et al., 2012). Interestingly, even in the normal healthy population, MMN indexes cognition. Dividing their subjects into high- and low-ability groups by means of a comprehensive psychometric assessment, Bazana and Stelmack (2002) observed that the MMN peak latency for tone-frequency change in a backward-masking MMN paradigm was considerably longer in the low- than high-ability subjects. Importantly, the MMN peak latency showed a substantial factor loading on the general factor of intelligence (the g factor) in the battery of the ability tests employed. Subsequently, De Pascalis and Varriale (2012) found that low-level auditory discrimination, as indexed by MMN, contributes to individual differences in fluid intelligence, concluding that MMN provides a valuable tool for examining intelligence in individuals who are not able or willing to comply with psychometric testing.

Moreover, Sculthorpe et al. (2009) found in normal healthy adults that 'higher mental ability' was associated with a larger MMN amplitude than 'lower mental ability' for occasional repetitions of two tones separated in frequency by either one or six semitones (Alain et al., 1994). For corroborating results, see Troche et al. (2009, 2010). Consistent with this, Schroeder et al. (1995) found that smaller MMN amplitudes were associated with cognitive decline. In addition, Houlihan and Stelmack (2012) reported that their 'high-ability' adults had a larger amplitude MMN in response to an occasional auditory feature-conjunction change than that of their 'low-ability' adults. Consistent with this, Light et al. (2007) found a strong association between the MMN amplitude for tone-duration increment and cognitive performance in normal healthy adults, concluding that sensory-level central nervous system (CNS) information processing, as reflected by MMN to auditory change, in clinically healthy individuals is strongly associated with cognitive and real-world psychosocial functioning of these individuals. Similar results were obtained in children by Liu et al. (2007) who reported that children with a higher level of general intellectual functioning showed MMNs with larger amplitudes for syllable change than those with a lower level of general intellectual functioning.

Further support for the MMN-cognition relationship was provided by pharmacological results, both with drugs enhancing and with those dampening cognition. Nicotine has well-known cognition-enhancing effects, observed in aged rodents and both in (as yet) healthy smokers and non-smokers (Martin et al., 2009; for a review, see Inami et al., 2005). In normal healthy subjects, a transdermal administration of nicotine shortened the MMN-peak latency (Inami et al., 2005) and an oral administration of nicotine enhanced the MMN-peak amplitude for a change in tone-interval duration (Martin et al., 2009), tone duration (Baldeweg, 2006), and consonant-vowel syllable (Harkrider & Hedrick, 2005). Moreover, nicotine enhanced the vMMN amplitude for change of the length of a vertically oriented bar (Dunbar et al., 2007). Studies of nicotinic agonists being developed for the treatment of cognitive deficits in schizophrenia and Alzheimer's disease, (e.g. α7 nicotinic agonists) also appear to enhance MMN (Preskorn et al., 2014). As already noted, a single dose of memantine, a noncompetitive NMDA receptor antagonist approved for the treatment of Alzheimer's disease, enhances MMN in both healthy non-psychiatric subjects and schizophrenia patients (Swerdlow et al., 2016).

Consistent with this, some substances such as alcohol adversely affected cognition as well as diminished the MMN amplitude (Jääskeläinen et al., 1995, 1996a, 1996b, 1996c). In addition, nitrous oxide (Pang & Fowler, 1999), triazolam (Clark et al., 1979), and chlorpheniramine (Serra et al., 1996), all impairing cognitive function, diminished the MMN amplitude.

1.18 **MMN and personality**

Several recent studies reported MMN correlates of the different dimensions of personality. It was shown by Hansenne et al. (2003) that the harm-avoidance (HA) dimension of Cloninger's (1994) model of personality was negatively correlated with the MMN amplitude for occasional longer-duration tones in an ignore condition in normal healthy adults, concluding that MMN is related to the behavioural inhibition system (BIS; Gray, 1976; closely related to HA of Cloninger's model). According to Hansenne et al. (2003), this is consistent with clinical studies conducted in patients with schizophrenia and in those with anxiety disorders (in whom MMN is affected). This is also consistent with Clark et al. (1996) who found enhanced frontal P3a amplitudes, indexing involuntary attention switch, in patients with generalized anxiety. The HA dimension corresponds to the tendency toward an inhibitory response, with individuals high in HA being pessimistic, fearful, shy, and easily fatiguable (Cloninger & Svrakic, 1997). Interestingly, Hansenne (1999), in their previous study, found a negative relationship between the P3 amplitude and the HA score in normal healthy subjects, permitting Hansenne et al. (2003) to conclude that, taken together, the results of these two studies suggest opposite effects of

BIS on P3 and MMN, and hence on controlled and automatic processing, respectively. Automatic processes are improved whereas controlled processes are impaired with the activation of BIS.

In addition, Wang et al. (2001) also found that MMN was related to personality. They assessed personality by using the Zuckerman (1994) model of personality. Their results showed that the (frontal) MMN amplitude was positively correlated with Neuroticism-Anxiety and negatively with Experience Seeking. Subsequently, Franken et al. (2005) found that the MMN amplitude for tone-frequency change was larger in high- than low-impulsive normal healthy subjects. Impulsivity is an important feature of a number of psychiatric disorders such as attention deficit hyperactivity disorder (ADHD), some personality disorders, and deviant behaviours such as criminal behaviour and aggression (Moeller et al., 2001). Impulsive persons are characterized with a preference for immediate gratification, risky activities, and novel sensations.

Impulsivity is regarded as being closely related to other personality constructs such as extraversion, novelty seeking, and sensation seeking (Zuckerman & Kuhlman, 2000). Most of the processes affected in High Impulsivity refer to cognitive top-down control processes: the lack of voluntary inhibitory control, and only a few authors relate Impulsivity to bottom-up processing, one of whom being Dickman (1993, 2000) who, in his 'attentional-fixation' theory, proposed that persons with high impulsivity relatively easily shift attention away from its current fixation. Importantly, the previously reviewed results of Franken et al. (2005) show that impulsivity is also linked to non-motor cognitive processes, with impulsive persons exhibiting enhanced pre-attentive processing of deviant stimuli, that does not depend on the execution of responses. The latter results are also in line with those of Sasaki et al. (2000) who, in their long-ISI condition, found a positive correlation between the late MMN amplitude and extraversion. Moreover, these results are also consistent with those of Zhang et al. (2001) who found increased MMN amplitudes in subjects at high risk for alcoholism as heavy drinkers and individuals at high risk for alcoholism are also high in impulsiveness (Granö et al., 2004). Hence, the results of Franken et al. (2005) showing that central auditory processing is modulated by normal fluctuations in impulsivity have implications for the study of psychopathology-related impulsivity, too. The authors concluded that personality variables, such as impulsivity, are variables that mediate the relation between psychopathology and psychophysiological parameters.

More recently, Matsubayashi et al. (2008), using MMNm, also found connections between personality variables and automatic central auditory processing in normal healthy subjects. The temperament and character inventory (TCI) was used to assess individual personality traits. It was found that the persistence score predicted the amplitude of the phonetic MMNm for the left hemisphere in a combined sample of males and females and that of the tone-duration MMNm for the left hemisphere in males. In addition, reward dependence predicted the peak latency of the tone-duration MMNm for the left hemisphere in males, and cooperativeness, the amplitude of the tone-frequency MMNm for the right hemisphere in females. These results suggest, according to the authors, that gender and personality traits have an effect on the individual variability of MMNm and may provide useful information to establish MMN/MMNm as a clinical tool for monitoring auditory cortical function on an individual basis.

1.19 **Overview and conclusions**

Brain events underlying auditory perception. (a) MMN makes it possible to determine the duration and width of the sliding TWI used by the brain in forming auditory percepts (Yabe et al., 1998, 1999; Näätänen et al., 2007; Näätänen & Winkler, 1999; Shinozaki et al., 2003); (b) MMN thus contributed to the solution of the binding problem in audition, shedding light on the feature integration that is a central prerequisite for unitary auditory percepts (Näätänen & Winkler, 1999; Näätänen et al., 2007, 2010); (c) by showing that auditory perception is directly based on memory-trace formation, MMN makes an important contribution to our understanding of both memory-trace formation, and (d) the relationship between perception and sensory memory in audition; (e) MMN also permits determination of the neurophysiological processes underlying auditory scene analysis, i.e. those controlling auditory stream formation and the segregation of parallel auditory input from different sources into separate auditory streams (for a review, see Näätänen et al., 2007).

Auditory short-term memory. (a) In addition to shedding light on the central principles governing the formation of short-term memory traces in audition, (b) MMN studies also confirmed the crucial role of the NMDA receptors in memory-trace formation (Javitt et al., 1996; Umbricht et al., 2002); and (c) showed that memory-trace formation occurs at a stage subsequent to cortical afferent responses and anteriorly to their locus, with the locus of memory-trace formation depending on the dimension of sound change (Näätänen et al., 2010; Paavilainen et al., 1991; see also Näätänen & Rinne, 2002); (d) Hence, MMN also enables mapping of the functional neuroanatomy of sensory memory in audition, (e) permits one to determine the duration and other properties of these memory traces (Näätänen et al., 2007), and (f) might also contribute to our understanding of the neurophysiological relationship between auditory short-term and long-term (or permanent) memories.

Auditory long-term memory. (a) With certain MMN paradigms, one can also probe long-term auditory memory traces, such as such as those of familiar melodies or voices, and determine their properties (Jacobsen et al., 2005; Roye et al., 2007); (b) The discovery of language-specific speech sound memory traces was also based on MMN/MMNm recordings, with these traces being located to the left temporal lobe by using MEG (Näätänen et al., 1997; Shestakova et al., 2002). MMN studies also suggested that the spoken language can be correctly perceived only when the corresponding speech-sound memory traces (recognition patterns) are sequentially activated by the corresponding speech-sound input, in analogy to piano keys (Näätänen, 1999); (c) MMN also enables one to unravel the brain basis of higher order linguistic phenomena such as the representations of words, sentences, grammatical rules, and even semantic meanings (Shtyrov & Pulvermüller, 2007; Pulvermüller & Shtyrov, 2006, Pulvermüller et al., 2008; Pulvermüller

& Assadollahi, 2007); (d) MMN also enables one to objectively monitor the progress of speech-sound perception as a function of exposure to a given language environment or language-training program. This helps one determine what kind of an auditory or auditory-linguistic training programme would be optimal.

Music perception and musicality. MMN also provides a tool for the objective evaluation of the different components of music perception (and talent) such as frequency, interval, and rhythm perception as well as the recognition of different abstract musical patterns. These brain prerequisites of music perception and production, and their improvement as a function of practice, can be measured by using MMN with no behavioural task, and even in small infants, by employing the paradigm developed for the objective evaluation of musical talent and skills by Vuust et al. (2011, 2012b; see also Tervaniemi et al., 2001).

Involuntary attention and conscious perception. MMN also played an essential role in describing the sequence of brain events underlying attention switch to infrequent change in unattended stimulation (Escera et al., 1998, 2000, 2003). This sequence of brain events is initiated by the emergence of a pre-perceptual change-detection signal in the auditory cortex, which activates the right-hemispheric frontal mechanism controlling for the direction of attention, resulting in attention switch to, and conscious perception of, stimulus change (Giard et al., 1990; Rinne et al., 2006). Hence, MMN also revealed an automatic cerebral warning mechanism for environmental changes of great biological significance. Furthermore, these studies also reconstructed the route from unconscious to conscious processes in response to auditory change, i.e. the brain mechanism of conscious perception in audition that brings sound change in sensory input into the focus of conscious awareness (for a review, see Näätänen et al., 2011).

Selective attention. MMN data were also essential in unravelling the brain mechanisms of auditory selective attention, showing that the selective-attention mechanism uses, in focusing selective attention to the desired auditory input channel, sensory information contained by memory traces involved in MMN generation (Alho et al., 1987a, 1987b, 1992, 1994; Näätänen & Michie, 1979; Näätänen, 1982, 1985, 1990, 1992; 2010; see also Hansen & Hillyard, 1983; Hillyard et al., 1973; Rissling et al., 2014).

Primitive sensory intelligence in audition. MMN studies revealed the occurrence of high-level automatic sensory-cognitive processes such as anticipation, extrapolation, rule extraction, pattern recognition, generalization, and even simple concept formation, in auditory cortex ('Primitive Sensory Intelligence'; Näätänen et al., 2001, 2010; see also Bendixen et al., 2007, 2009, 2012; Carral et al., 2005; Schröger et al., 2007). In contrast to the attention-dependent cognitive processes, these automatic cognitive processes occur even in infants (Carral et al., 2005; Ruusuvirta et al., 2004) and in different animal species such as rabbit (Astikainen et al., 2000), rat (Ruusuvirta et al., 1998; Astikainen et al., 2011), guinea pig (Kraus et al., 1994a), pigeon (Schall et al., 2015), dog (Howell et al., 2012), cat (Csépe et al., 1987a, 1987b) and mouse (Ehrlichman et al., 2008). For a review, see Näätänen et al. (2010). Furthermore, recent vMMN studies revealed the occurrence of analogous automatic sensory-cognitive processes even in vision (for a review, see Kimura et al., 2011). Consequently, as already mentioned, these intelligent auditory-cortical processes, with similar automatic processes in other sense modalities (Stefanics et al., 2011), appear to provide the perceptual-cognitive core of cognitive processes shared by a large range of different species, different states of consciousness, and different developmental stages as proposed by Näätänen et al. (2010).

Chapter 2

How to record and analyse MMN

2.1. **Principles in MMN elicitation**

MMN is usually recorded in the oddball paradigm in which 'standard' stimuli, repeated at short stimulus onset asynchronies (SOAs), are occasionally interspersed with 'deviant' stimuli which elicit MMN. MMN is traditionally measured from difference waves obtained by subtracting the event-related potential (ERP) to standards from that to deviants. The whole difference wave, however, may not necessarily represent a 'pure' MMN alone, for a deviant stimulus may also activate new or fresh afferent elements because of the longer SOAs between consecutive deviants than those between consecutive standards. Although measuring a MMN that is unconfounded with fresh afferent elements may not be an issue for clinical research if the response properties fulfil other desirable properties (e.g. high test-retest reliability, sensitivity to clinical, cognitive, or therapeutic features), it should be noted that frequency, intensity- and duration-increment deviants may also suffer from this potential problem. Therefore, in determining the (genuine) MMN amplitude, measurement windows should be chosen from the early post-N1 time zone. On the other hand, the duration- and intensity-decrement MMNs and the stimulus-omission MMN are relatively free of this type of problem. Furthermore, more novel paradigms have been developed for estimating the contribution of the new afferent elements to the difference wave. In these paradigms (Schröger & Wolff, 1998b; Jacobsen & Schröger, 2003; Jacobsen et al., 2003), the deviant stimulus is presented in a block with no repetitive standard stimuli which are instead replaced by a number of different infrequent stimuli, each presented at the same low probability as the deviant stimulus in the oddball paradigm, say, at 10%.

A possible way to reduce the N1 amplitude, and to shorten the block duration, is to present the stimuli with no silent break between them. Schröger et al. (1994) presented a continuous sequence of identical patterns of five tones differing in frequency, with the standard pattern being composed of brief tones of 500-638-720-920-1040 Hz, occasionally replaced with a deviant pattern in which tones one and three were interchanged but was otherwise identical to the standard pattern. It was found that the deviant patterns elicited MMN even though the auditory stimulation was continuous, i.e. no silent between-pattern interval indicated the beginning of the next tone pattern. It was concluded that the MMN mechanism is not necessarily timed by an 'external' reference but rather uses 'internal units' extracted from the repetitive structure inherent in the continuous flow of acoustic signals. Subsequently, Pihko et al. (1995) presented their subjects with a continuous sound consisting of two alternating frequencies of the same short duration. It was found that an occasional shortening of one of the tones elicited MMN with a peak latency that was shorter with shorter-duration deviants in a graded manner. The total recording time was only 11 min. These results were confirmed in adults by Kalyakin et al. (2009) and in children by Cong et al. (2009). In a similar vein, Winkler & Schröger (1995) showed that MMN was elicited by duration deviants in a paradigm with two alternating short tones of different frequencies. Moreover, Lavikainen et al. (1995) found that a minor frequency change of a brief duration in a continuous tone elicited MMN, together with N1.

The MMN amplitude is decreased by increasing the deviant-stimulus probability (Ritter et al., 1992). This is partially due to the standard stimulus being more often replaced by a deviant stimulus (and then being unable to contribute to the trace strength equally often) than with a smaller deviant-stimulus probability. Another factor that warrants consideration in the context of eliciting 'pure' MMNs, however, is the fact that with shorter deviant-stimulus SOAs, the deviant stimuli start to develop a trace of their own (cf. Donchin's (1981) influential context-updating hypothesis of P3; see also Sutton et al., 1965; Javitt et al., 1996; Sams et al., 1984; Winkler et al., 1996a, 1996b; Sussman & Winkler, 2001), which in turn inhibits MMN generation with regard to the original standard (Näätänen et al., 1987; Ritter et al., 1992). Therefore one should split the deviant stimuli to either side of the standard stimulus. For instance, Ritter et al. (1992) presented their 20%-probability frequency deviants of 5% on both sides of their 1000 Hz standards, i.e. 10% at 1050 Hz and 10% at 950 Hz. In fact, an early account of MMN (Näätänen, 1984) explained the MMN elicitation in terms of the deviant stimulus starting to develop a representation of its own in the sensory memory system already engaged by the representation of the standard.

Subsequent studies (Sato et al., 2000; Haenschel et al., 2005) found that the frontally recorded MMN is more sensitive to probability manipulation than the auditory cortex (i.e. mastoid electrode) MMN. When two deviants happen to occur consecutively, then MMN to the second deviant is smaller in amplitude than that to the first deviant (Müller et al., 2005b). This decrease of the MMN amplitude is, however, markedly smaller if the second deviant deviates from the standard in an attribute different from the first deviant (Müller et al., 2005b; Nousak et al., 1996; Sams et al., 1984). Further, with larger magnitudes of stimulus deviation, the contribution of new afferent elements may be enhanced, depending on the type of auditory deviation used, but the genuine MMN, too, is usually enhanced in amplitude and its peak latency is shortened (Tiitinen et al., 1994; for a review, see Näätänen et al., 2007).

It is also noteworthy that some threshold duration has to be exceeded by the standard stimulus to provide sufficient sensory data for the formation of a precise memory trace. This duration (which may be longer for more complex stimuli) for simple stimuli is of the order of 50–100 ms (Paavilainen et al., 1991), roughly corresponding to the stimulus duration needed for the N1 amplitude to reach its maximum (Näätänen & Picton, 1987). This correspondence supports the hypothesis of the reciprocity of the N1 and MMN generators (Näätänen, 1984; Cowan et al., 1993) according to which N1 reflects trace formation (the amount of sensory input to the trace system by a stimulus), a prerequisite for MMN elicitation by deviant stimuli. When a memory trace for a stimulus already exists, then the N1 amplitude is small and stimuli differing from that represented by the trace will elicit MMN. On the other hand, if there is no trace, then the N1 amplitude is large (being generated by a strong trace-formation process) and no MMN is elicited by a deviant stimulus (Paavilainen et al., 1993). With more complex standard stimuli, the MMN amplitude for deviants may be larger. It was found by Tervaniemi et al. (2001) that MMN elicited by a frequency change was larger in amplitude with spectrally complex sounds than with simple sinusoidal tones as standard stimuli. In addition, the rate at which standards are presented is, of course, of importance for trace formation. With shorter SOAs between the standards, the MMN amplitude gets larger (Näätänen et al., 1987; Sabri & Campbell, 2001; Javitt et al., 1998).

2.2. **Different MMN paradigms**

MMN can be recorded in a variety of stimulus paradigms for studying different aspects of central auditory processing, including auditory discrimination, sensory-memory duration, trace formation, temporal resolution, and distraction.

Auditory discrimination

Auditory discrimination has been traditionally studied by employing the classical oddball paradigm in which usually one type of deviant stimulus only is delivered in a block. Recently, more time-effective stimulus paradigms with multiple types of deviant stimuli were introduced such as the 'optimal paradigm' of Näätänen et al. (2004). In this paradigm, only every second stimulus is a standard while the rest of the stimuli are deviants of different types (frequency, duration, intensity, locus of the origin, and gap deviants, each at 10%; Fig. 2.1). Importantly, MMNs obtained are of the same order of magnitude

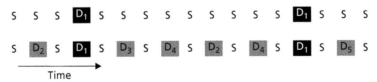

Fig. 2.1 A schematic illustration of the oddball (top) and the multi-feature (bottom; Optimum-1) paradigms. Whereas in the oddball paradigm, 1-2 deviants have traditionally been presented, the multi-feature paradigm can include several deviant types. In this paradigm, the deviants alternate with the standards so that every other stimulus is a standard and every other one a deviant sound. The rationale of the multi-feature paradigm is that each deviant stimulus strengthens the memory traces for those sound features it shares with the rest of the stimuli. For example, if the frequency of the sound changes, the remaining unchanging features, e.g., duration, intensity, strengthen the respective representations.
Based on Näätänen et al. (2004).

as when each deviant is presented in the traditional single-deviant oddball paradigm (at the same 10% probability). This novel 'multi-feature' paradigm enabled recording of the discrimination profile of an individual in only 15 min using five different auditory attributes, with similar data quality to that in the traditional single-deviant oddball paradigm. Subsequent research demonstrated that this paradigm can even be successfully used in infants and older children (Lovio et al., 2009; Petermann et al., 2009; Sambeth et al., 2009; Partanen et al., 2013c) and with speech stimuli (Lovio et al., 2009; Pakarinen et al., 2009; Partanen et al., 2013c, 2013d; Davids et al., 2009). It should be noted, however, that this 'optimal' and other multi-feature auditory oddball paradigms described here have not undergone the same level of extensive validation (short- and long-term reliability, sensitivity to drug effects, relationships to important domains of cognitive function) as the classic and simpler oddball paradigms, particularly in clinical research applications (Light et al., 2012).

In Pakarinen et al.'s (2007) multi-level MMN paradigm, each of the four types of stimulus deviations used occurred at six different magnitudes of stimulus change. As expected, all the 24 different sound changes elicited MMN and, further, the MMN amplitude was increased and peak latency decreased with an increasing magnitude of stimulus change (Fig. 2.2). Importantly, the MMN amplitude and peak latency predicted the subject's accuracy and speed in detecting these deviants among standards in a separate behavioural discrimination task (see also Pakarinen et al., 2009). A further modification of the original 'optimal' paradigm is the time effective three-deviant version of Fisher et al. (2011a, 2011b) with duration, frequency, and intensity deviants, which resulted in considerable time savings.

Moreover, Vuust et al. (2011, 2012b) extended the 'optimum paradigm' to a musical context by developing a novel multi-feature MMN paradigm (with pitch, intensity, timbre, sound source location, rhythm, and pitch slide deviants) integrated into a complex musical context (the Alberti bass, an accompaniment commonly used in the Western musical culture in both classical and improvisational music genres providing a harmonic background for a melody). The authors found MMNs for all the six different deviant-stimulus types in this paradigm lasting for 20 min, concluding that this short objective measure can putatively be used as an index for auditory and musical talent and development. Nonetheless, while it is an important validation of the concept that MMNs *can* be elicited in this paradigm in healthy subjects, it is unknown whether such a paradigm would be suitable for use in clinical trial applications.

Sensory-memory duration

With an increasing SOA, MMN is attenuated in amplitude and its peak latency is prolonged (Alain et al., 1994; Schröger & Winkler, 1995), disappearing when the memory-trace duration is exceeded (Näätänen et al., 1987; Lindín et al., 2013). Therefore, MMN serves as a potent probe of the sensory-memory trace duration, providing a possible index of general brain plasticity. In young healthy subjects, this duration is of the order

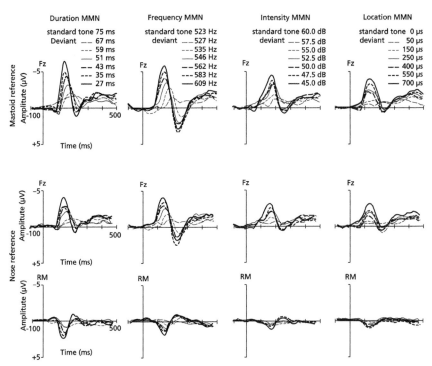

Fig. 2.2 Top panel: MMN, recorded with a variant of the multi-feature paradigm, to duration, frequency, intensity, and perceived sound-source location change as a function of the magnitude of stimulus change in recordings referenced to the mean of the two mastoid electrodes.
Lower panel: The same waveforms referenced to the nose electrode and shown from the Fz and the right mastoid (RM).

Reprinted from Clinical Neurophysiology, 118(1), Pakarinen, S., Takegata, R., Rinne, T., Huotilainen, M. & Näätänen, R. 2007, *Measurement of extensive auditory discrimination profiles using the mismatch negativity (MMN) of the auditory event-related potential (ERP)*, 185–177, Copyright 2007, with permission from Elsevier.

of 10 s (Böttcher-Gandor & Ullsperger, 1992) but is considerably shortened with aging (Pekkonen et al., 1993, 1996; Coope et al., 2006; Grau et al., 1998) and, in particular, in Alzheimer's disease (Pekkonen et al., 1994).

Grau et al. (1998) designed an ingenious paradigm to effectively determine the sensory-memory trace duration. Trains of three stimuli of 75 ms in duration were delivered at 300 ms SOAs while the consecutive trains were separated by a 'probe interval'. This interval was, in different stimulus blocks, either 0.4 s or 4 s, and was equiprobably terminated by a standard or a deviant. The results demonstrated that with this paradigm, one can determine sensory-memory duration in less than a half of the time needed with the conventional MMN paradigm. Further confirmation for the Grau paradigm was provided by the excellent MMN data of Glass et al. (2008a, 2008b) from their studies on the developmental trajectory of the memory-trace duration in the early childhood.

Memory-trace formation

In the beginning of a stimulus block, the standard stimulus has to be repeated for a couple of times before a deviant stimulus can elicit MMN (Cowan et al., 1993; Winkler et al., 1996a, 1996b). Moreover, the MMN amplitude gets larger with an increasing number of standards preceding a deviant (Sams et al., 1983; Imada et al., 1993; Javitt et al., 1998; Baldeweg et al., 2004; Haenschel et al., 2005; Matuoka et al., 2008) and with a shorter SOA between the standards (Näätänen et al., 1987; Sabri & Campbell, 2001; Javitt et al., 1998; Alain et al., 1994). For supporting fMRI results, see Sabri et al. (2004). The so-called roving paradigm is well suited for investigating the formation of the memory trace. In this paradigm, when the deviant stimulus is presented, it will thereafter be repeated whereby it starts to serve as a standard stimulus. Therefore, one can determine, for instance, how many repetitions are needed to elicit an MMN, i.e. how many sounds are needed to form a sufficient memory trace for discriminating the deviant stimulus. In addition, MMN elicitation early in a stimulus block may be facilitated by the standard stimulus of the block being identical to that of the preceding block (Cowan et al., 1993).

The presence of a sensory-memory trace can usually be determined only indirectly, i.e. by presenting deviant stimuli in a sequence of standard stimuli, as there usually is no ERP sign of memory-trace formation (besides the attenuation of the amplitudes of the exogenous ERP components with stimulus repetition). However, in 2002, Näätänen and Rinne (2002) described a new type of a negative component, apparently a correlate of memory-trace formation. Using a randomized sequence of tones of different frequencies, the authors found a 'repetition negativity' which was elicited by a few consecutive repetitions of a tone in a randomized sequence of tones with different frequencies. This negativity was also observed when complex-tone stimuli were used. (However, in some stimulus paradigms, the repetition effect may also be of a positive polarity; Haenschel et al., 2005). Näätänen and Rinne (2002) concluded that the repetition negativity might reflect a central principle governing the formation of long-term sensory memory representations: from an almost endless variation of auditory input, more enduring representations are developed only for those sounds that are repeated after a brief interval and at least a couple of times.

Temporal resolution

MMN provides an excellent index of temporal resolution, i.e. of the ability of the central auditory system to precisely track the rapidly varying stimulus patterns typical, for instance, for consonants. Auditory temporal resolution (the minimal time interval between two consecutive events that can be perceived as separate) can be objectively determined by using paradigms with stimuli including a gap in the middle. This probably is the only way of determining temporal resolution in infants and in different patient groups. In the MMN-based determination of temporal resolution of Desjardins et al. (1999), gap stimuli (deviants) were constructed by using two 2000

Hz Gaussian-enveloped tone pip markers with peak amplitudes separated, in different stimulus blocks, by 4, 5, or 7 ms. The standards were energy- and duration-matched tone pips with no gap. It was found that the gap-detection thresholds measured with MMN matched well with the behaviourally measured thresholds. (For corroborating ERP and MEG results, see Uther et al., 2003). Subsequently, Trainor et al. (2001) showed that with this procedure, auditory temporal thresholds can be determined in individuals at different ages and that MMN is elicited even in the absence of attention and does not require a behavioural response. This means it can be measured in a similar way across the whole life span. For example, Bertoli et al. (2002, 2005) found that even in healthy elderly persons, MMN to a short gap in a brief tone was attenuated in amplitude, indexing their increased difficulties in correctly perceiving rapid speech-sound patterns, such as consonants (Chapter 7).

Temporal window of integration

Temporal window of integration (TWI) duration can be estimated both with behavioural and MMN measures. It was shown that about 150–200 ms from stimulus onset are needed for the completion of the trace development, and thus for a fully elaborated percept to emerge (Scharf & Houtsma, 1986; Cowan, 1984; Massaro, 1975; Winkler & Näätänen, 1994; Winkler et al., 1993). With MMN, this can be probed by varying the constant SOA of a stimulus block in which an infrequent stimulus omission elicits MMN only when the constant SOA is shorter than 150 ms (Yabe et al., 1997, 1998; see also Tervaniemi et al., 1994). Yabe et al. (1997) proposed that auditory input is processed in circa 150–170 ms temporal segments; therefore stimulus omission from this time segment initiated by the preceding stimulus elicits MMN, whereas stimulus omission occurring thereafter does not.

Shinozaki et al. (2003), recording MMNm to infrequent omissions of the second tone in repetitive tone pairs composed of two closely spaced tones of different frequencies, extended the concept of the TWI to also involve the spectral proximity of stimuli. Their 'spectro-temporal window of integration' (STWI) only integrates those stimuli falling in the same TWI that are also rather similar in frequency (see also Yabe et al., 2001), while accepting larger differences in the early than late phase of TWI, i.e. TWI became progressively narrower as time from window onset elapsed. Shinozaki et al. (2003) concluded that their study provides:

> the first neurophysiological evidence of the two-dimensional (spectro-temporal) window of integration existing in the human brain. Two stimuli presented in close succession in the time-by-frequency surface might be presented in the auditory system as a unitary integrated event. This auditory spectro-temporal integration should play an indispensable role for the neural processing of complex signal sequence such as vocalizations, speech and music. (p. 570)

Consistent with this, Yabe (2002) suggested that the deviance-detection sensitivity non-linearly decreases toward the end of TWI.

Backward masking

Auditory masking refers to any observation such that information in an auditory test stimulus is reduced by the presentation of another (masking) stimulus (Massaro, 1975). The perception of sequentially presented sounds may be hindered by backward masking, with a subsequent sound preventing or decreasing the perception of an immediately preceding sound, apparently by affecting its memory-trace formation and maintenance (Massaro, 1975). Backward masking can be assessed both behaviourally and by using MMN: a masker presented shortly after each stimulus of the oddball paradigm causes MMN to deviants and the subject' ability to discriminate stimuli behaviourally to disappear in parallel (Winkler & Näätänen, 1995; Winkler et al., 1993). By using this type of paradigm, it was found by Kujala et al. (2003) that backward masking is enhanced in individuals with dyslexia. In addition, in chronic alcoholism, the MMN-data pattern also suggests the presence of increased backward masking, which is associated with the patients' working memory deficit (Ahveninen et al., 1999).

Perceptual streaming and stream segregation

In conditions with different frequent stimuli occurring in parallel streams, MMN may show modularity, essential, for instance, in listening to a certain speaker in the presence of concurrent speakers (Bregman et al., 1990). When two sound sequences, one to the left ear and the other to the right ear, are presented at a rapid rate, then deviants in each stream elicit MMN relative to the standards of the same ear only, there being no, or very little, across-ear 'cross-talk' (Ritter et al., 2000). This means that there can be two or several parallel stimulus sequences with separate MMN elicitation in the same stimulus block. A comparison of MMNs elicited in either one, two, or three concurrent auditory streams, defined by spatial position and frequency, showed that the MMN amplitude was smaller when there were three than one or two streams (Nager et al., 2003). This result reflects, according to the authors, the capacity limits of auditory sensory memory, resulting in less accurate traces with an increasing number of concurrent stimulus streams.

Separate streams can also be created within the same locus of sound origin by introducing a major frequency difference between two concurrent stimulus sequences, with each sequence being delivered at short SOAs (Sussman et al., 1999; Yabe et al., 2001a, 2001b; Shinozaki et al., 2000; see also Ritter et al., 1995; Gomes et al., 1997; Brattico et al., 2002). Moreover, a moving sound source (e.g. the consecutive steps of a walking person) also forms a sound stream, and if there is a deviation in that moving source, MMN is elicited, even in the presence of continuous loud environmental noise (Winkler et al., 2003).

The streaming paradigm might be useful, for instance, for determining why the elderly in particular find it difficult to listen to a certain speaker in a restaurant table at the presence of concurrent speakers. This problem may originate from a deficient stream segregation. In such a case, stream-specific MMNs would not be elicited (see Müller et al., 2005a, 2005b); hence, MMN might provide an index for pre-perceptual stream segregation supporting the perception of the speech message of a given speaker in the presence of multiple parallel sound sources.

Distraction

Voluntary selective attention enables our cognitive system to protect task-related processing from irrelevant information while enhancing the perceptual representation of information that is currently important. New information or changes outside the current focus of attention may, however, break through this shield as involuntary attention mechanisms cause attention to be automatically allocated towards unexpected or new information. Schröger and Wolff (1998b) developed a novel paradigm to study this interplay between shielding and receptiveness of the central auditory system. In its classic version, subjects perform a two alternative forced-choice duration-discrimination task on a sequence of short and long sounds. Additionally, the stimulus sequence contains infrequent changes on a task-irrelevant dimension (e.g. frequency) which can occur equiprobably on a short or long sound. Performance on the duration-discrimination task was impaired by irrelevant frequency changes (deviants), resulting in prolonged RTs and decreased hit rates compared to performance after standards (Schröger & Wolff, 1998b). This behavioural impairment has been replicated with different dimensions of stimulus change and in different populations (e.g. Ahveninen et al., 2000). The comparison of ERPs elicited by deviants and standards revealed several different stages of deviance-related processing as follows: (1) involuntary change detection reflected by MMN; (2) involuntary attention shift to the deviant stimulus (P3a); and (3) the subsequent reorienting of attention to the task-relevant aspect of stimulation (the reorienting negativity (RON); Schröger & Wolff, 1998b).

In the distraction paradigm developed by Schröger (1996), tones of 80 ms in duration were presented via headphones to the left or right ear. Each left-ear stimulus (S1) was followed by a right-ear stimulus (S2) with an SOA of 200 ms. The interval between the offset of a right-ear stimulus and the onset of the next left-ear stimulus was 820 ms. Left-ear stimuli (80 dB sound pressure level (SPL)) had a frequency of 700 Hz (standard) and were randomly replaced by a frequency deviant consisting of a 50 Hz ('small deviant') or 200 Hz ('large deviant') change, randomly a frequency increment or decrement. Right-ear stimuli had a frequency of 1500 Hz and an intensity equiprobably either 80 or 70 dB SPL. The subject was instructed to attend to right-ear stimuli and to press a button to low-intensity right-ear stimuli and to withhold a response to high-intensity right-ear stimuli. In this and similar stimulus paradigms, the task performance was poorer after an irrelevant deviant than standard stimulus in the opposite ear. (For a review, see Escera et al., 2000.)

The auditory distraction paradigm provides a powerful tool for investigating and monitoring the cognitive system in its interactions between bottom-up (involuntary) and top-down (voluntary) processing of task-relevant and irrelevant information. These processes may be altered in a variety of different clinical populations including children with developmental disorders, older adults with cognitive decline, or patients with brain lesions affecting perception and cognition (Alho et al., 1994a, 1994b; Deouell et al., 2000a, 2000b; Bäckman et al., 2000; Gumenyuk et al., 2005; Kaipio et al., 1999, 2000, 2001). Currently, the description of the behavioural deficits of such patients includes terms such as 'distractible' or 'disinhibited' on the one hand, and 'inattentive' or 'apathetic' on the other hand. However, there are hardly any standardized tools for either quantifying the deficit, or more importantly, addressing the subcomponents of the deficit in neural as well as cognitive terms. If the distraction paradigm is to be used for investigating different clinical populations, then the test should be as brief as possible and consist of a feasible and easily comprehensible primary task without sacrificing sensitivity, and should prefer-ably examine processing characteristics for different deviations to obtain a comprehensive view of the underlying causes of the deficits (for a review, see Grimm et al., 2008).

Primitive sensory intelligence

As already reviewed, there seems to exist a common core, i.e. automatic sensory-cognitive processes that form the basis for higher-order cognitive processes. This evidence, based on the MMN/MMNm data, indicates that in audition, complex cognitive processes occur automatically and mainly in the sensory-specific cortical regions. These processes include stimulus anticipation and extrapolation, sequential stimulus-rule extraction, and pattern and pitch-interval encoding. Recently, analogous evidence from the visual modality has also become available (for a review, see Kimura et al., 2011). Currently, it is not known to what extent these forms of sensory intelligence are preserved or affected in different severe psychiatric disorders. By employing paradigms tapping these sensory-cognitive processes, MMN might open new avenues for understanding, evaluating, and monitoring the ongoing disease process and for different attempts at remediation.

Novel paradigms have been developed to evaluate these sensory-cognitive functions. Saarinen et al. (1992), in a pioneering study, presented tone pairs to their subjects in-structed to ignore auditory stimuli. The tone pairs randomly varied in frequency, with the constant feature of the standard pairs being an abstract, or second order, one: the standard pairs were ascending ones (the second tone being higher in frequency than the first tone), whereas the deviant pairs were descending ones. Thus, the abstract attribute defining the standards was the rule governing the frequency relationship between the two tones forming a pair. Nevertheless, MMN was elicited by deviant pairs, showing that the pre-attentively formed sensory representations were capable of encoding the abstract attribute ('ascending pair'), i.e. of deriving a common invariant feature from a set of phys-ically varying events.

More recently, Paavilainen et al. (2007) presented their subjects with a sequence of four equiprobable tones: short–low, short–high, long–low, long–high, with the rule then being that short tones were followed by low tones and long tones by high tones. MMN was elicited, in subjects instructed to ignore stimuli, by violations of the sequential rules, e.g. when a high tone followed a short one. Interestingly, subjects were able, in a subsequent active detection condition, to detect correctly only about 15% of the rule-violating stimuli, and none of them was able to describe the rule verbally. Subsequently, Bendixen et al.

(2007; see also 2009, 2012; Bendixen & Schröger, 2008; Bendixen et al., 2010; for a review, see Bendixen et al., 2012) developed a sensory-intelligence paradigm that was even more taxing to these automatic processes. They found MMN to these highly complex rule violations. Importantly, when the rule was unexpectedly changed during an ongoing stimulus block, then only two to three exemplars of stimuli obeying the new rule sufficed for rule updating: MMN was elicited by subsequent stimuli that violated the new rule.

2.3 **Conclusions**

(1) The central auditory system automatically carries out even complex cognitive processes forming a sensory-cognitive basis for higher-order cognitive processes.

(2) These automatic cognitive processes include sequential stimulus-rule extraction and pitch-interval encoding. These various features can be extracted using MMN elicited in typical or cleverly designed auditory paradigms.

(3) It is possible that these processes are affected in different cognitive brain disorders providing new avenues for understanding and treating these different disorders. Additional studies are needed to evaluate the psychometric properties of MMN and other features extracted from these promising novel paradigms.

Chapter 3

The development of MMN

3.1 Introduction

The central nervous system goes through immense changes during early development, starting with an overproduction of neurons and synapses during foetal development, which is followed by a selective death of neurons (apoptosis) and the elimination of synapses (pruning) (e.g. Freberg, 2006). Pruning may eliminate about 40% of cortical synapses after the first year of life. The survival of neurons and synaptic connections is dependent on neurotrophins and neural activity. Only those synapses which belong to functionally active neural assemblies will survive.

The myelination of the neurons in humans begins at about 24 weeks after conception, but a burst of myelination occurs at around the time of birth, continuing until early adolescence. The myelination starts from the spinal cord, successively continuing in hindbrain, midbrain, and forebrain. Further, the sensory areas become myelinated before the motor areas. The last area completing the myelination is the prefrontal cortex.

During neural development, the auditory event-related potential (ERP) changes, whereby some components emerge and the existing ones change in amplitude and latency. The auditory ERP of infants is dominated by a large, slow positivity, which becomes earlier and sharper in waveform by the toddler stage (e.g. Morr et al., 2002). During infant development, the N2 and N4 emerge after the P1 (Choudhury & Benasich, 2011), and the peak latencies of these responses gradually become shorter with age (Jing & Benasich, 2006). The N1 may be absent or small in children younger than 10 years of age, particularly if the stimulation rate is fast, growing in amplitude during adolescence (Ponton et al., 2002; Wunderlich & Cone-Wesson, 2006). The adult auditory ERP is, after brainstem potentials and middle latency responses, primarily composed of the P1, N1, and P2 components (for reviews, see: Näätänen & Picton, 1987; Näätänen, 1992).

3.2 Sound-change detection in infancy

A distinct response to changes in repetitive sounds appears to be present even in foetuses, recorded with flat bottom magnetoencephalography (MEG) devices or those specifically designed for investigating magnetic signals from the womb of pregnant women. Sound-change-elicited neural responses have been recorded from foetuses at 33–40 gestational weeks (Huotilainen et al., 2005; Draganova et al., 2005). A MMN-like response was found for a frequency change at about 320–330 ms from deviant-stimulus onset. Thus, the MMN provides an opportunity to investigate the very earliest stages of auditory processing, language development, and learning.

The first studies on newborn change-elicited responses were published in the early 1990s. These studies reported negative responses for frequency changes at about 300 ms (Alho et al., 1990) and for vowel changes at about 200–250 ms (Cheour-Luhtanen et al., 1995) from stimulus-change onset. However, some later studies reported predominantly positivities (mismatch responses, MMR) rather than negativities for sound changes in infants (e.g. Dehaene-Lambertz & Baillet, 1998; Leppänen et al., 1997, 1999; Morr et al., 2002; Trainor et al., 2003; Jing & Benasich, 2006; Partanen et al., 2013a; Partanen et al., 2013c). There may be several reasons for the contradictory results concerning the change-elicited response in the childhood. Stimulus parameters, for example, the type and magnitude of stimulus deviance (Cheng et al., 2015) as well as age (Trainor et al., 2003) or maturity (Leppänen et al., 2004) may affect the results. Furthermore, the MMR may be hidden under a slow positive response typical of infants, or different signal processing approaches may affect the results (Trainor et al., 2003). The instability and low signal-to-noise ratio of infant data might also lead to inconsistent results. Therefore, it is of utmost importance always to ensure that the responses under inspection are significantly different from zero. Unfortunately, there are many infant studies which have ignored this test.

There are studies suggesting that positive MMRs mature towards the more adult-like negativity at the age of 4–9 months. Jing and Benasich (2006) investigated MMRs for changes of the fundamental frequency (100–300 Hz) of harmonic tones in 6-, 9-, 12-, 16, and 24-month-old children. They found a change-elicited response with a positive polarity at around 200–300 ms from change onset at 6-month-old infants, whereas at 9 months of age, a negative deflection (MMN) was found at around 170 ms after change onset. This negativity was also present at 12, 16, and 24 months of age.

Trainor et al. (2003) compared MMRs for a deviant sound with a silent gap, between 2-, 3-, 4-, and 6-month-old infants. This change elicited a positivity in 2–4 month-old infants whereas at the age of 6 months, an MMR with a negative polarity, i.e. an MMN, was found. Individual data suggested that MMRs resembling those recorded from adults were seen in some infants at the age of 3 months (31%), in a large number of infants by the age of 4 months (58%), and in most infants by the age of 6 months.

He et al. (2009a) investigated the effect of a fast (400 ms) and slow (800 ms) stimulus onset asynchrony (SOA) and small (1/12 octave) and large (1/2 octave) frequency changes on the MMRs of adults, 4-month-olds, and 2-month-olds. In adults and 4-month-olds, negative MMNs were found, with a peak latency that decreased with the shorter SOA and the amplitude which was larger for the larger deviance. However, in the 2-month-olds, only a broad positive MMR was observed.

MMRs with a positive polarity have been reported even in 6–7 year-old children. For example, Maurer et al., (2003) compared change-elicited responses at this age and in adults for large and small frequency and phonetic changes. For both types of changes, the authors found frontal positivity in children and negativity in adults. However, their SOA was 383 ms (stimulus duration 100 ms). It is quite possible that in children, the

MMN could not be detected due to this very rapid stimulation rate, since the MMN has been reported to emerge at around 300–400 ms after stimulus-change onset at the age of 4–7 years (Shafer et al., 2010). Furthermore, this MMN with negative polarity was reported to follow positivity, especially in children younger than 5.5 years, and commenced at 100–300 ms from change onset. Thus, with rapid stimulation rates, the later, negative MMN might be hidden whereas some earlier change-related positive components might remain visible even at the age of 6–7 years.

The developmental changes in the MMR in infants coincide in time with major changes in the neural assemblies in the central auditory system. The adult MMN might be generated in the supragranular layers of the primary auditory cortex (A1) so that the apical dendrites in superficial layer II are depolarized, as shown by intra-cranial recordings in monkeys (Javitt et al., 1994). In layer III, this is accompanied by a passive circuit-completing source. The adult MMN seems to be associated with the extra-lemniscal pathway projecting from the thalamus (caudomedial part) to the superficial layers of the auditory cortex.

In infancy, during the first postnatal months, the auditory cortex goes through major physiological changes. Its synaptic density reaches its maximum (Huttenlocher & Dabholkar, 1997) and energy metabolism increases (Chugani & Phelps, 1991) at about 3 months of age. However, investigations on axonal diameters, development of myelin sheaths, and increases in conduction velocity suggest that only layer I is fully functional by the fourth postnatal month (Moore, 2002; Moore & Guan, 2001). After the age of 4 months, the vertical axons that penetrate layers IV, V, and VI from thalamic loci and horizontal axons from neurons in these deeper layers become fully functional. These developmental changes might underlie the transition of the immature MMR with positive polarity into the negative adult-like MMN response.

3.3 **Complex auditory skills in infancy**

Infant perception and cognition are very challenging to investigate due to the obvious reason that behavioural measures are hard to obtain from infants, particularly from newborns, who sleep most of the time. Therefore, the MMR has been increasingly used in recent years to investigate infant cognition. These studies have revealed that the infant brain analyses auditory information in a quite sophisticated manner, being able to carry out complex operations in extracting information.

The ability to organize sound streams. In conditions when there are several sound sources, our central auditory system has to segregate these inputs in order to analyse the contents of the relevant sound stream. For example, when there are several concurrent conversations (in a cafeteria, party, or some other gathering), one has to be able to extract the contents of the speech of a person with whom the conversation is going on. This is possible since the auditory system can group sounds together based on their physical characteristics. This ability, called streaming (Bregman, 1990), helps us to follow, for example, a male speaker during a nearby conversation of female speakers.

It has been known for a long time that infants can recognize their mother's voice (DeCasper & Fifer, 1980), but what happens if there are additional sound sources while the infant's mother is talking? By observing head-turning or non-nutritive sucking indicators, it was shown that infants can segregate concurrent sound streams (McAdams & Bertoncini, 1997).

Using the MMR, it was determined whether this ability is present even in newborns (Winkler et al., 2003). Two-to-five-day-old infants were presented with single sound streams or concurrent streams with low- vs high-frequency sounds. In a *control condition*, frequent soft (61 dB sound pressure level (SPL)) and infrequent louder (76 dB (SPL)) tones were presented with a uniform SOA of 750 ms. In the *one-stream condition*, two intervening tones were added between consecutive tones of the control condition (whereby the SOA was 250 ms between the stimuli). These intervening tones, delivered randomly, had equiprobably a frequency of 1655, 1732, 1898, or 1986 Hz and an intensity of 66, 71, 81, or 86 dB (SPL), which resulted in 16 different tones. In the *two-stream condition*, the frequencies of the intervening tones were lowered to 250, 262, 287, and 300 Hz, while the other parameters were not changed. Additionally, there was a control condition inspecting the effect of the sound-presentation rate.

In the control condition, the infrequent louder tones elicited a positively displaced MMR. In the one-stream condition including intervening tones, this response was abolished presumably due to the loudness variation of the intervening tones. However, in the two-stream condition, in which the intervening tones were low in frequency, the MMR again was significantly elicited, as in the control condition. The data pattern observed, i.e. a distinct response for deviant stimuli in the control and two-stream conditions and the absence of this response in the one-stream condition, was similar to that in the adults included in this study. These results show that the newborn brain can segregate sound streams. In practice, this suggests that newborns have the neural mechanism which is required for keeping a track of one speaker while several individuals are concurrently talking.

Binding sound features together. Another important perceptual ability is to conjoin different sensory features. An example of such feature binding in the visual domain is face perception, an important ability for humans, which appears to exist early in infancy (Valenza et al., 1996). Ruusuvirta et al. (2003) aimed to determine whether auditory feature binding occurs in the newborn brain. Their stimuli were four tones, a loud low-frequency tone, a soft low-frequency tone, a loud high-frequency tone, and a soft high-frequency tone. Two of these stimuli occurred frequently and two rarely in the sound sequences. The stimuli were assigned to standards and deviants so that across the tone categories, there was a symmetrical probability distribution for the levels of both features. Due to this, it is not possible to discriminate the categories based on frequency or intensity alone. It was found that the deviant stimuli elicited significant MMRs in newborns. This result suggests that the newborn brain can make a distinction between sounds even when combinations of sound features serve as the cue for detecting differences between them. This indicates that the tones were processed as holistic entities of their features, suggesting the presence of functional feature-binding mechanisms in the newborn brain.

Sensitivity to music categories. Newborn neural abilities in music perception have also been tested. Virtala et al. (2013) investigated whether the newborn brain can categorize consonance vs dissonance and major vs minor chords. Their standards were consonant root major chords and deviants dissonant, inverted major, and root minor chords. Transposed chords at several frequency levels were used and, therefore, no MMR could result unless the central auditory system could categorize the stimuli. The results suggested the sensitivity of the newborn brain to dissonant and minor chords, whereas no significant responses were elicited by inverted major chords. Similar results were found in adults and musically trained children, too (Virtala et al., 2011, 2012). These results suggest that the newborn brain has adult-like abilities to extract interval structures and react to dissonant sounds.

Processing of invariant speech features. An important auditory skill in speech perception is the ability to extract the identity of speech sounds irrespective of the speaker, e.g. whether the speaker is a male, female, or child, and despite the prosodic variation in the speech. Also this skill is present in adults at a low level of perception, as reflected by the MMN (Shestakova et al., 2004). Further, Dehaene-Lambertz and Pena (2001) investigated whether this ability is present in newborn infants by recording MMRs for changes of syllables, /pa/ vs /ta/, which were uttered by four female speakers, and having, therefore, different fundamental frequencies (F0s) and durations. Significantly different responses for the standard and deviant syllables were found even in the presence of this speaker variation. This suggests that the central auditory system can early on extract the identity of speech sounds from the acoustically varying speech signal.

Extracting auditory rules. Our perception of the auditory environment relies on the ability to make predictions on the forthcoming sound events based on the regularities present in the preceding sound input (Bregman, 1990; Winkler, 2007). This occurs without our awareness, as shown by studies suggesting MMN elicitation for violations of such regularities during passive listening even when the participants cannot detect these violations in attentive conditions (van Zuijen et al., 2006).

The ability to detect regularities and extract rules from the sound environment may be fundamental for learning languages. For example, one task of an infant in learning the native language is to find word boundaries. The breaks between words are one cue, but not a reliable marker as such (Kuhl, 2004). In each language, syllables are combined and occur sequentially with certain probabilities. With proper neural computational skills, these relationships and probabilities can be learned, which leads to the detection of words.

The fundamental ability to extract regularities develops early or might even be innate, since violations of auditory rules elicit MMRs even in newborns. For example, Carral et al. (2005) presented to sleeping newborns tone pairs with an ascending frequency (low-high) at seven different frequency levels, infrequently changing the order of the tones (high-low). They found that the tone-order change violating the rule according to which

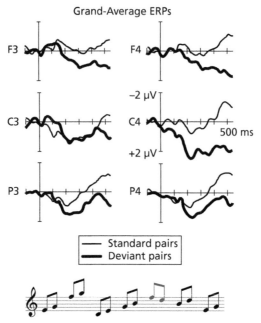

Fig. 3.1 Sleeping newborns can extract regularities from the auditory scene. Sleeping newborns were presented with tone pairs having an ascending frequency at 7 different frequency levels. Occasionally, the order of the tones within the pair was reversed. This change elicited a positively displaced MMR in newborns, suggesting that their brain could form a representation of the regular aspect, the rule that 'the 2nd tone is higher in frequency than the 1st one'.
Reproduced from Carral, V., Huotilainen, M., Ruusuvirta, T., Fellman, V., Näätänen, R. & Escera, C., *A kind of auditory 'primitive intelligence' already present at birth*, The European journal of neuroscience, 21 (11), 3201–3204, fig. 1, https://doi.org/10.1111/j.1460-9568.2005.04144.x Copyright © 2005, John Wiley and Sons.

the second tone is higher than the first one elicited distinct responses (Fig. 3.1). This indicates that the newborn brain can automatically extract regularities from auditory input.

3.4 **Plasticity in the infant brain**

The human infant learns native language surprisingly effortlessly. It was proposed by Kuhl (2004) that this ability is largely based on 'neural commitment' to language learning. The early stages of language learning are supported, or might even be based on, the infant brain's ability to detect patterns. Initially, the infant brain is not specialized to any language but discriminates sounds belonging to various languages (Kuhl, 2004). The exposure to the native language shapes the brain, which becomes tuned to this language. There is evidence for the development of the native-phoneme neural representations at the age of 6–12 months. MMN responses to native (Finnish /e/ vs /ö/) vs non-native (Estonian /e/ vs /õ/) vowel changes were compared in a cross-linguistic design (Cheour et al., 1998). At the age of 6 months, MMN indicated no facilitation for the discrimination of native (/ö/) vs Estonian (/õ/) vowel in Finnish infants whereas such a facilitation was found at the age of 12 months. In contrast, these two vowels elicited comparable MMNs in Estonian infants, whose language includes both of them. These results suggest that by the end of the first year of life, the infant's speech system adapts to the mother tongue and at the same time becomes less sensitive to sounds not belonging to the native language.

Besides plasticity associated with natural learning of the mother tongue, the effects of training on the infant brain have also been determined. One important question is how a foreign language exerts an influence on the infant brain at the age when it is getting specialized to the native language. Conboy and Kuhl (2011) tested how a foreign language, Spanish, affects the language system of infants from monolingual English-speaking families. Baseline recordings were carried out at the age of 41 weeks, yielding MMNs to a deviant syllable typical of the English vs Spanish language while a syllable common to these two languages served as the standard stimulus. After this baseline MMN recording, the infants participated, at the age of 42–46 weeks, in 12 language training sessions each including a 25-minute play session during which the language used was Spanish. The MMN recording described above was carried out again about 1–2 weeks after the last training session.

In the baseline recording at the age of 9 months, a significant MMN was found for the English contrast only, with the MMN for the Spanish contrast being insignificant, which is compatible with the idea that tuning to one's native language is underway at this age. However, after the training period including exposure to the Spanish language, MMNs for both speech contrasts significantly differed from zero. Furthermore, at an earlier latency range, the MMN for the native contrast had enhanced in amplitude and become significantly different from zero. Thus, these results, first of all, show that even a brief exposure causes learning of foreign speech sounds in infants whose brain is at the developmental stage of getting tuned to the native language. The results of this study, showing also an enhancement of an MMN-like response for the native language during this period, support the suggestion that improvements in native language learning continue during the exposure to a foreign language. However, interpretation of these interesting results must be cautious since no control group receiving either no or placebo training was included in this study. Therefore, it is difficult to disentangle possible rapid developmental effects from those specifically caused by the training.

How early on are we able to form memory traces and for how long can they last? Do we have memories preceding our birth? Foetuses are not detached from the world surrounding them: they receive information on the flavours of the food their mother is eating; they receive tactile information by moving and touching in the womb; and the mother's voice and other nearby sounds reach the ears of the foetus. The learning capacity of the foetal brain was investigated by studies employing auditory training during the foetal stage and measuring neural responses after the birth (Partanen et al., 2013a) and then again after several months (Partanen et al., 2013b). In the first of these studies (Partanen et al., 2013a), Finnish pregnant mothers played a CD containing a pseudoword /tatata/ and its variants /tatota/ and /tatata/ with a higher or lower F0 in the middle syllable. They played the CD to their unborn babies starting from pregnancy week 29 and continuing until birth. After these infants were born, their MMRs were compared with those recorded from a control group of infants who had not heard such material. MMRs were recorded for the pseudowords and their variants as well as for duration and intensity changes in the middle syllable of the pseudoword. Additionally, there was a control condition with harmonic tones equally unfamiliar for the two groups of infants.

Since Finnish is very rich with vowels and also contains vowels of different lengths, it could be expected that vowel and vowel duration changes would elicit a significant MMR in both groups. Indeed, the MMR for vowel changes was significantly elicited in both groups and the MMR for the vowel duration change was significant in the training group and nearly significant in the control group. These results are consistent with previous studies showing that newborns have MMRs for vowel changes (e.g. Kujala, A. et al., 2004; Partanen et al., 2013c).

Finnish speech, at least in the Greater Helsinki area where the participating families were living, has a descending or monotonic prosody. Therefore, the F0 change in the middle of the pseudoword, included in the training material, is a feature which foetuses in this area would very seldom hear. Therefore, it could be expected that there is a difference in the MMRs of the two infant groups for this change after their birth. The data clearly supported this expectation. Firstly, the MMR was significantly elicited for this change in the training but not in the control group. Secondly, there was a group difference in the amplitude of this response, with the MMR-related activity being stronger in the training than control group (Fig. 3.2). This result implies that the infant brain can become tuned to the auditory features of the environment even prior to birth. A subsequent study, investigating foetal learning of melodies, determined whether the memory traces formed prior to birth are long-lasting (Partanen et al., 2013b). It was found that the neural response to a melody was stronger in newborns who had been exposed to it in the womb than in newborns without such exposure. Moreover, this amplitude difference still existed in a follow-up recording after 4 months (Fig. 3.2). This suggests that the memory traces of sounds formed prior to birth can last for as much as several months.

These results suggest that sound environment affects the foetal brain, which may have both positive and negative consequences on the developing auditory system. Some sounds, like music, have positive influences on neural function (Särkämö et al., 2013), whereas some sound material, such as noise, may be harmful (for a review, see Kujala & Brattico, 2009). Excessive background noise in, for example, work places has long-term detrimental effects on adult central speech processing and attention (Kujala, T. et al., 2004; Kujala & Brattico 2009). Studies using animal models have shown that an unstructured auditory environment, containing primarily noise, impairs the development of auditory-cortex organization. Noise-rearing of rat pups had an influence on the response-selectivity of their neurons and prevented the emergence of the normal topographic organization of sound representations in the auditory cortex (Chang & Merzenich, 2003). Therefore, a noisy environment during pregnancy or the noise of the intensive care of prematurely born babies may have an influence on the auditory-system development. On the other hand, the results of Partanen et al. (2013a) on the enhancement of MMR amplitudes after

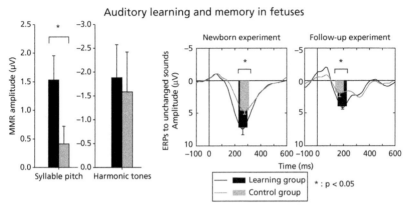

Fig. 3.2 The infant brain forms memory traces prior to birth. A group of fetuses were exposed to auditory input from the 29th pregnancy week until birth. After birth, MMRs were recorded for these 'training' stimuli (pseudoword /tatata/ with occasional changes in the middle syllable; on the left). In the Figure, the average MMR amplitudes (with standard errors of the means) are shown to frequency changes in the middle syllable from this group (black bars) and a control group (grey bars) not exposed to these stimuli. The frequency change elicited a robust and significant MMR in the exposed group but not in the control group, suggesting an enhanced accuracy in discriminating this change in the exposed group. In a subsequent study (on the right) the duration of memory traces acquired at the fetal stage was determined. Newborns, who had repetitively heard a melody prior to birth had a stronger response for this melody than a control group for which it was novel. In a follow-up study after four months, this amplitude difference was still found.

Data from Partanen, E., Kujala, T., Näätänen, R., Liitola, A., Sambeth, A., and Huotilainen, M., *Learning-induced neural plasticity of speech processing before birth*, PNAS, 220, 15145–15150, DOI: doi:10.1073/pnas.1302159110, 2013 and Partanen, E., Kujala, T., Tervaniemi, M. & Huotilainen, M., Prenatal music exposure induces long-term neural effects, PloS one, 8 (10), e78946, DOI: https://doi.org/10.1371/journal.pone.0078946, 2013.

exposure to pseudowords prior to birth imply that auditory abilities could be supported early on. Indeed, rat studies have also shown that a structured sound environment including, for example, music, is beneficial for the development of the auditory cortex (Kim et al., 2006) and cognitive abilities (Aoun et al., 2005).

These results showing the capacity of the foetal brain for learning lead to an important question: are these learning effects transient or do memories of the learnt material persist in the infant brain? This was investigated by exposing the foetuses to the melody of 'Twinkle, twinkle, little star' starting from pregnancy week 29 until the birth of the babies (Partanen et al., 2013b). The responses for the melody were recorded after birth from these babies and control babies who were not exposed to this melody. The neural response, a positive peak at around 250 ms from sound onset, for this melody was larger in amplitude in the training than control group. Moreover, at the end of the follow-up period when the infants were 4 months of age, the significant amplitude difference between the groups still existed. These results suggest that the foetal brain can form memory traces which may be last long, at least for several months. Thus, the environment starts to shape the brain even before birth and the auditory experiences at that time form long-lasting memory traces.

3.5 MMN development from toddler stage to school-age

The MMN peak latency. There are relatively few studies on the MMN development from the toddler stage to school age. In 2–3 year-old children, MMNs were recorded with the multi-feature paradigm (see Pakarinen et al., 2007) for five types of acoustic deviants—frequency, duration, intensity, location, and a sound including a gap—with frequency and duration deviants having a small, medium, or large magnitude of deviance (Putkinen et al., 2012). MMNs with a negative polarity differing significantly from zero were found for all the duration deviants, for the gap and intensity deviants, and for the largest frequency increment deviant. Another study (Niemitalo-Haapola et al., 2013), also employing the multi-feature paradigm, recorded MMNs for speech-sound changes at the age of 2 years. It was found that all the deviant stimuli used (consonant, vowel, and vowel duration change, and syllable frequency and intensity change) elicited significant MMNs. Thus, at the toddler stage, the central auditory system can discriminate multiple acoustic and speech-sound feature differences quite well.

The MMN peak latency changes during the childhood development. Glass et al. (2008b) studied MMN for a tone-frequency change (1000 vs 1200 Hz) in 2-, 3-, 4-, 5-, and 6-year-old children. The MMN was significant in conditions with various SOAs in the time windows as follows: at the age of 2: 140–248 ms; age of 3: 132–248 ms; age of 4: 132–232 ms; and age of 6: 108–212 ms. Thus, in this study, the MMN peak latency was fairly stable at the ages of 2–4 years, but became shorter, corresponding to peak latencies reported in adulthood, by the age of 6 years. Consistent with this, a peak latency shortening for MMNs, elicited by tone-frequency changes (1000 vs 1100 Hz), was reported in a study comparing 5–8 and 8–10-year-olds and adults (Gomot et al., 2000). The peak latency was at the age of 5–7 years 200 (+/- 29) ms, at the age of 8–10 years 163 (+/-26) ms, and in the adults 138 (+/-21) ms. Some studies have reported somewhat longer peak latencies for 5–7 year old children. A peak latency range of 265–336 ms was reported for MMNs elicited by frequency, duration, intensity, and gap deviants in 5–7-year-old children (Petermann et al., 2009), and a peak latency range of 270–335 ms for MMNs elicited by a vowel, consonant, vowel duration, frequency, and intensity change of a syllable in 6-year-old children (Lovio et al., 2009).

The MMN peak latency further shortens by age as suggested by a study on 7–12 and 13–16-year-old children and adults (Bishop et al., 2011). The average peak latency for a large tone-frequency deviant (1000 vs 1200 Hz) was in the child and teenager groups around 180–190 ms and in adults around 160 ms. For /da/ vs /bi/ syllable change, the average MMNs peaked at about 160 ms in the children and teenagers, whereas the peak latency in adults was about 140 ms.

The MMN amplitude. The amplitude of the MMN is very sensitive to stimulus and experimental parameters and, therefore, the most reliable approach to determine its developmental trajectory is to compare MMN amplitudes obtained with identical experimental parameters in different age groups. An MMN recorded from 2-, 3-, 4-, 5-, and 6-year-old children for a tone-frequency change from 1000 to 1200 Hz showed no significant effect of age on this amplitude (Glass et al., 2008b). This suggests that the discrimination of large acoustic differences of tones appears to be stable between the ages of 2 and 6 years.

Another study (Bishop et al., 2011) compared the MMNs (100–250 ms after change onset) and late discriminative negativities (LDN) (350–550 ms after change onset) elicited by large (1000 vs 1200 Hz; /ba/ vs /bi/) and small (1000 vs 1030 Hz; /ba/ vs /da/) stimulus differences in age groups of 7–12, 13–16, and 35–56 year olds. Large and small tone changes elicited MMNs significantly differing from zero within the typical 100–250 ms time window in adults and teenagers, whereas in children the MMN was significant only for a brief time period for the larger deviant. For syllable changes, the MMN was distinct for the larger deviancy in this time window in all groups. However, for the smaller change, it was absent in children, significantly differed from zero for a brief time in teenagers, and robust in adults. For the LDN, the results were the opposite, with the LDN amplitude being enhanced for smaller deviances and diminished during development, suggesting that these two components reflect at least to some extent different types of processing.

The developmental trajectories of the MMN amplitudes seem to be to some extent distinct for the different deviant sound features, as shown by studies employing the multi-feature paradigm which enables one to compare MMNs elicited by multiple sound-attribute changes occurring in the same stimulus sequences. When MMNs for changes in frequency, duration, intensity, location, and for a sound including a gap were investigated in 2–3-year-olds (Putkinen et al., 2012) and compared with adult MMNs for these sound attributes (Näätänen et al., 2004) similarities and dissimilarities were found. The sound duration and gap deviants elicited MMNs which had relatively similar parameters in these two age groups, whereas differences between the groups were found in MMNs for frequency changes. While a 10% change in the fundamental frequency of a harmonic tone elicited a robust MMN significantly differing from zero in adults, it elicited no significant MMN in the children.

Distinct changes in the MMN amplitudes for different types of sound changes even occur between the age-ranges of 4–6 and 7–12 years. This was evident in a study using a pseudoword (/tatata/) with a vowel (a->o), vowel duration, consonant duration, frequency, and intensity changes in the middle syllable (Partanen et al., 2013d). The older child group had significant MMNs for all other sound deviances except for the sound-frequency changes, whereas in the younger children, significant MMNs were elicited by other deviants except for the vowel change.

MMN and sensory-memory duration. In addition to the ability to accurately discriminate sounds, short-term memory functions are vital for information processing and learning. For example, we need short-term memory in order to comprehend sentences or to process grammar, as well as when we try to learn new words (Baddeley et al., 1998). Short-term memory deficits, in turn, are a marker of language impairment and may predict a delayed language development in children who have a language disorder (Botting & Conti-Ramsden, 2001). Therefore, it is important to determine the developmental trajectories of different memory functions.

Glass et al. (2008b) determined the development of sensory-memory duration by recording MMN for frequency changes (1000 vs 1200 Hz) in 2-, 3-, 4-, 5-, and 6-year-old children varying the presentation interval of the stimuli. They reported MMNs in each age group and found that the sensory-memory duration increases from 1–2 s in 2–3 year-olds to more than 2 s in 4-year-olds and to 3–5 s in 6-year-olds, as indicated by the presence of the MMN. Thus, the sensory-memory capacity appears to tremendously increase during the preschool age.

MMN components and their role in cognition. Change-elicited responses in children usually include two components, an early component at the range of around 200–350 ms (e.g. Shafer et al., 2000; Lovio et al., 2009, 2010; Kuuluvainen et al., 2016) and a late component at the range of around 400–450 ms (Korpilahti et al., 2001; Hommet et al., 2009; Bishop et al., 2011; Liu et al., 2014; Kuuluvainen et al., 2016). A few publications report even an earlier MMN component, commencing at 100–200 ms (Lee et al., 2012).

The role of these components in speech vs non-speech processing and their associations with language and cognitive measures was systematically investigated in 63 typically developing 6-year-old children by recording responses to syllables with a change in the consonant, vowel, vowel duration, syllable frequency, and syllable intensity, and their non-speech counterparts (Kuuluvainen et al., 2016). Also, cognitive and language functions were tested as follows: performance and verbal intelligence quotients (IQ), phonological and general language skills, reading skills, working memory, and rapid naming.

Firstly, it was found that the earliest change-elicited response (elicited at 100–250 ms; called early discriminative negativity, EDN, by Kuuluvainen et al., 2016) and the MMNs (elicited at 200–350 ms) were stronger to speech than non-speech sound changes, whereas the LDN (elicited at 350–500 ms) was stronger for the vowel than its counterpart change only. Thus, these responses suggest that at the age of 6, there are native-language speech sound representations, which are most robustly reflected by the first two change-elicited responses.

Secondly, there were several associations between these responses and cognitive and language measures. For example, larger EDN amplitudes in the speech than non-speech condition were associated with better phonological skills, and larger LDNs to vowels vs their counterparts over the left hemisphere were associated with higher verbal IQ (VIQ) scores. Furthermore, stronger left-hemispheric LDNs for speech than non-speech stimuli were connected with better verbal short-term memory.

Evidently, these three change-elicited negativities that can be detected from 6-year-old children reflect distinct processes. The first two components are connected with speech processing, being enhanced for native speech sounds similar to the adult MMN (Näätänen et al., 1997; Kuuluvainen et al., 2014). LDN showed similar behaviour, but only for the vowel and its counterpart stimuli. However, its speech-related enhancement was associated with high performance IQ (PIQ) scores and when this enhancement was left-hemispheric, it was associated with high VIQ and verbal short-term memory performance. These LDN connections with verbal cognitive functions are consistent with results showing, for example, that left-lateralized LDNs to speech sound changes in preschoolers at the age of 6–7 years predict later reading skills (Maurer et al., 2009), which are thought to be based on the integrity of speech (Snowling & Melby-Lervåg, 2016) and verbal working memory functions (Smith-Spark & Fisk, 2007).

3.6 **Conclusions**

(1) During the development from infancy to adulthood, auditory ERPs develop from a predominantly slow positivity into a waveform including the P1-N1-P2 complex in the adulthood. New components emerge and their peak latencies become shorter.

(2) The MMN/MMR is present even prior to birth. In newborns, both negatively (MMN) and positively (MMR) displaced change-elicited responses have been reported. The positive MMRs typically invert the polarity during the first 6 months of life. Infants at the age of 3–4 months may have a large variance in the polarity of this response. The polarity of the MMN/MMR may also be influenced by the experimental or analysis parameters.

(3) The MMN latency and amplitude change during the development. Fairly stable MMN peak latencies have been reported between the ages of 2–6 years, after which the MMN latency becomes shorter during school age. The MMN amplitude becomes larger during the development from school age to adulthood. Furthermore, the developmental trajectory of the MMN amplitude is somewhat different for different sound features.

(4) In children there are several MMN-like components, two of which (MMN, LDN) have been frequently reported and an early one (EDN) in few publications. These components are associated with different language and cognitive functions in 6-year-old children.

(5) MMR/MMN studies have shown that the infant brain can process surprisingly complex information, even soon after birth and during sleep. For example, the newborn brain can conjoin different sound features, segregate sound streams having different acoustic properties, and extract regularities from auditory input. These results suggest that infants have the core abilities needed for, for example, selective attention and language and music perception.

(6) Besides opening a new window to the auditory 'skills' of the infant brain, the MMR/MMN has illuminated learning and plasticity of the infant brain, for example, the acquisition of native- or foreign language speech sounds. Moreover, even learning prior to birth was revealed with MMR recordings. This important finding implies that the sound environment shapes the brain of an unborn infant.

Chapter 4

Developmental disorders

4.1. Developmental dyslexia

In modern society, academic skills play a major role in enabling people to lead a normal and successful life. Skill in reading is naturally the cornerstone for learning and acquiring knowledge at school and interacting in modern communities in which so many functions are computerized. Backwardness in reading not only compromises learning and jeopardizes a successful future career, but it also repeatedly causes feelings of failure at school, affecting self-esteem and motivation.

The smooth and seamless orchestration of a complex neural network, primarily involving regions in the left hemisphere, is needed for reading (Norton & Wolf, 2012). For successful reading, multiple cognitive and linguistic processes have to function both accurately and automatically. Written visual input first arrives at the primary visual cortex, in which the primary orthographic analysis occurs, continuing in the occipito-temporal region. The temporo-parietal areas are responsible for the integration of visual and auditory information. The inferior frontal gyrus, in turn, contributes to the higher-level functions of reading and language, such as semantic search and working memory.

Dysfunction in this neural network contributes to problems in reading-skill acquisition. A failure to acquire fluent reading skills despite normal intelligence, unimpaired senses, and adequate education is called developmental dyslexia or specific reading disability. It is a common developmental disorder, estimated to affect 5–17% of school age children (Shaywitz et al., 1990). Affecting the child's ability to acquire information, it has a serious impact on his/her psychosocial and educational outcome.

Genes associated with dyslexia. Dyslexia runs in families, and its genetic nature has been established in family and twin studies (for a review, see Kere, 2011). Specific genes contributing to the genetic risk of dyslexia have been identified with genetic mapping and molecular cloning. Genetic linkage studies on diverse populations and language groups have resulted in consistent and replicable genetic mapping results suggesting an association between dyslexia and certain positions in the genome (loci). These loci serve as a starting point for a more detailed analysis, which has resulted in the identification of susceptibility genes of dyslexia, such as *DYX1C1, DCDC2, K1AA0319, C2Orf3, MRPL19,* and *ROBO1.* The genes known so far do not sufficiently explain the risk for dyslexia; thus, much more research is needed to achieve a more complete picture. However, they are already of great help in identifying neurodevelopmental processes which have a pertinent contribution to the development of dyslexia.

Theories on the origins of dyslexia. Despite extensive research on its neural and cognitive basis, there still are fundamental disagreements on the underlying neurobiological factors in dyslexia. One of the key problems in identifying the causal factors underlying dyslexia is the complexity of the disorder: a variety of deficits and brain systems can be linked to the condition. In addition, the dyslexic population is heterogeneous in terms of the types of deficits. Dysfunctions in this population have been described in the neural basis of different sensory processes, including vision (Stein, 2001) and audition (Wright et al., 2000), and even the tactile modality (Grant et al., 1999), as well as motor functions, such as controlling eye-movements or keeping balance (Stoodley & Stein, 2013). Cognitive functions of individuals with dyslexia also diverge from the average. For instance, working- and short-term memory problems are common (Berninger et al., 2008). Furthermore, dyslexia is often associated with naming problems, which are an indicator of an insufficient automaticity or speed of information flow between neural circuits relevant for reading, such as visual and speech networks (Norton & Wolf, 2012). Co-morbidities complicate this picture further. For example, attention deficits, such as attention deficit and hyperactivity disorder (ADHD), are common in dyslexia (Willcutt & Pennington, 2000).

Bradley and Bryant (1978) observed that children with reading difficulties were poorer than normal-reading children in detecting a deviant sound in the beginning, middle, or end of successively presented four words (e.g. weed, peel, need, deed), which suggests the presence of phonological processing deficits in these children. Based on this phonological hypothesis of dyslexia (Liberman, 1973; Snowling, 2000), it was suggested that the phonological processing impairment could result from a more basic auditory deficit in perceiving rapid acoustic changes (Tallal, 1980; Farmer & Klein, 1995). This suggestion has been tested in a number of behavioural and neuroscientific studies with variable results. Studies comparing the performance of reading-impaired and unimpaired participants in phonological and wide range of auditory tasks (e.g. temporal-order judgement and repetition, frequency and intensity discrimination, gap detection, and the detection of frequency and amplitude modulation, and illusory movement) suggested predominantly a phonological impairment in dyslexia (Ramus et al., 2003). It was found that whereas all dyslexic participants had deficits in phonological processing, only 39–45% of them had problems in carrying out these non-linguistic auditory tasks. Furthermore, in those dyslexic individuals who had auditory discrimination problems, the problems were not limited to temporal discrimination.

Taken together, while a large variety of perceptual deficits are associated with dyslexia, it is evident that impairments of sound processing, particularly in the language domain, play a major role. The main temporal-lobe generators of the MMN overlap the perisylvian areas in which anatomical anomalies have been reported in dyslexia (Ramus, 2004), which speaks of an important role for MMN in neuroscientific dyslexia research. Since attention deficits are associated with dyslexia and as they may be one confounding factor in determining what dyslexics do and do not perceive, MMN can be used to disentangle how central auditory processing is compromised in this disorder. Furthermore, recording

MMN and other event-related potentials (ERPs) helps to determine which auditory processing stages do not function properly.

Associations between dyslexia, genes, and MMN

Evidence of the associations between dyslexia, genes, and the MMN is accumulating. The detection of these connections and understanding their nature illuminates the origins and causes leading to dyslexia, which is a complex disorder affected by multiple genes and having a large phenotypic variation. These connections were explored, for example, by carrying out a genome-wide association analysis in 200 dyslexic participants (8–19-years old) between genetic markers and MMN elicited by a change from /ba/ to /da/ (Roeske et al., 2011). It was found that rs4234898, a marker on chromosome 4q32.1, was significantly associated with MMN's late component. The authors chose not to analyse the first MMN component in order to avoid the possible confounding contribution of N1 in their analysis. Another study (Czamara et al., 2011) determined the associations between MMN and *DCDC2* and *KIAA0319*, the candidate genes of dyslexia on chromosome 6, also imputing rare variants in this region. These candidate genes are expressed in left-hemispheric temporal-occipital brain regions which are involved in processes such as grapheme-phoneme associations (van Atteveldt et al., 2004) and speech functions related to the development of reading and spelling (Blau et al., 2009). Their participants also were 8–19 year-old dyslexic individuals and /da/ (standard) and /ba/ (deviant) were used as stimuli. They included in the analyses both the early and late MMNs. They found that four rare variants were significantly associated with the later MMN component.

These results are very promising, further supporting the strong connection between MMN and dyslexia and suggesting that this response has a great potential as a biomarker of dyslexia. However, it would be important to include also normal-reading participants in the analyses to determine whether the findings are specifically related to dyslexia and do not merely reflect some general aspect of speech sound processing. Furthermore, the connections between MMN, dyslexia, and genes should be investigated more extensively, including also other candidate genes and all MMN components in children, of which three have been identified in 6-year olds (Kuuluvainen et al., 2016). Furthermore, these three components are distinctly associated with various cognitive and language measures (Kuuluvainen et al., 2016). Therefore, new insight would be gained on dyslexia by determining the connections between the different candidate genes, MMN components, and behavioural test results.

Sound discrimination

MMN studies have supported the theory according to which individuals with dyslexia have phonological–auditory impairments. Recent studies have even suggested associations between genetic markers of dyslexia and CV-syllable elicited MMNs (Roeske et al., 2011). Diminished MMN amplitudes have been systematically reported in individuals with dyslexia for stop consonant changes in syllables (Schulte-Körne et al., 1998; Lachman et al., 2005; Sharma et al., 2006; Bitz et al., 2007; Hommet et al., 2009) and for frequency changes of sounds (Baldeweg et al., 1999; Kujala et al., 2003; Renvall & Hari, 2003; Kujala et al., 2006). For sound-duration changes, some studies have reported diminished (Corbera et al., 2006; Huttunen-Scott et al., 2008) and some normal-like MMN amplitudes (Baldeweg et al., 1999; Kujala et al., 2000). Delayed MMN peak latencies have also been reported in dyslexia (Kujala et al., 2006; Hommet et al., 2009).

The multi-feature paradigm, enabling the comparison of MMNs elicited by multiple different deviant types, revealed that adults with dyslexia may have larger than normal MMNs for some sound changes (e.g. sound-source location) while having diminished MMN amplitudes for some other change types (e.g. frequency) (Kujala et al., 2006b). When frequency and duration MMNs elicited in this and oddball paradigms were compared with each other, MMNs were smaller for changes in the multi-feature than oddball paradigm in dyslexic but not in normal reading adults (Kujala et al., 2006b). This might suggest abnormal memory trace formation in people with dyslexia for stimuli in acoustically variable streams, which is the natural context of auditory and speech perception.

Some studies aimed at shedding light on the debate as to whether dyslexia is specifically associated with impairment in phonological processing or with a more general auditory deficit. For example, Schulte-Körne et al. (1998) used MMN to compare the discrimination of speech and non-speech stimuli in dyslexic and control adolescents. Their speech stimuli were syllables (with /da/ as the standard stimulus and /ba/ as the deviant stimulus) and sine-wave tones (1000 Hz as the standard and 1050 Hz as the deviant stimulus). The authors found that MMNs for the tone stimuli did not differ between the groups, whereas the syllables elicited a smaller-amplitude MMN in dyslexic than control adolescents. The authors interpreted this result as reflecting a deficit specific to the phonological system rather than a general failure in processing auditory information in dyslexia.

There are two major problems in this study, however. Firstly, sine-wave tones differ from syllables not only in terms of being non-speech sounds but they also differ a great deal in spectral and temporal complexity. Thus, it is impossible to tell whether the different pattern of results obtained with the two stimulus types are caused by the stimuli belonging to 'speech' vs 'non-speech' categories or simply by their different degrees of complexity. Secondly, subsequent MMN studies suggested that individuals with dyslexia might even have problems in discriminating small pitch separations (Baldeweg et al., 1999; Renvall & Hari, 2003; Kujala et al., 2003; Kujala et al., 2006). For example, Baldeweg et al. (1999) found, using a standard tone of 1000 Hz and deviants of 1015, 1030, 1060, and 1090 Hz, that all changes but the largest elicited smaller MMNs in the dyslexic than control subjects and that these stimuli also were less accurately discriminated in an active deviance detection task by the subjects with dyslexia. Furthermore, the degree of phonological impairment correlated with the frequency-discrimination test results and MMN elicited by frequency changes. Consequently, these results show that individuals with dyslexia suffer from increased difficulties in processing small pitch differences and, further that their phonological impairment is associated with the frequency discrimination deficit as reflected by MMN.

An elevated vulnerability to the masking effects of successive sounds has also been observed in dyslexia: a temporal change, a too-early occurring third sound in a four-tone
sound pattern, elicited an MMN in normal-reading adults but not in those with dyslexia
(Kujala et al., 2000). However, when the first and last sounds of the sound pattern were
removed, this too-early sound elicited comparable MMN responses in these two groups.
These results indicate that the first and last sounds in the patterns caused higher than
normal masking effects in the auditory system of the subjects with dyslexia. A further
study showing that the MMN of dyslexic subjects is affected more by sounds following
than preceding the critical sound material suggests a stronger backward than forward
masking effect in dyslexia (Kujala et al., 2003). Abnormally small MMNs for various
acoustic changes and its vulnerability to masking effects in dyslexic subjects implicate
impaired early bottom-up auditory mechanisms in sound discrimination.

Abnormal native-language processing

In early childhood, our speech system becomes specialized to our native-language speech
sounds. This *native language neural commitment* (Kuhl, 2004) develops in early infancy,
being evident at the age of 6–12 months as enhanced MMN amplitudes for native vs foreign speech sounds (Cheour et al., 1998a). This specialization for the native language is
evident both in behavioural discrimination measures and MMNs. One might not be able
to make a distinction between two foreign sounds, whereas a native speaker of the language including these sounds can discriminate them effortlessly. Consistent with this, unfamiliar speech contrasts elicit no or only small MMNs whereas acoustically equally large
native-language contrasts elicit robust MMNs (Näätänen et al., 1997; Winkler et al., 1999).

Bruder et al. (2011) hypothesized that individuals with dyslexia might have an atypical
development of native-language speech-sound representations. The authors compared
MMNs elicited by native and unfamiliar vowel changes between children with or without
dyslexia. In children with normal reading development, an expected MMN enhancement
was found for the native vowel change compared with the unfamiliar one. However, in
dyslexic children, no MMN amplitude differences were found between the two types
of changes. Furthermore, this group had a smaller MMN amplitude for the prototypical vowel change than the control group, whereas no group differences were found for
MMNs elicited by the unfamiliar change. These results suggest impaired tuning to the
speech sounds of the native language in dyslexia. Abnormal native-language development
in dyslexia was also suggested by a study comparing MMNs for phonotactically high vs
low probability words in dyslexic and normal-reading children (Bonte et al., 2007). The
normal-reading children showed a larger MMN amplitude for the words with high than
low phonotactic probability, whereas dyslexic children showed no such pattern. These
results suggest abnormal tuning of the central auditory system for statistical regularities
related to phoneme combinations in dyslexia.

These results suggest that the native language is abnormally represented in the central
nervous system in dyslexia, supporting the theory of underdeveloped phonetic representations in these individuals. Furthermore, the results indicate that the selective tuning for

language regularities is aberrant in dyslexia. As these deficiencies are reflected in MMN, it indicates that low-level fundamental language processes are dysfunctional in this disorder.

Impaired stages of auditory processing

ERPs reflecting distinct stages of information processing enable one to pinpoint the levels where the dysfunctional processes emerge. Evidence has been obtained on several impaired sound-processing stages in dyslexia. Abnormal processing has been shown even in subcortical structures, with the peak latencies of brain stem responses being longer in poor than good readers (Banai et al., 2009). Kujala et al. (2006a) used a passive and an active target-detection condition to determine auditory dysfunctions at pre-attentive and attentive processing stages in dyslexia. The deviant sound used in this study was a duration deviant since it was shown that MMNs may be normal-like for duration changes in dyslexic adults when sounds are presented as discrete events in the oddball paradigm (Baldeweg et al., 1999). It was hypothesized that the identification of duration deviants might be hampered in dyslexia when these deviants are embedded within complex sound material. This would emerge either as an aberrant MMN, reflecting problems at the early stage of processing caused by masking effects of the surrounding sounds (Kujala et al., 2000, 2003), or at later stages associated with attentional processing, in components like the N2b or P3. Subjects were presented with pseudowords composed of three syllables (/tatata/) and tonal patterns of a comparable structure in separate conditions. Deviant stimuli were occasional longer-duration vowels/tones occurring randomly in one of the three segments. The MMN was recorded in a passive condition and the N2b and P3a while subjects were detecting deviants indicating with a button press in which segment the deviant occurred.

It was found that the MMN was normally elicited by the large duration deviants in dyslexic adults, which is consistent with the results of Baldeweg et al. (1999) showing normal-like MMNs for large duration deviants in dyslexic participants. However, when the task was to attend to the stimulation, deviant sounds elicited an N2b in control but not in dyslexic subjects. This N2b absence was associated with deviant-sound identification impairment in a concurrent target-detection task. When the types of errors were analysed in more detail, it was found that dyslexic subjects did detect the pseudowords and tone patterns that included a deviant segment but they could not identify the segment position.

These results together with the diminished MMN amplitudes and delayed MMN and brainstem peak latencies in dyslexia suggest that various stages of central auditory information processing may be affected in this disorder. Furthermore, they also suggest that even sound changes that are discriminable for individuals with dyslexia in a simple context may be hard for them to detect in a normal-like more complex context, such as words.

Impaired audiovisual processing

According to the phonological deficit theory on dyslexia (Vellutino et al., 2004), the connection between reading difficulties and poor phonology is proposed to originate from degraded phonological representations, which lead to unstable associations between speech sounds and the corresponding letters. This suggestion is supported by observations indicating poor matching of acoustically and visually presented pseudowords but a normal-like matching of these words within each modality in dyslexia (Fox, 1994; Siegel & Faux, 1989; Snowling, 1980).

The low-level neural processing of audiovisual integration can be tapped with MMN (Widmann et al., 2004; Froyen et al., 2008; Mittag et al., 2011). These studies suggested a modulation of MMN by visually presented input. For example, larger-amplitude MMNs were elicited by speech sound changes when concurrent letters were presented than when scrambled images were shown instead (Mittag et al., 2011). These results suggest that MMN in the audiovisual condition was composed of both the activation elicited by the mismatch between the speech sounds and the mismatch between the visually shown letter and the deviating speech sound.

This audiovisual MMN paradigm was used to investigate letter–speech sound integration in dyslexia. It was found that when an easily discriminable /a/-/o/ vowel contrast was used, it elicited a normal-like MMN in dyslexia, not differing from that of control participants. However, when these vowels were presented together with visually shown letters, the effect of enhanced MMN, found in normal-reading individuals (Froyen et al., 2008), was not found in dyslexic children (Froyen et al., 2011). Another study, with a larger set of stimuli (syllables with a consonant, vowel, and vowel duration changes and syllable frequency and intensity changes) found corroborating results, suggesting no modulation of the MMN by visually presented letters in dyslexic participants (Mittag et al., 2013).

These results support the notion of impaired processes associated with the integration of visually presented letters and corresponding speech sounds in dyslexia. However, audiovisual integration of other types of stimuli, in addition to letters and speech sounds, was also shown to be abnormal in dyslexia. For example, this was shown by recording neural responses from dyslexic and control children during an audiovisual matching task (Widmann et al., 2012). Visual patterns composed of rectangles were presented on the computer screen, each followed by a sound sequence which was either congruent or incongruent with the visual pattern. If a sound was incongruent with one of the visual elements, the child's task was to press a designated response key and if the visual and auditory patterns were congruent, then another response key. It was found that at an early latency (140–180 ms from the onset of incongruency), a negative response (composed presumably of MMN and N2b) was significantly different for congruent and incongruent trials in control but not in dyslexic children. At a later latency (216–256 ms), both groups had a significant difference in the responses for these trial types, but the incongruent-minus-congruent difference waves were significantly smaller in dyslexic than control children. This response significantly correlated with the score and the reading time of short and long words, with the amplitude being larger in children having high than low reading scores.

Taken together, these results support the notion of impaired audiovisual integration in dyslexia. However, they also indicate that this integration deficit is not limited to letters and speech sounds. Even the crossmodal integration of nonlinguistic stimuli seems to be associated with reading since the neural responses related to incongruences of visual rectangle patterns and tone sequences were significantly associated with reading-skill measures.

MMN as an early marker of dyslexia

Since MMN can be recorded even from infants and foetuses (Draganova et al., 2005; Huotilainen et al., 2005), it is helpful in searching for early markers of abnormal auditory perception. The MMN signs of central auditory system deficits are evident in children with a familial risk for dyslexia before school age (Lovio et al. 2010) and even in infancy (Molfese, 2000; Leppänen et al., 2002). For example, Leppänen et al. (2002) found differences in mismatch response (MMR, the infant counterpart of MMN) amplitudes of 6-month-old infants with or without a familial risk for dyslexia. They recorded MMRs for small and large duration changes of stop consonants within a pseudoword. The small consonant-duration change elicited an MMR in the control infants but not in the at-risk infants. Furthermore, the large consonant-duration change elicited an MMR in both groups of infants but the MMR for this large stimulus change was smaller in amplitude in the at-risk than control group over the left hemisphere, whereas no group differences were found over the right hemisphere. These results indicate that infants at-risk for dyslexia are impaired in discriminating stop-consonant durations. Furthermore, this deficit seems to be more severe in the left than right temporal lobe. These results are encouraging for they suggest that central auditory impairments could be identified even in the early infancy.

Showing a connection between MMN and the risk for dyslexia at a very early age is important for using MMN for the early identification of auditory dysfunctions, which serves as a basis for developing intervention programmes. The next important step was to show that the MMN measures do have a predictive power for future reading skills. Maurer et al. (2009) determined whether MMNs recorded in preschool children, with or without a familial risk for dyslexia, predicted their reading ability in the second, third, and fifth school grade. In addition to recording the MMN (its late component) for phoneme and tone changes, skills related to reading acquisition (phonological and preliteracy abilities, letter and word reading) were tested in these preschoolers. It was found that across all the three grades included in this study, both the behavioural measures and the degree of left-lateralization of the phoneme-MMN predicted future reading skills in the whole sample (Fig. 4.1). The MMN had an additive predictive value on the behavioural measures, increasing the explained variance. Furthermore, the improved prediction by the phoneme-MMN remained significant in the subgroup which was diagnosed as dyslexic at school age (n = 21). Syllable-segmentation accuracy and the MMN lateralization significantly predicted reading skills averaged across all three grades. Moreover, the phoneme MMN was the only significant predictor of reading skills for the third and fifth grades.

Consistent with these results, MMRs recorded even from younger children, those at the age of 17 months, were associated with later language and reading skills (van Zuijen

phoneme IMMN in kindergarten

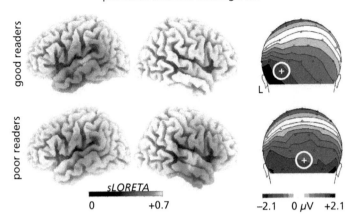

Fig. 4.1 The IMMN elicited by phoneme changes predicts future reading skills. IMMNs were recorded for phoneme changes from about 6-year old preschool children and the amplitudes were correlated with reading-skill measures obtained at the school-age. It was found that children who became better readers at school had a more left-lateralized IMMN than children who became poor readers.

Reprinted from Biological Psychiatry, 66, Maurer, U., Bucher, K., Brem, S., Benz, R., Kranz, F., Schulz, E., van der Mark, S., Steinhausen, H. C., and Brandeis, D., *Neurophysiology in preschool improves behavioral prediction of reading ability throughout primary school*, 341–348, Copyright (2009), with permission from Elsevier.

et al., 2012). The MMRs of infants with or without a risk for dyslexia were recorded for stimuli similar to those used by Kujala et al. (2000), including a temporal change in a tone pattern (a tone occurring earlier in the deviant stimulus). Their language development was investigated at the age of 4 and 4.5 years and their skills related to literacy in the second grade. The results showed that, firstly, the temporal change elicited an MMR in the control group whereas no MMR was found in the infants at risk for dyslexia. Secondly, there was a significant association between the MMR amplitude and the preliterate language-comprehension skills and later fluency in reading words. Furthermore, a subsequent study by van Zuijen et al. (2013) determined in more detail how MMR is associated with later reading skills in dyslexia. MMRs were recorded for consonant changes in brief pseudowords in 2-month-old infants with and without a risk for dyslexia who at the second grade performed a word reading fluency test. In order to determine whether the MMR could predict later reading skills, the children were grouped based on this reading test. It was found that fluently reading control children had frontally maximal MMR in infancy whereas MMR of fluently reading children at risk for dyslexia was more parietally preponderant. However, in the at-risk group performing poorly in the reading test the MMR was absent.

The results from these three studies are very promising, suggesting that there is a connection between the MMN/MMR amplitude in the childhood and future language and reading skills. So far, the primary means in early identification of possible future reading deficits has been to behaviourally test preliteracy abilities, such as phonological awareness and letter knowledge. The results of Maurer et al. (2009) showed that MMN significantly adds to these measures and, further, those of van Zuijen et al. (2012, 2013) demonstrated that even infant MMRs have predictive value for future language and reading skills. In future, it would be of utmost importance to improve the MMN recording and analysis methods for obtaining its parameters more reliably from individuals than is currently possible. Reaching sufficient reliability in MMN quantification would promote its use as a measure in individual diagnostics, thereby improving the early identification of reading-related deficits.

Intervention effects on dyslexia and MMN

MMN both reflects cortical sound-discrimination accuracy as well as changes in this accuracy as a result of, for instance, training (Näätänen et al., 1993; Menning et al., 2000; Atienza & Cantero, 2001) or exposure to special language or auditory environments (Cheour et al., 1998a; Koelsch et al., 1999; Winkler et al., 1999). Furthermore, MMN is an appealing means for determining cortical plasticity in recovery (from, e.g. stroke) and the effectiveness of intervention (Ilvonen et al., 2003; Särkämö, et al., 2010). Thus, it reflects neural plasticity of brain processes associated with early cortical sound discrimination. MMN has been successfully used as an index of plastic cortical changes after systematic intervention in developmental disorders. Dyslexia often persists until adulthood despite the extensive exposure to literary material even in countries with high educational standards. Therefore, simplified intervention programmes might be helpful in ameliorating dysfunctional cognitive sub-processes involved in reading. One such approach, which improves general skills in structuring and integrating visual and auditory information, was helpful in improving reading skills in children with dyslexia (Kujala et al., 2001). This intervention programme includes no speech or linguistic material. Visual symbolic information is presented on a computer screen, followed by a sound sequence. In one of the exercises, the child has to judge which of the two visual patterns (sequences of rectangles) presented on the screen matches with a sound pattern. In the other exercise, one visual pattern is presented on the screen, followed by a sound sequence, with the child's task being to press the space bar at the moment when the last sound should occur.

The effects of this intervention programme on reading skills and cortical plasticity were determined in Finnish first-grade children with problems in reading-skill acquisition. Two groups, matched in gender, intelligence quotient (IQ), and reading-skill test results, were formed at the end of the autumn semester. Children in the training group were using the programme twice a week for 10–15 minutes over a period of 7 weeks in the spring semester. The effects of the intervention programme were evident in several ways. After the intervention, the children in the training group had better reading-skill scores than their untrained controls. Auditory plasticity was evident in two ways. Firstly, after the intervention, the training group was faster than the control group in responding to deviant target stimuli, which were order reversals in a tone pair composed of brief 500 Hz and 750 Hz tones. Secondly, the amplitude of the MMN elicited by these tone-order reversals increased only in the training group. Furthermore, a correlation was found between the changes in the MMN amplitude and those in the reading-skill scores when all children were included in the analysis.

Evidently, this non-linguistic audiovisual training improved reading skills in the trained children and caused plastic changes in their central auditory system. This result is surprising in the light of the current view according to which dyslexia primarily stems from an impairment of phonological processing (Ramus et al., 2003; Bishop & Snowling, 2004). Perhaps several subsystems of the brain involved in reading are affected in dyslexia (Norton & Wolf, 2012). The audiovisual training programme used by Kujala et al. (2001) might have ameliorated one component of the neural network employed in reading, which is responsible for the effective integration of sequential audiovisual information. These results hence suggest that at least some individuals with dyslexia have non-phonological deficits contributing to their reading impairment.

While it is important to support the reading skills of children with reading skill acquisition not progressing normally at school, the prevention of reading difficulties with early intervention would be even more ideal. It would alleviate learning delays and diminish problems related to slow advancement in learning to read, such as feelings of inferiority compared with normally progressing peers, which also leads to motivational problems. Low motivation, in turn, can seriously further delay reading skill acquisition and may eventually affect school performance in general.

Fortunately, there are encouraging results on intervention effects on preschoolers. Lovio et al. (2012) investigated the effects of an intervention programme called GraphoGame (Lyytinen et al., 2007, 2009) on pre-reading skills (with reading and writing tests, assessment of phonological skills, letter knowledge, and letter recognition) and MMN (for vowel, vowel duration, and consonant changes in syllables and syllable frequency and intensity changes) of preschool children. In this game, orthographic items (letters) are presented on the screen in balls falling from the top of the screen to the bottom. Concurrently, a speech sound is presented through earphones and the child has to click with the mouse the letter corresponding to the speech sound. The game becomes more demanding when the child's performance improves, proceeding via several subsequent levels of the same format (e.g. phonemes, syllables) onto non-word items.

The children participating in the study were not performing at the level of their age in reading-related tasks and some of them additionally had a familial risk for dyslexia. The children were pseudorandomized into two training groups so that the main characteristics (age, gender, reading-related test scores, and familial dyslexia risk) did not significantly differ from each other. One of the groups played GraphoGame and the other the control game, which is a game giving training in number knowledge and basic addition and subtraction. The games are matched in terms of game type, motivational aspects, and visual appearance. The training was carried out over 3 weeks (5–20 min training per session, total of 3 hours) and was implemented in the child's kindergarten. The control group did exercises with the number-knowledge control game following exactly the same play format.

Both groups showed progress in the follow-up period. However, the group which was training with the GraphoGame improved more in the reading-skill tests and had more prominent changes in the MMN than the control group playing mathematical exercises (Fig. 4.2). The group with GraphoGame exercises improved in all the six subtests on reading-related skills, whereas the control group improved in three of them only. Furthermore, whereas the MMN changes were insignificant in the control group, the MMN amplitude was enhanced for the vowel and vowel-duration change but not for the rest of the stimuli in the training group. This is what was expected, since in the GraphoGame exercises, one has to match the speech sounds to the letters. There was also a connection between the changes in the measures of reading-related skills and MMN. A significant correlation was found between the change in letter knowledge and letter recognition scores and the change in the amplitude of the MMN elicited by the vowel deviant.

It is quite encouraging indeed that even such a short training improves skills needed for acquiring reading competence and concurrently modulates the neural basis of language in preschool children. An improved reliability in detecting early signs of reading and language deficits with combined behavioural and MMN measures (Maurer et al., 2009) and effective intervention for children at high dyslexia risk could remarkably alleviate difficulties in reading-skill acquisition.

Conclusions

(1) The discrimination of speech sounds and acoustic differences between sounds, such as frequency is abnormal in dyslexia, as suggested by a number of MMN studies. Studies assessing the connection between neural and behavioural processing suggested that the diminished MMNs were associated with poor perceptual sound discrimination and reading skills. These results suggest multiple problems in accurately perceiving differences in basic sound features in dyslexia, which can be expected to impair auditory and speech perception.

(2) The MMN amplitudes are diminished to changes occurring within sound patterns in dyslexia. These results suggest an elevated vulnerability of the central auditory system of dyslexic individuals for acoustic masking effects.

(3) Native-language speech sound representations, which are thought to be pertinent for reading-skill development, were poor in individuals with dyslexia as evidenced by MMNs recorded for native and foreign speech-sound contrasts. Also the detection of statistical regularities, needed for language perception, is impaired in dyslexia as suggested by MMN results.

(5) Audiovisual integration, an obligatory process in reading, was also impaired in individuals with dyslexia at the level of MMN. The results suggesting deficient integration of letters and speech sounds is compatible with the current leading theory according to which the main cause of dyslexia is poorly associated letters and speech sounds.

(6) It was found that the absence of MMN in infancy or its abnormal lateralization pattern in preschool children predicts poor reading performance at school. This suggests

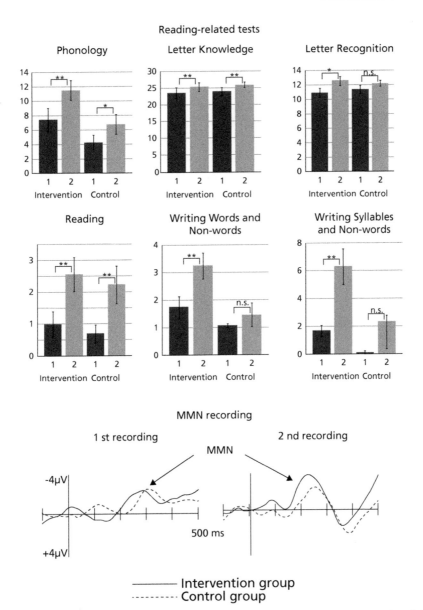

Fig. 4.2 Effects of GraphoGame intervention on pre-reading skills and MMN. Top: results of the first assessment are with dark grey and the second assessment with light grey. The first two bars represent the results of the intervention group and the third and fourth bars those of the control group. The intervention group improved in all tests whereas the control group improved in only half of the tests. Bottom: the MMNs for vowel changes before and after the training. No group differences were found before the intervention, whereas after it the MMN amplitude is stronger in the intervention than control group.

Reprinted from Brain Research, 1448, Lovio, R., Halttunen, A., Lyytinen, H., Näätänen, R. and Kujala, T., *Reading skill and neural processing accuracy improvement after a 3-hour intervention in preschoolers with difficulties in reading-related skills*, 42–55, Copyright (2012), with permission from Elsevier.

that the MMN serves as an early marker of central auditory problems associated with dyslexia and a strong association between low-level auditory discrimination processes and reading skills.

(7) This strong association is further supported by studies showing a concurrent modulation of MMN with the reading-skill improvement caused by intervention in dyslexia. Crucially, associations were found between changes in reading skills and MMN amplitudes. Thus, MMN is dynamically associated with reading skills reflecting plastic changes occurring during reading-skill improvement.

(8) The robust association between MMN and dyslexia, as suggested by infant MMN and later reading skills as well as MMN modulation along with dyslexia alleviation after intervention, is further supported by association analyses between MMNs in dyslexic individuals and dyslexia candidate genes. Research employing the approach of determining connections between genes, dyslexia, and MMN, as well as cognitive and language measures, would illuminate the origins of reading deficits, which are still not sufficiently known.

4.2. Specific language impairment

Specific language impairment (SLI) is a common developmental disorder, affecting about 3–10% of children (Tomblin et al., 1997). It may have a serious impact on the child's psychosocial and educational outcome. SLI is diagnosed if the child's oral language is delayed compared with other, nonverbal cognitive abilities and there is no other apparent neurological or sensory reason (Leonard, 1998). Particularly phonological and morphological production is affected in this disorder, but the problems may also emerge at various other levels of language processing, such as in grammar or telling stories (Bishop, 2006). For example, the speech of a 7–8-year-old child with SLI might resemble that of a 3-year-old, including simplified sounds and words in ungrammatical strings. The type and severity of these problems varies, but there are often deficits both in understanding and producing language. The difficulties in understanding language may become evident when the child has problems in using toys to demonstrate what is meant by 'the man is chased by a dog', confusing who does what to whom.

Poor performance in pseudo-word repetition tasks is characteristic in SLI; it has been interpreted as reflecting phonological and verbal short-term deficits (van der Lely & Howard, 1993; Gallon et al., 2007). It has been proposed that a more general deficit in perceiving auditory input might underlie the phonological deficits (Tallal & Gaab, 2006). According to this hypothesis, impairment or slowness in processing auditory spectro-temporal cues leads to weak representations of speech sounds. Children with SLI are poorer than typically developing children in processing spectro-temporal acoustic cues occurring at rapid pace (for a review see Tallal, 2004). An association between the ability to perceive rapid acoustic variation and language problems was suggested by a study (Benasich & Tallal, 1996) determining auditory discrimination accuracy in infancy in children with vs without a risk for SLI and comparing these results with later language outcomes. Infants were taught to make a distinction between two sound sequences, one with alternating low- and high-pitched tones and the other repeating a low-pitched tone, after which the threshold for discriminating the two sequences with the fastest sound-presentation rate was assessed. It was found that this threshold predicted the language outcome at the age of 2 years. Those infants who had low thresholds, i.e. needed a slower pace of presentation in order to discriminate the two sound streams, also had poorer language outcome at the age of 2 years.

Early atypical language development might cause SLI. It was proposed that during normal development, infants automatically focus their attention to relevant speech features, weighting features of speech sounds that are vital for semantic distinctions (Jusczyck, 1997). The weighted representations help to segment the speech stream into words. Dysfunctions in focusing on relevant speech features or in the automaticity or this process leads to poor segmentation skills, inadequate phonological representations, and delayed word learning.

The origins for this kind of atypical development are thought to stem from several interacting risk factors of the genetic and environmental origin (Bishop, 2006). SLI tends to run in families and, moreover, monozygotic twins who have an identical genetic makeup get more similar SLI diagnoses than dizygotic twins who share 50% of those genes which vary between different individuals. Furthermore, it was shown that the genes rather than the environment the twins share have a significant effect. The heritability, that is, the proportion of the trait variance that can be attributed to genetic factors, is around 0.5–0.75 in school-aged children. Rather than being inherited in a simple manner, SLI is a complex genetic disorder. The range of language dysfunctions associated with SLI is influenced by a number of distinct genes.

Some scholars treat SLI and dyslexia as manifestations of the same underlying dysfunction differing in severity and developmental stage, whereas others suggest that despite some phenotypic similarities, they are distinct disorders (Bishop & Snowling, 2004). The early language development may be delayed in children with a family history of dyslexia and dyslexic individuals may display deficits in oral language tasks involving no reading or writing. SLI children, in turn, may have similar core phonologic impairments as those with dyslexia. However, in SLI, semantic and syntactic deficits are widespread, influencing fluent reading-skill acquisition and reading comprehension.

While it is possible to classify some children as belonging to one of these disorders, the language- and reading-related difficulties of many children are somewhere in the continuum between SLI and dyslexia (Bishop & Snowling, 2004). A study determining phonological deficits in SLI and dyslexia proposed a multidimensional model (Ramus et al., 2013). It reported that these disorders do not always co-occur and that some children with SLI do not have phonological deficits. Furthermore, they show a partly different profile in phonological representations vs skills than those with dyslexia.

Sound discrimination in SLI

Both speech and non-speech sound discrimination have been investigated with MMN in children with SLI. One of the first studies using MMN to this end (Korpilahti &

Lang, 1994) determined whether cortical frequency (500 vs 553 Hz) and duration (50 vs 110 or 500 ms) discrimination is impaired in SLI (called dysphasia in that article). MMN for the frequency change was significantly diminished in children with SLI (see also Holopainen et al., 1998). Also the MMN amplitude for the large duration change was significantly smaller in the SLI than control group, whereas the group difference failed to reach statistical significance for the MMN elicited by the small duration change. Consistent with these results, another study found a diminished MMN for a tone change from 700 to 750 Hz in children with SLI (Rinker et al., 2007). Furthermore, their MMN scalp topography was more right-ward lateralized than that of control children.

Differences between children with vs without SLI have also been reported for a component called late MMN, MMN2, or late discriminative negativity (LDN), elicited after the typical MMN time window (150–300 ms) of school-aged children. For example, Bishop et al. (2010) found that this response was significantly smaller in children with than without SLI for a smaller deviance (1030 vs 1000 Hz), whereas no group difference was found for a larger deviance (1200 vs 1000 Hz).

However, not all studies on SLI reported diminished MMNs for acoustic differences between tone stimuli. Uwer et al. (2002), comparing MMNs for tone frequency and tone duration changes in children with receptive or expressive SLI and those with no SLI found insignificant MMN differences between the three groups for these changes. The F0 difference between the standard and deviant stimulus was quite large in this study, 1000 vs 1200 Hz, which might not be sufficiently challenging for the central auditory system of children with SLI. Furthermore, the difference between the duration deviant and standard sounds was 175 vs 100 ms, which is much smaller than the one that yielded group differences in the study of Korpilahti and Lang (1994), who showed group differences for large but not for small duration changes.

Overall, these results suggest that at least some SLI subgroups have dysfunctions in the low-level auditory discrimination which is not limited to speech processing. Furthermore, the size of the deviance has an impact on the results. Large-magnitude deviances appear not to differentiate the groups with or without SLI, whereas smaller deviances are hard to discriminate for the central auditory system of children with SLI. However, MMNs to very small deviances might not differentiate the groups either since they could be difficult to discriminate also for the auditory system of children with no SLI.

Diminished MMNs/LDNs have been reported both for consonant (Uwer et al., 2002; Davids et al., 2011) and vowel changes (Shafer et al., 2005; Datta et al., 2010) in SLI. New information on the nature of the speech-processing deficit in SLI was found by applying both MMN recording as well as discrimination and identification tests. For an /e/-/i/ contrast of short vowels (with 50 ms duration), a significant MMN was found both at an early (100–300 ms) and late (300–500 ms) latency window in the control group, whereas only the late response was significant in the group with SLI (Shafer et al., 2005). This pattern of results was also found in an attentive condition during which the children had to detect rare target tones in the vowel sequences. The behavioural tests revealed that the children with SLI were unimpaired in tasks requiring discrimination of the vowels but impaired in vowel identification. The discrimination task only requires the recognition of a feature difference between the stimuli but not the perception of features critical for categorizing the vowels. Therefore, these results were interpreted as reflecting incorrectly weighted phonological memory representations in SLI.

Based on these results, Datta et al. (2010) hypothesized that longer speech sounds might be easier to process for the central auditory system in SLI. They used short (50 ms) and long (250 ms) /e/ and /i/ stimuli in their MMN recording and behavioural test. Early-latency MMNs (at 190–250 ms) were indeed found both in children with and without SLI when the stimulus duration was 250 ms. However, the behavioural tests revealed a similar pattern of results for the 250 ms stimuli as was found for the 50 ms stimuli: the two groups did not differ in vowel discrimination but in vowel identification the SLI group performed more poorly than did their controls. Thus, while the lengthening of the vowels improved the pre-attentive cortical discrimination in SLI, it did not lead to improved vowel cat-egorization. This could reflect deficient matching of incoming acoustic information with phonological categories or problems in maintaining a memory trace for a sufficient time for completing this matching.

The atypical cortical sound discrimination in SLI is evident also in the MMN peak la-tencies. A delayed MMNm (magnetic counterpart of MMN) and its strong connection with language measures in SLI was demonstrated by magnetoencephalographic (MEG) recordings (Roberts et al., 2012) employing speech (/u/ and /a/) and non-speech (300 and 700 Hz tones) sounds. An index for the general MMNm was obtained by combining the data for both stimulus types and hemispheres. It was found that whereas there were no group differences in the M100 peak latencies, the MMNm was significantly delayed in the SLI group. Moreover, this delay was strongly associated with receptive and expres-sive language measures (Clinical Evaluation of Language Fundamentals—Fourth edition; CELF-4). The classification accuracy of the MMNm between the groups was 89.1%, with the sensitivity for SLI being 84% and specificity 92%.

Effects of masking on audition in SLI

In natural listening conditions, there usually are several concurrent sound sources. Quite often we also listen to speech while there are competing sounds coming from the envir-onment. Therefore, the sounds and speech we are listening to are at least partially masked by other sounds. It has been shown that masking sounds affect the perception of children with SLI and typically developing children differently. When the masking noise was pre-sented concurrently, before, or after tones to be detected, it was found that children with SLI needed a higher intensity of the tones than the control children did to detect them in the presence of the masks (Wright et al., 2007). The backward-masking condition was particularly challenging for the children with SLI, there being no overlap in this condition in the performance of the groups.

Marler et al. (2002) found corroborating results in their psychophysics experiment showing that particularly backward masking elevates the tone-detection thresholds in children with SLI. In addition, the authors determined neural correlates of masking effects with MMN. The duration of the standard stimulus was 108 dB (SPL) and that of the deviant one 88 dB (SPL), with the masking sound being a narrow-band noise masker with the duration of 150 ms. Group differences were found both in the MMN amplitude and latency, with the MMN of the children with the SLI being diminished and delayed. Unfortunately, there was no control condition in this study without a masking stimulus, and, therefore, one cannot conclude that the MMN differences observed between the groups are genuinely caused by the masker. However, the MMN and psychophysics results together do support the hypothesis of elevated masking effects in the central auditory system of individuals with SLI, with the MMN results further indicating that masking both impairs and slows down cortical discrimination.

Early-age neural indices of SLI

The results discussed in the foregoing were obtained in school-aged children, from the age of 5 years up to 10–13 years. Since SLI runs in families (Nudel et al., 2014), its neural indices may exist even in early childhood. Indeed, abnormal change-elicited responses have been reported in infants at risk for SLI. For example, MMRs were recorded for vowel-duration changes of syllable /ba/ in 2-month old infants with or without a familial background of SLI (Friedrich et al., 2004). This deflection was significantly delayed in the infant group at risk for SLI. These results, consistent with those obtained in school-aged children (Roberts et al., 2012), suggest slower than normal cortical auditory processing in SLI. The early onset of this deficit could potentially contribute to slowed language development in these children.

An association between the infant MMN and future language problems was demonstrated by a follow-up study (Weber et al., 2005) recording the MMN for word stress patterns at the age of 5 months and thereafter determining the language skills at the ages of 1 and 2 years. The word-production rate was assessed in these children, since a low production rate is thought to predict future language problems. Based on the results of this test, the subgroups for inspecting MMN at the age of 5 months were formed. It was found that MMN for the stress-pattern change was smaller in amplitude in the group of children with a low than high word production rate at the toddler stage (Fig. 4.3). These results suggest that the MMNs in infancy reflect later language skills at least at the group level.

Connections between language problems and MMN were not shown for speech stimuli only but also in studies employing tones and probing frequency discrimination or the sensory-memory duration. For example, MMRs were recorded for paired 100 Hz tones with within-pair intervals of 70 ms or 300 ms, with the deviant being a 300 Hz second tone in the pairs. MMRs were recorded from infants having a familial history of language problems at the ages of 6, 9, 12, 16, 24, 36, and 48 months (Choudhury & Benasich, 2011). At the ages of 3 and 4 years, the relationship of the language skills and ERPs was determined. Infants at risk for the SLI had smaller MMR amplitudes at 6 and 9 months than control infants; however, somewhat surprisingly, this predominantly left-hemispheric

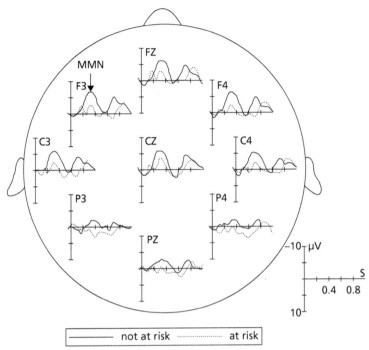

Fig. 4.3 Diminished MMNs in infants at risk for SLI. Deviant minus standard difference waves from 5-month old infants with (dashed line) or without (continuous line) a familial risk for SLI. The standard stimulus was a pseudo word and the deviant one included a change in stress pattern.

Reprinted from Cognitive Brain Research, 25, Weber, C., Hahne, A., Friedrich, M., & Friederici, A. D., *Reduced stress pattern discrimination in 5-month-olds as a marker of risk for later language impairment: Neurophysiologial evidence*, 180–187, Copyright © (2005), with permission from Elsevier.

difference was found for changes in the short inter stimulus interval (ISI) condition only. Furthermore, in this condition, a negative change-elicited response that the authors called N2, obtained at 6, 9, and 12 months, predicted performance in the language tests when the children were 3–4 years old, such that a smaller amplitude and a longer latency were connected with a poorer performance in language tests.

Grossheinrich et al. (2010), in turn, determined the association between the sensory-memory duration at the age of 5 years and earlier language skills, assessed at the age of 2 years. They recorded MMNs for frequency changes (1000 Hz vs 1200 Hz) in short (500 ms) and long (2000 ms) ISI conditions. They employed the time-effective paradigm of Grau et al. (1998) in which a train of four stimuli were presented with an ISI of 500 ms. In the long-ISI condition, the first tone after a 2000 ms interval was either a standard or a deviant. The presence of MMN to deviant stimuli after this long interval would indicate that there still was a memory trace for the preceding four tones. The MMNs of the late talkers was diminished, but only in the long-ISI condition requiring the retention of the memory trace for 2000 ms. The authors also classified the late talkers into two groups when they were 5-years old, of which one had reached the performance level of the control group in language tests, whereas the other was still performing poorly in these tests. It was found that the MMNs were not different between these two groups, which might indicate that the MMN reflects some risk factor for SLI present early on and persisting irrespective of the future language development. Furthermore, an association between the MMN amplitude and neuropsychological test results was found. This relationship emerged for the subtest 'word order', in which a list of words is uttered to the child who should point out pictures of these items in the presented order.

Effects of intervention on SLI and MMN

The low-level auditory impairment, as reflected by MMN and other ERPs, can be alleviated by intervention in SLI. The effects of language intervention on neural speech processing were determined in 5-year old children with the SLI with MEG recordings (Pihko et al., 2007). There were two matched groups, one performing language exercises and the other one physical exercises. Language tasks included speech, articulation, and phoneme discrimination exercises, rapid processing, and phonological and linguistic awareness training. The physical exercises included a variety of motor activities. The children participated in the training sessions in groups for 8 weeks, three times a week, with each session lasting for 20–30 minutes.

Magnetic responses were recorded before and after the training period for two stimulus sets as follows: standard /da/, deviants /ba/, and /ga/ and standard /su/, deviants /so/, and /sy/. The effects of training were evident both on standard-stimulus elicited P1m responses and MMNm to deviants as well as on behavioural discrimination test results. The P1m for /da/, /ba/, and /ga/ but not for the rest of the syllables were enhanced in both groups after training but significantly more in the language-intervention group. Furthermore, the left-hemisphere MMNm for the /sy/ deviant was enhanced after training in the language-intervention group but not in the control group. In the syllable-discrimination test, the performance of the language-intervention group improved for the /da/-/ba/ and /su/-/so/ pairs, which originally were the most difficult to discriminate.

These results show that it is possible to alleviate speech-perception deficits in SLI children even in early childhood. This is an important observation since it implies that the language skills of these children can be supported prior to their school start, which would facilitate learning and diminish the negative consequences of learning delay. The intervention effects were associated with enhancements of the P1m and MMNm for syllable stimuli, suggesting the amelioration of low-level language dysfunctions.

Conclusions

(1) Diminished MMN amplitudes have been reported in children with SLI for frequency and duration changes in sounds as well as consonant and vowel changes in speech stimuli. This suggests abnormalities in discriminating both acoustic and phonetic aspects of auditory information in SLI.

(2) Also differences in MMN scalp distributions and latencies have been reported between participants with vs without SLI. For example, delayed MMNms were found
in SLI, which were strongly associated with receptive and expressive language
measures.

(3) Evidence was also found on an elevated vulnerability of the central auditory system
of children with SLI to masking effects of successive sounds, as reflected in MMN
and test performance. These results imply that children with SLI have difficulties in
detecting the identity of sounds occurring in rapid succession.

(4) Auditory deficits in SLI are evident early on, since atypical MMNs have been reported
in infants at risk for this disorder due to family history of SLI.

(5) The MMN recorded in infancy was found to be significantly associated with language
skills assessed later in childhood, suggesting that the MMN may serve as an early indicator of language difficulties.

(6) With appropriate intervention the neural basis of speech processing and discrimination can be improved in children at risk for SLI, as suggested by changes in MMNm
due to the intervention.

4.3. **Autism spectrum disorders**

Autism spectrum disorders (ASD) are characterized by aberrant features in social interaction, communication, behavioural traits, and narrow interests. The autism spectrum involves a triad of co-occurring deficits in communication, socialization, and imagination
(see Happé & Frith, 1996, for a review). Social communication is qualitatively impaired
and there are restricted and repetitive patterns of interests and behaviour. The severity of
these deficits vary within the spectrum, with the most severe cases striving for extreme
isolation and being obsessively resistant to change.

ASD involves neurodevelopmental variants, with the main diagnostic subgroups traditionally being autism (Kanner, 1943) and Asperger syndrome (AS; Asperger, 1944) (WHO
1993; American Psychiatric Association 1994). The diagnostic criteria were recently revised (DSM-5), and the term ASD is now used for describing the diagnoses included in
'pervasive developmental disorders' in ICD-10 and DSM IV. In DSM-5, ASD includes
diagnoses which were previously classified as follows: autistic disorder, AS, childhood
disintegrative disorder, and pervasive neurodevelopmental disorder not otherwise spe-
cified. In ASD, there are developmental disorders in which the symptoms are on a continuum from mild to severe manifestation (Lauritsen, 2013).

ASD runs in families (Eapen, 2011), with the heritability estimates as high as 80%
(Lichtenstein et al., 2010). According to twin and family studies (Eapen, 2011), first-
degree relatives have a more than a 20-fold increase of risk, and the concordance rate for
monozygotic twins is 70–90% and that for dizygotic twins about 10%. So far, about 500
genes have been identified which are associated with various forms of this spectrum, with
each gene accounting for just a minor fraction of the cases belonging to ASD (Baudouin,
2014). Thus, ASD appears to be a constellation of infrequent disorders, converging to a

narrower set of symptoms emerging at the behavioural level. There is considerable overlap in the genes and genomic loci between ASD and some other disorders, like intellectual deficiency, schizophrenia, epilepsy, and ADHD (Eapen, 2011).

Language development may vary to a great deal within the spectrum, for example, between individuals with autism and AS. According to the traditional classification, children who could have autism show abnormalities and remarkable delays in the language development. These children may remain nonverbal or have only little functional language (Gillberg & Coleman, 2000). In autism, semantic-pragmatic deficits are widespread (Rapin & Dunn, 2003), entailing, for instance, an impaired understanding of nonliteral language and poor conversation skills. In language and communication difficulties, one key area of problems in ASD is the social and metaphorical use of language (Lord & Paul, 1997). Words are often used in a literal manner. For example, an individual with ASD might interpret 'on the wall' as on top of the wall instead of hanging on the wall, and there might be errors in using pronouns—for instance, a child with autism may use 'you' to refer to him/herself. Also echolalia is frequent; if asked a question, the child may repeat it instead of answering.

Furthermore, problems in speech prosody, both conceiving the intentions conveyed with prosody and producing prosody, are common (McCann & Peppé, 2003; Paul et al., 2005). However, there is an extensive variety in describing the types of prosodic abnormalities in ASD in the literature and some unquantifiable terms, such as 'singsong', 'wooden', and 'bizarre', have been used in describing this prosody (Baron-Cohen & Staunton, 1994). Prosodic stress is abnormally placed, tending to occur at the beginning of utterances (Baltaxe & Guthrie, 1987). Investigations on continuous speech in young adults with ASD have identified that phrasing is dysfluent or inappropriate and, further, that the placement of stress is abnormal: for instance, in an utterance, there can be a failure in emphasizing a contrastive word (Shriberg et al., 2001).

The primary dysfunction in ASD is impairment in social interactions, whereas deficits in communication are thought to be their secondary consequences (Mundy & Neal, 2001; Wing, 1988). However, central auditory processing impairments might also contribute to the language deficits found in ASD (Bomba & Pang, 2004; Rapin, 2002). Structural and functional abnormalities in ASD in brain areas belonging to the language- and sound-processing network are consistent with this notion. For example, an abnormal asymmetry of frontal and temporal language areas was demonstrated with magnetic resonance imaging (MRI) in this disorder (De Fosse et al., 2004; Herbert et al., 2002; Rojas et al., 2002). Furthermore, regional cerebral blood flow (rCBF) recordings carried out during rest indicated hypoperfusion of the superior temporal gyrus of both hemispheres (Gendry Meresse et al., 2005; Ohnishi et al., 2000; Zilbovicius et al., 2000). During sound listening or sentence comprehension tasks, diminished activation was also found in the left-hemisphere language-related areas in individuals with autism (Boddaert et al., 2003, 2004; Müller et al., 1999). Moreover, bilateral voice-selective areas in the superior temporal sulci were not activated when adults with autism heard vocal sounds, but showed a normal activation pattern for non-vocal sounds (Gervais et al., 2004).

In addition to language and communication impairments, individuals belonging to ASD often have aberrant perceptual abilities (e.g. Leekam et al., 2007). It has been suggested that individuals with ASD have a detail-focused cognitive style (Happé & Frith, 2006), originally described by Kanner (1943) as 'inability to experience wholes without full attention to its constituent parts'.

The aberrant perception in ASD involves all sensory modalities, but most prominently the auditory domain (Dahlgren, 1989). The atypical auditory functions involve both hyper- and hyposensitive features. A child with ASD may appear to be inattentive to her/his name, may even ignore loud sounds, or might seek for auditory stimulation by producing sounds. Furthermore, individuals with ASD have elevated problems in perceiving speech in noisy environments (Alcantara et al., 2004).

While the behaviours described in the foregoing indicate hyposensitivity to sounds, some other behaviours rather suggest auditory hypersensitivity. Sounds may cause distress to individuals with ASD, and some of them seem to have superior hearing abilities. Musical savants with ASD have also been reported (Heaton et al., 1999; Mottron et al., 1999), and an increased prevalence of perfect pitch has been suggested (Rimland & Fein, 1988). Furthermore, superior pitch-discrimination and memory skills (Bonnel et al., 2003; Heaton, 2003, 2005; Heaton et al., 2001, 2008; Mottron et al., 2000; O'Riordan & Passetti, 2006), as well as enhanced loudness perception (Khalfa et al., 2004) have also been reported.

Since these various perceptual abnormalities apply to different subgroups of ASD, individuals belonging to this spectrum clearly form a very heterogeneous group. For example, frequency discrimination was enhanced in 20% in a group of 72 adolescents with ASD (Jones et al., 2009). This heterogeneity might stem from the complex genetic aetiology. Tens to hundreds of genes contribute to the risk of autism (Betancur, 2011).

Orientation to sensory events also seems to be abnormal in ASD. This is evident even in very young children. For example, at the age of 6–12 months, their social orienting was abnormal, whereas their orienting to non-social stimuli resembled that observed in infants with typical development (Maestro et al., 2002). Abnormal orientation both for social and non-social auditory stimuli was also observed in preschoolers with ASD, but this abnormality was more pronounced for social stimuli (Dawson et al., 2004). A higher preference for non-speech sounds than speech sounds was also shown in ASD (Blackstock, 1978; Klin, 1991).

MMN and other ERPs are very attractive tools for investigating this spectrum of disorders, involving a variety of aberrations in the central auditory function. Furthermore, it is challenging to investigate individuals especially at the lower-functioning end of the spectrum, since they have communication problems or can even lack speech altogether. Therefore, unique information can be obtained with MMN which can be recorded even from individuals who do not cooperate in behavioural tests.

Sound discrimination in ASD

Studies using MMN have suggested both hypo- and hypersensitive sensory processing in ASD, which is consistent with clinical observations (Bonnel et al., 2003, 2010; Mottron et al., 2006; O'Neill & Jones, 1997). The different studies report partly conflicting results, which may result from the heterogeneous clinical features of the ASD group (the degree of mental retardation, language skills) or stimuli and paradigm used.

Changes in MMN amplitude and latency. Some studies have suggested hypersensitive discrimination of frequency and hyposensitive discrimination of sound duration in children with ASD. Lepistö et al. (2005, 2006) recorded MMNs from children (aged 7–11 years) with autism with no mental retardation and in children with AS for several change types of stimuli within the same stimulus blocks: vowel identity, duration, and frequency, and their non-speech counterparts. MMNs were smaller in amplitude in children with autism than in their controls for duration changes of vowels and their non-speech counterparts (Lepistö et al., 2005). Further, in children with AS, the results were similar for duration changes of the vowel counterparts whereas for duration changes of vowels, the effects did not reach statistical significance (Lepistö et al., 2006). Children with AS also participated in a behavioural discrimination test, yielding results that were consistent with the MMN results: the hit rate in these children was lower and the reaction time tended to be longer than those in control children for duration differences of both speech and non-speech sounds. Frequency changes of both speech and non-speech stimuli elicited enhanced MMN amplitudes in autism (Lepistö et al., 2005) and frequency changes of non-speech stimuli in AS (Lepistö et al., 2006). Further, the same stimulus paradigm was also used to study adults with AS to determine whether these effects persist from childhood to adulthood (Lepistö et al., 2007). It was found that the MMN was enhanced in amplitude in these participants both for frequency and duration changes (Lepistö et al., 2007). Thus, hypersensitive sound discrimination might become predominant in the adulthood in AS (see also Kujala et al., 2007a).

Results consistent with the studies reporting enhanced MMN amplitudes, suggesting hypersensitive auditory processing in ASD were also found by Gomot et al. (2002, 2011). These authors reported shorter than normal MMN peak latencies in 5–11 year-old children with autism. Furthermore, this shortened MMN peak latency, followed by an enhanced P3a, correlated with resistance to change, which is an important feature in autism (Gomot et al., 2011). This was evident in a subgroup of autistic children with the highest scores in Revised Behavior Summarized Evaluation Scale (BSE-R) reflecting intolerance of change, whose MMN amplitude and latency abnormalities were also more pronounced (Fig. 4.4).

However, there also are a number of studies reporting hypo- rather than hypersensitive frequency discrimination in ASD. These studies showed diminished or delayed MMNs or MMNms for sound-frequency or vowel changes (formants of which are composed of different sound frequencies). In 8–32-year-old low-functioning and moderately or severely language-impaired autistic patients (Tecchio et al., 2003), the MMNm for a change of tone frequency from 1000 to 1200 Hz was absent. Another study (Dunn et al., 2008) reported that a similar frequency change elicited diminished MMN amplitudes in 6–12-year-old children with autism matched with typically developing children in their non-verbal IQ. However, the MMN recordings were carried out with a noisy background with the sound

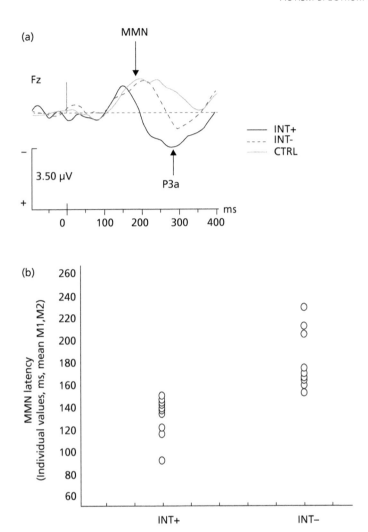

Fig. 4.4 Grand-mean MMN waveforms in two subgroups with ASD and in control children. In children with ASD, the MMN peak latency was shorter and the P3a amplitude larger than those in control children. These effects were more pronounced in the subgroup of children with ASD and high intolerance to change (INT+) than in children with low intolerance to change (INT−). The individual latency values are shown with circles for the two ASD groups on the bottom.

on in the video which the participants were watching. This could explain the diminished MMNs in children with autism, since noise diminishes the MMN amplitude (Kujala & Brattico, 2009) and has a more pronounced effect on auditory perception of individuals with than without ASD (Alcantara et al., 2004).

However, some other studies, carried out in silent electroencephalography (EEG) recording conditions, also reported MMNs reflecting hyposensitive frequency discrimination in ASD. It was shown, for example, that 11-year-old children with AS had delayed MMNs for frequency changes of tones (280 Hz vs 320 Hz; Jansson-Verkasalo et al., 2005) and diminished MMN amplitudes for syllable-frequency changes (Kujala et al., 2010). Furthermore, MMNm peak latencies were longer than normal both for tone (300 vs 700 Hz) and vowel (a vs u) changes in 8–17-year-old (Oram Cardy et al., 2005) and 6–15-year-old children with autism with no mental retardation (Roberts et al., 2011). However, a more detailed inspection of the data revealed that this delay was the most pronounced in children with autism also having language impairment (Roberts et al., 2011). Furthermore, in adults with autism with a performance IQ of 52–99, hyposensitive discrimination was suggested by a delayed MMNm peak latency for vowel changes in the left hemisphere (Kasai et al., 2005). Importantly, this delay correlated with the severity of autism.

The MMN results in ASD are variable and to some extent even contradictory. However, these results seem to reflect the actual variation of the phenotypes in ASD, since there are subgroups with different MMNs, and the MMN results may correlate with some traits in ASD. This is consistent with the variability in the perceptual abilities reported in ASD. For example, in a group of 72 adolescents with ASD, enhanced frequency discrimination skills were reported in 20% of them (Jones et al., 2009). Complex genetic aetiology might explain this heterogeneity. Autism might be a manifestation of tens or even hundreds of genetic and genomic disorders (Betancur, 2011).

Aberrant MMN sources. In ASD, not only the amplitude and latency patterns of MMN are abnormal, but also the neural networks contributing to MMN seem to be affected. MMN topographies with posterior distributions in ASD in comparison with those in control groups were reported (Gomot et al., 2002; Lepistö et al., 2005; Jansson-Verkasalo et al., 2005). These results either suggest increased activity in posterior temporo-parietal areas or decreased activity of the frontal MMN generators. Gomot et al. (2002) used scalp-current density mapping in their study of MMNs for frequency changes in children with autism, which improves the identification of local neural activities. Their results suggested that MMN has a posterior and more lateral scalp distribution in these children than those who are developing typically, which was interpreted by the authors as resulting from hypoactive frontal areas. These results are consistent with reports suggesting that the frontal lobe metabolism is abnormal (George et al., 1992; Zilbovicius et al., 1995) and neurotransmitter synthesis insufficient (Chugani et al., 1997) in autism. Furthermore, since some studies have shown parietally enhanced and frontally normal-like MMN amplitudes for frequency changes in children with autism (Lepistö et al., 2005), the temporo-parietal MMN generator activity might be abnormally strong in these children. However, this result should be confirmed, for example, by modelling sources of magnetic or electric signals. MMN generator sources have indeed been reported in the parietal areas (Lavikainen et al., 1994; Levänen et al., 1996), in addition to the temporal and frontal areas (Alho, 1995; Kujala et al., 2007). Due to these multiple sources, it is difficult to deduce how their contributions might underlie the observed MMN scalp topography.

MMN was also abnormally lateralized in ASD. In children with AS, MMNs were generally diminished in amplitude over the left hemisphere for speech and non-speech sound changes (Lepistö et al., 2006). In adults with the AS, in turn, the MMN amplitudes for frequency changes of speech sounds were enhanced over the right and midline scalp areas relative to those over the left hemisphere, whereas the MMN scalp distribution in their controls was more symmetrical (Lepistö et al., 2007). Consistent with the MMN amplitude results suggesting abnormal discrimination processes in the left hemisphere in autism, MMNm peak latencies were longer than normal in the left hemisphere of adults with autism (Kasai et al., 2005).

However, diminished amplitudes of the MMN, presumably originating from the right hemisphere, were also reported in individuals with ASD. These studies used words including prosodic changes, which are predominantly processed in the right hemisphere (Gandour et al., 2004). MMNs were smaller in amplitude for prosodic changes in words over the left hemisphere of adults with AS than those in control participants (Kujala et al., 2005). Furthermore, right-hemisphere preponderant MMNs were reported for prosodic changes in word stimuli in healthy children, whereas children with AS had a symmetrical MMN scalp distribution (Korpilahti et al., 2007).

These results show that the neural assemblies processing auditory input are abnormally distributed in in several ways ASD. The evidence speaks for both left- and right-hemisphere dysfunctions as well as for abnormal activity in parietal and/or frontal areas. The results suggest a lower than normal activity of the left hemisphere and deficient prosody processing in the right hemisphere. Furthermore, the frontal areas display abnormally low activity and the parietal areas possibly abnormally high activity in ASD.

The neural basis of speech perception in ASD

Besides deficits in processing of acoustic features of sounds, individuals with ASD have various problems in processing speech. The pattern of deficits related to speech varies remarkably within this spectrum, with the individuals with AS primarily having deficits related to the pragmatic aspects of speech, such as prosody, whereas in autism, speech deficits may be severe and widespread. Semantic-pragmatic deficits are quite universal in the ASD (Rapin & Dunn, 2003).

The human speech system is remarkably flexible and efficient in speech analysis. It can, for instance, effortlessly and rapidly analyse the speech of a person never met before, even though the way each individual speaks varies enormously. This is very demanding as such and, yet, we can manage this task even when speech is degraded by, for example, background noise. The demanding task of rapid and effective neural speech analysis is based on the speech system's capacity to extract relevant invariant features from speech (Bishop, 1997).

In autism, speech-perception processes are not fluent, which might result from enhanced low-level perceptual processing leading to a detail-oriented style of processing (Happé & Frith, 2006; Mottron et al., 2006). The theory of the detail-oriented information-processing style in autism is mainly based on observations made with regard to visual processing in individuals with autism, suggesting that they are superior in visual search, disembedding skills, and discrimination learning (for reviews, see Dakin & Frith, 2005; Happé & Frith, 2006). In the auditory domain, the higher than normal sensitivity to some acoustic features may be associated with detail-oriented processing (Bonnel et al., 2003; Heaton 2003, 2005; Mottron et al., 2000; O'Riordan & Passetti, 2006), also reflected in neurophysiological responses, in particular MMN (Gomot et al., 2002, 2011; Lepistö et al., 2005, 2008).

The enhanced low-level and detail-oriented processing style may lead to a too-focused processing of the intrinsic acoustical differences between speech sounds that belong to the same phonetic category (Gustafsson, 1997; O'Riordan & Passetti, 2006). This may result in problems in extracting relevant invariant phonetic features from speech. This, in turn, might hamper the formation of proper phonetic categories in the central speech system, which may impair language development in autism.

The assumption of abnormal phonetic invariance detection in autism was assessed by recording MMN in conditions including acoustic variation vs no variation (Lepistö et al., 2008). In the *varying-frequency condition*, a repetitive vowel was presented, continuously varying in frequency, with occasional changes of the vowel identity (e.g. from a repetitive /a/ to /u/). In the *constant-frequency condition*, the same vowels were presented as in the varying-frequency condition, but the frequency of the vowels was constant. Consistent with the postulated superior low-level perceptual skills in autism (e.g. Mottron et al., 2006), a centro-parietally enhanced MMN amplitude was found in the *constant-frequency condition* in children with autism. However, in the *varying-frequency condition*, these children had a smaller MMN response than that in typically developing children. The results also suggested that this effect might be specific to speech: namely, in control conditions, no such effect was found for MMNs to frequency changes when the identity of the repetitive vowel continuously varied (i.e. vowel category changed all the time) vs did not vary.

It was also found that the groups had very different processing patterns in conditions with stimulus variation. In children with autism, MMNs were larger in amplitude for frequency changes of vowels with varied identity than for changes of vowel identity when vowels were varying in frequency. In contrast, the results of the control children were exactly the opposite. These results suggest that the neural apparatus of typically developing children is more adept in extracting linguistically relevant than irrelevant features from sound streams, which does not seem to apply to children with autism.

Evidently, children with ASD seem to have a profoundly different stimulus-processing style than that of their typically developing peers, and further, these differences originate from the early pre-attentive stages of speech processing. This detail-oriented perception, i.e. a difficulty in perceiving wholes without fully processing their fundamental parts (Happé & Frith, 2006; Mottron et al., 2006), might be defective when one has to extract invariant information. In natural speech-listening conditions, this might lead to difficulties in extracting phonetic information required to effectively perceive and understand speech.

Orienting to speech in ASD

Several aspects of speech analysis in general occur effortlessly and without focused attention, for instance, the early speech-feature, lexical, syntactic, and grammar processing (Pulvermüller & Shtyrov, 2006), which can be probed with MMN. However, attention is mandatory for successful communication, which is the core problem area in ASD. There is ample evidence that individuals with ASD have aberrant attention to speech and other social stimuli. This is evident even in early infancy, for example in 32–52-month-old children (Kuhl et al. 2005). A change from a repetitive /wa/ to a deviant /ba/ syllable elicited a smaller-amplitude MMN in children with ASD than that in healthy children (Kuhl et al., 2005). Furthermore, the children with ASD who preferred non-speech sounds, determined with head-turning responses, had no MMNs whereas children preferring speech had MMNs which did not differ from those of the control children. Thus, the absence of MMN to speech sounds in infants with ASD is associated with inattentiveness to speech, which might lead to poor acquisition of speech-related skills.

Neural responses associated with orientation towards stimuli have also indicated that individuals with ASD tend to be abnormally inattentive to speech. A potentially significant change in the sound stream elicits P3a when this event attracts attention (Escera et al., 2000). P3a follows MMN, indicating that a stimulus has opened a channel to conscious perception. In ASD, this channel functions quite aberrantly. This was evident, for example, in a study comparing P3a in children with vs without autism for vowels, their non-speech counterparts, and simple sinusoidal tones (Čeponienė et al., 2003) while children were attending to a video film. It was found that vowel changes elicited a smaller P3a amplitude in these than typically developing children, whereas no group differences were found for changes of the non-speech stimuli. Consistent with these results, Lepistö et al. (2005) reported smaller than normal P3a amplitudes in children with autism for speech-pitch and phoneme changes, but not for non-speech pitch changes or for speech or non-speech duration changes. A similar tendency was found in children with AS (Lepistö et al., 2006). In adults with AS, impaired attention switching to speech was also found. In the same stimulus paradigm as that used by Lepistö et al. (2005, 2006), these adults showed a larger P3a amplitude to non-speech than speech changes, an effect not found in their controls (Lepistö et al., 2007). Furthermore, the adults with AS had a smaller P3a amplitude for speech-sound changes than controls, whereas the non-speech-P3a was larger in adults with AS than that in their controls. These results imply that the neural processes leading to the orienting of attention towards speech sounds do not function normally in ASD.

Moreover, reduced P3a responses were found in children with autism for novel non-speech sounds when they occurred in streams of speech sounds but not when they occurred in streams of non-speech sounds (Whitehouse & Bishop, 2008). These results suggest that attention to sound streams composed of speech is suppressed so that novel sounds within these streams are abnormally detected in autism, irrespective of whether or not they are speech. Thus, the type of the sound stream, not the type of the sound change, affects the responsiveness to auditory changes in autism.

The effect of attention on change-related responses in autism has also been investigated. It was found that whereas the P3a amplitudes were smaller for changes among unattended speech than non-speech streams, those for speech changes increased to the normal level when children with autism attended to auditory stimuli (Whitehouse & Bishop, 2008). However, this study included in its sample children with high-functioning autism who had conversational speech skills. Furthermore, those children were excluded who could not correctly detect targets of the attentive task with 80% accuracy, leading to the rejection of almost half of the children with autism. Thus, these results concern a subgroup of children with autism with normal-like attentive abilities and cannot, therefore, be generalized to the entire population with autism.

The studies reviewed in the foregoing suggest that whereas MMN seems to be more affected by the type of sound change (e.g. pitch or duration) than by sound quality ('speechness') (Lepistö et al., 2005, 2006) in ASD, P3a reflecting attention-switching appears to be affected by sound quality. It was found that P3a was diminished in amplitude or absent for changes in speech-sound sequences but was relatively normal for changes in non-speech sound sequences in ASD (Čeponienė et al., 2003; Lepistö et al., 2005). In early childhood, this tendency might hinder the development of language and communication skills. It was suggested that typically developing infants prefer speech sounds, which grants them a special status in auditory perception (Jusczyk & Bertoncini, 1988). This facilitates the selection of acoustic signals relevant for communication, promoting language learning. If this bias towards speech is insufficient, then the child might not efficiently process the speech signal, which could lead to the underdeveloped neural representations of speech and inefficient speech analysis.

Conclusions

(1) MMN studies have suggested both hypo- and hypersensitive processing of changes in autism spectrum, as reflected in diminished vs enhanced amplitudes or delayed vs speeded latencies. The type of acoustic change (e.g. frequency/duration) and the make-up of the inherited genes underlying the phenotype presumably contributes to these findings. These neurophysiological results are consistent with the observed heterogeneous pattern of stimulus processing in the autism spectrum, in which both low and high sensitivity to sensory stimuli has been found.

(2) This suggestion is supported by studies showing an association between different perceptual phenotypes in the autism spectrum and MMN. In this spectrum,

children with a preference for non-speech sounds had diminished MMNs for syllable changes, whereas no such effect was found in children who preferred speech sounds. Furthermore, short MMN peak latencies were associated with the resistance to change. Delayed peak latencies, in turn, were connected to the most severe types of autism or language delay.

(3) Detail-oriented processing style as suggested by enhanced and speeded MMNs for acoustic changes in the autism spectrum might be improper for extracting invariant information, which is a necessary skill for identifying speech sounds which are normally heard in wide acoustic variation (e.g. due to speech prosody or different speakers). Indeed, whereas changes of vowels in a repetitive sound stream elicited robust, even larger than normal, MMNs in children with autism, these same changes elicited smaller MMNs in these than control children when the frequency of the vowels varied. This suggests that during normal listening conditions including acoustic variation, children with autism have difficulties in detecting the identity of speech sounds, which can be expected to impair speech perception.

(4) Several studies have reported differences in MMN scalp topographies between groups with vs without ASD. The MMNs had a more posterior scalp topography in individuals with ASD than in their controls, consistent with the suggestion of abnormal frontal-lobe metabolism. Also, diminished left-hemispheric MMNs for both speech and nonspeech sound changes or stronger right–left asymmetry in ASD than control participants were reported. These results suggest that auditory discrimination functions are abnormally distributed in the neural networks subserving audition in ASD.

4.4. **Oral clefts**

Nearly two-thirds of main craniofacial malformations are oral clefts (Johnston et al., 1990), with the incidence being 0.5–2 per 1000 live births (Hagberg et al., 1998). Oral clefting is a consequence of a failure of a union of oro-facial structures during the embryonic stage, which results in a cavity in the roof of the mouth. It is not considered to be a syndrome or a disease, but rather a manifestation of an underlying disease or syndrome (syndromic clefts), or an isolated phenomenon (nonsyndromic clefts). However, pathological conditions have increasingly been reported in association with clefts that were previously considered nonsyndromic, including central nervous system (CNS) abnormalities, endocrine dysfunctions, heart and eye deficits, language and learning disorders, craniosynostosis, and midfacial deficits (Shprintzen, 1995). The clefts directly cause impairments of speech, and they also compromise infant feeding and result in middle ear disease, peripheral hearing loss, and orthodontic problems. There are several variations of oral clefts. According to one widely used subdivision, there are isolated clefts of palate (CP) and clefts of the lip and palate (CLP), which includes cases of cleft lip/alveolus.

It was suggested that oral clefts have a multifactorial causation, resulting from inherited predisposition which is coupled with unfavourable environmental influences (Habib, 1978). According to the current view, the aetiologies can be grouped into four main categories as follows: (1) chromosomal and (2) genetic disorders, as well as (3) teratogen- and (4) mechanically induced clefting (Shprintzen, 1995). Teratogen- (e.g. alcohol, corticosteroids, retinoic acid, anticonvulsant drugs, and some psychoactive drugs) and mechanically (amniotic tearing, twin pregnancy, and uterine tumour) induced clefts are very rare. Chromosomal abnormalities include excessive genome defects involving multiple genes or even a whole chromosome. The individuals affected often cannot survive or if they do, they suffer from major brain and body malformations, and mental retardation.

The majority of the syndromes associated with clefts have a genetic origin, including a deletion or duplication of one or several neighbouring genes. Most of them include CP but not CLP. The CATCH 22 syndrome, which results from a small deletion on chromosome 22 (therefore being also called the 22q11 deletion syndrome), is the most frequent syndrome involving clefts (Goldberg et al., 1993). This syndrome includes over 30 clinical features, with the most typical being CP, cardiac anomalies, velopharyngeal insufficiency, learning and language disabilities, characteristic features of face, and disturbances of personality. There are several candidate genes, such as *TGFA* and *RARA*, which have a role in the fusion of mouth and roof tissues, the malfunctions of which can lead to oral clefting (Brewer et al., 1999; Sakata et al., 1999).

A range of learning and language disabilities and an elevated risk for psychiatric disorders are associated with oral clefts. Children with nonsyndromic oral clefts usually have a general IQ within normal limits but at the lower end, whereas their language and learning skills are clearly poorer than average (Čeponienė et al., 2002). Besides deficient speech, up to 46% of children with nonsyndromic oral clefts have a specific language disability (Broder et al., 1998). In general, the results on cognitive and language skills in patients with oral cleft are quite diverse. However, the most common result was that these skills are poorer in children with CP than in those with CLP (Estes & Morris, 1970). Whereas children with CP are often impaired in language comprehension, association, and reading, those with CLP have expressive language deficits such as poor speech intelligibility or phonetic inventory (Richman, 1980; Richman & Eliason, 1984). For example, at the age of 10–13 years, the incidence of reading disability in CP is 33%, whereas in CLP it corresponds to that of the general population (9%) (Richman et al., 1988). Thus, the deficits of children with CP are more harmful for cognitive development than those of children with CLP. The poorer language skills in CP than CLP are evident even at the toddler stage (Scherer & D'Antonio, 1997).

An additional fact hindering the language development in children with oral clefts is their high risk of hearing loss. The majority of these children get a middle ear disease due to the dysfunction of the Eustachian tube (Gould, 1990), which continues until the beginning of school age. Therefore, they are suffering from variable degrees of auditory deprivation at the developmental stage when they should acquire the core language skills, which may be one reason for their language deficits.

CATCH 22 is most commonly associated with CP (Ryan et al., 1997). The IQ of children with this syndrome is at the lower end of the normal range and virtually all of them suffer from cognitive disabilities and need tutorial assistance (Golding-Kushner et al.,

1985; Kok & Solman, 1995). These children have deficits in language, communication, associative reasoning, mathematics, and motor coordination. Furthermore, psychiatric disorders have a high prevalence in this population. Thirty per cent of adults with this syndrome have schizophrenia (Murphy et al., 1999), whereas in childhood, social impairments, anxieties, and attention deficits have been reported (Swillen et al., 1999).

Sensory memory in oral clefts

MMN has been used for investigating auditory sensory memory in children with oral clefts, since adequate sensory memory is essential for a number of cognitive functions, including higher levels of memory processes and fluent speech functions. Cheour et al. (1997) varied the stimulus-onset asynchrony (SOA) in sequences of 1000 Hz standard and 1100 Hz deviant tones in different conditions and recorded MMN from 6–10-year-old children with a 22q11 deletion syndrome with normal peripheral hearing and from healthy control children. The MMN elicited with all the SOAs used (450 ms, 800 ms, 1500 ms) significantly differed from zero in control children, suggesting that their auditory sensory memory could maintain the memory trace for as long as 1.5 seconds. However, in children with 22q11, MMNs were significantly elicited only with the shortest SOA, suggesting that the duration of the memory trace was shorter than 800 ms. Furthermore, the MMN amplitude was significantly smaller in the children with the 22q11 deletion syndrome than that in the control children, in the two conditions with the shortest SOAs. These results suggest that the auditory sensory-memory trace maintenance is weaker in children with the 22q11 deletion syndrome than that in normal healthy children.

A further study showed that this sensory memory deficit is not limited to this more severe type of oral clefts but rather applies to CP as well (Cheour et al., 1998b). In children with both cleft types, MMNs were significantly elicited by stimuli presented with 450 ms and 800 ms SOAs only. Furthermore, the MMN amplitude in children with the 22q11 deletion syndrome was smaller than that in controls for the 800 ms and 1500 ms SOAs whereas in children with CP, a smaller MMN amplitude relative to that in the controls was found for the 1500 ms SOA only. This suggests that the dysfunction in the sensory-memory trace maintenance was present in both groups but was more severe in the 22q11 deletion syndrome. A subsequent study (Cheour et al., 1999) suggested that the impairments at sensory memory are evident as early as in infancy in children with CP. In this study, MMN-like responses were found in all nine healthy neonates for frequency changes of tones presented with a 800 ms SOA, whereas only three out of nine neonates with CP had this type of a response, with the rest of them having a positively displaced change-related response, which could be a sign of an immature MMN in these infants.

The results suggesting MMN diminution for stimuli presented with long intervals in children with oral clefts were replicated by Yang et al. (2012) in larger infant groups at the age of about 15 months. Furthermore, their results suggested that the auditory impairment is of cortical origin. In this study, 34 infants with nonsyndromic cleft lip and/or palate and 34 healthy infants were included. By using otoscopy and tympanometry, it was ensured that the middle ear of all these infants was functioning normally. The auditory brainstem and middle latency potentials did not significantly differ between the groups. However, the area of the MMN amplitude, obtained for frequency changes of stimuli presented at about 1000 ms intervals, was significantly smaller in children with oral clefts than that in control children. These results suggest that in children with oral clefts, auditory information is normally transmitted in the subcortical structures when there is no peripheral hearing loss. However, at the cortical level, sound discrimination is compromised, at least for stimuli occurring at a relatively slow pace.

The effect of cleft type on sensory memory

The association between different cleft types with different degrees of cognitive disabilities raises the question of whether the cleft type also has an effect on the extent of sensory-memory dysfunction. This question was addressed in a study including 78 children at the age of 7–9 years with different types of nonsyndromic oral clefts with no higher hearing thresholds than 25 dB (Čeponienė et al., 1999a). Their MMNs, obtained for frequency changes with different SOAs, were compared with those of age-matched healthy children. Based on clinical examination, several subgroups of the children with oral clefts were created.

With the shortest SOAs, which were 450 and 800 ms, MMNs significantly differing from zero were found in all groups. However, with the longest, 1500 ms, SOA, the MMNs in the oral cleft groups were less robust and they were insignificant in the group with the clefts of the soft palates only (CPO3). In this SOA condition, there was a significantly smaller MMN amplitude in the children with than without oral clefts. Furthermore, a Group × SOA interaction showed that the groups differed from each other in the condition with the longest SOA. As Fig. 4.5 shows, all groups with oral clefts had smaller MMN amplitudes than the control group, there also being differences in the average MMN amplitudes between the subgroups of oral clefts. The subgroup of cleft lip with or without a defect in the alveolar arch (CL/A) had the largest average MMN amplitude of the oral cleft groups, whereas the amplitudes diminished for the cleft types which were more posteriorly located, closer to the pharyngeal wall. When the MMNs obtained only with the longest SOA were included in the analysis, their amplitudes were significantly smaller in children with overt CP, submucous clefts, and CLP than those in healthy children.

These results replicate the findings obtained in the studies described earlier in this chapter, indicating sensory-memory dysfunction in oral clefts and, further, they suggest that the severity of this dysfunction depends on the cleft type. The MMN amplitudes of the children with the CP only were significantly diminished. Consistent with this, children with this cleft type have more severe problems in the symbolic usage of language than children with some other cleft types (cleft lip with or without a defect in the alveolar arch, unilateral CLP; Richman, 1980). For symbolic language use, in turn, well-functioning memory systems, including working and short-term/sensory memory are mandatory. For example, well-functioning sensory memory, as reflected by MMN, was associated with the functioning of the phonological loop of working memory (Čeponienė et al., 1999b). Therefore, memory dysfunction as reflected by the MMN in subgroups of children with oral clefts may contribute to their language-related impairments.

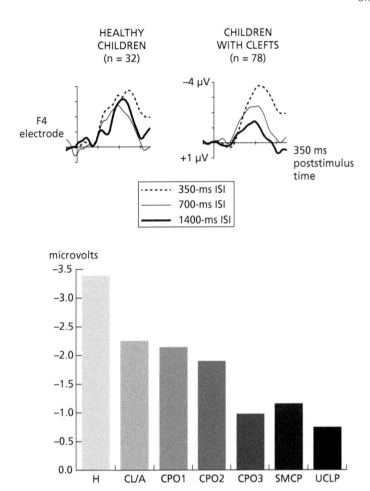

Fig. 4.5 MMN responses (top) elicited by three stimulus rates in healthy 7-10 year old children (left) and in those with oral clefts (right). Average MMN amplitudes (bottom) in the condition with a 1400 ms inter-stimulus interval in healthy children and in those with oral clefts classified on the basis of the anterior-posterior degree of clefting. Subgroups of the children with oral clefts were created as follows: cleft lip with or without a deficit in the alveolar arch (CL/A), complete unilateral cleft of lip and palate (UCLP), and clefts of the palate only (CPO). The group with CPO was still divided into subgroups of clefts extending to foramen incisivum (CPO1), those extending to the region between the foramen incisivum and soft palate (CPO2), clefts in the soft palate only (CPO3), and submucous clefts of the soft palate (SMCP).

Reprinted from Clinical Neurophysiology, 110, Čeponienė, R., Hukki, J., Cheour, M., Haapanen, M. L., Ranta, R., & Näätänen, R., *Cortical auditory dysfunction in children with oral clefts: relation with cleft type*, 1921–1926, Copyright (1999), with permission from Elsevier.

The origin of the MMN abnormality in oral clefts

The cognitive and language dysfunctions of children with oral clefts might be affected by the middle ear effusions which are highly prevalent in these children during infancy and early childhood (Broen et al., 1998). Such a condition degrades sound reception which deprives the child's developing central auditory system from adequate input, which may result in underdeveloped receptive and expressive language functions (Friel-Patti & Finitzo, 1990). However, it was suggested that the incidence of middle-ear disease would not be associated with certain cleft types in a systematic way, and would, therefore, not explain the connections of the memory and language dysfunctions to the oral cleft subtype (Čeponienė et al., 1999a). It was therefore proposed that both cleft and neural dysfunction could be genetically transmitted (Čeponienė et al., 1999a).

To test the viability of the hypothesis of a common genetic background of oral clefts and neural dysfunctions, MMNs of infants with oral CLP, with CP only, and healthy infants were recorded as neonates and at 6 months later (Čeponienė et al., 2000). The MMN amplitudes obtained from these infants both when they were newborns and at 6 months of age were significantly smaller in the group with CP only than in healthy infants. This cleft group also had significantly smaller MMN amplitudes than the group with CLP as newborns. The MMNs of these infants, in turn, did not significantly differ from those of healthy infants. These results suggest that even as newborns, the children with CP only, with language disabilities more severe than those of children with CLP, have diminished MMN amplitudes. These results support the proposed genetic origins of language and neural dysfunctions of certain oral cleft types.

22q11 and cognitive function

Syndromic oral clefts caused by a microdeletion at the region of 22q11, involving malformations of the palate, face, and heart, are associated with cognitive deficits and a high incidence of psychiatric disorders (Ryan et al., 1997). These individuals may have communication impairments and a mild to moderate learning disability. Furthermore, they have an elevated risk for psychiatric disorders, with the risk for schizophrenia being markedly increased, occurring in 30% of adults (Murphy et al., 1999). In childhood, these oral clefts are associated with social impairments, anxieties, and attention deficits (Arnold et al., 2001; Swillen et al., 1999).

Since language and working memory deficits are associated with schizophrenia and MMN is abnormal in these patients and in some of their relatives (Michie et al., 2002), MMN along with measures of language function and working memory were used as candidates for endophenotypes in the 22q11 deletion syndrome (Baker et al., 2005). This study, including teenagers and young adults with this syndrome and IQ-, gender-, and age-matched healthy participants, found significant group differences both in expressive language, working memory, and MMN amplitude, which was reduced for both speech and non-speech sounds in individuals with 22q11 deletion syndrome.

The pattern of MMN results in individuals with 22q11 deletion syndrome resembled that found in schizophrenic patients. Firstly, the MMN reduction in these individuals was seen at the frontal scalp but not at electrodes primarily measuring the temporal lobe component of MMN. A similar MMN pattern has been reported for idiopathic schizophrenia (Baldeweg et al., 2002; Sato et al., 2003; Todd et al., 2003), which might reflect poor connectivity between the temporal and frontal areas. Secondly, the MMN amplitude was more severely reduced for duration than frequency changes in the 22q11 deletion group, which is consistent with findings in schizophrenic patients (Michie et al., 2000; Umbricht & Krljes, 2003). Thirdly, despite reductions in the MMN amplitude, both this group and schizophrenic patients (Todd et al., 2000) performed at a normal level in a behavioural tone-discrimination task. This dissociation between the MMN and discrimination-test results is compatible with the view that the temporal lobe MMN primarily contributes to discrimination processes whereas the frontal-lobe MMN is involved in other functions (Shalgi & Deouell, 2007), probably mediating attention switch to change (Näätänen & Michie, 1979; Rinne et al., 2000).

Conclusions

(1) Several studies consistently reported absent or diminished MMNs to changes in sounds presented at long intervals in participants with oral clefts but normal-like MMNs when the interval was shorter. This suggests impaired sensory memory maintenance in oral clefts.

(2) The type of oral clefts have an influence on the MMN amplitude. The subgroup of children with a cleft lip with or without a defect in the alveolar arch (CL/A) had the largest average MMN amplitude of the oral cleft groups, whereas the amplitudes diminished for the cleft types which were more posteriorly located, closer to the pharyngeal wall. These results suggest that the severity of the dysfunction depends on the cleft type.

(3) Diminished MMN amplitudes were found even in newborns with oral clefts, with the oral cleft type affecting the MMN. The MMN amplitude was smaller in infants with the most severe oral cleft, CP only, than in infants with oral CLP and in healthy infants.

(4) When MMNs and language and working memory functions of adults and teenagers with the 22q11 deletion syndrome and IQ, gender, and age-matched control participants were compared with each other, differences were found in all of these measures. The participants with 22q11 deletion syndrome had diminished MMN amplitudes for both speech and non-speech sounds and poorer expressive language and working memory functions.

Chapter 5

Aging

5.1 Introduction

With aging, MMN/MMNm is generally attenuated in amplitude and its peak latency is prolonged (Czigler et al., 1992; Pekkonen et al., 1996; Kiang et al., 2009; Kisley et al., 2005; Rimmele et al., 2012; Bertoli et al., 2002; Ruzzoli et al., 2012). Alain and Woods (1999) reported that the MMN amplitude (collapsed over tone-frequency and -pattern deviants) progressively decreased by 0.06 μV per year and the MMN peak latency was prolonged by 0.06 ms/year. In a study of duration-change MMN conducted in 147 healthy adults and 257 schizophrenia patients, Kiang and colleagues (2009) also detected an average reduction of 0.06 to 0.8 μV per year in each of the groups. Notably, Kiang and colleagues found that the severity of MMN impairment in schizophrenia (d≈1.0) was comparable across age bands. Such characterization of age effects in both healthy subjects and neuropsychiatric patient populations has implications for biomarker development via normative efforts that consider demographic factors and stimulus parameters (cf. Light et al., 2012; Light et al., 2015). With regard to stimulus parameters, the duration-change MMN is more affected by aging than the frequency-change MMN (Pekkonen et al. 1996b). Consistent with this, Kisley et al. (2005) concluded, on the basis of their MMN results, that the processing of temporal stimulus features deteriorates more with aging than that of the other stimulus features such as frequency or loudness. For a meta-analysis of the aging effects on MMN, see Cheng et al. (2013). In the visual and somatosensory modalities, a similar aging effect can also be observed, with vMMN (Lorenzo-López et al. 2004; Tales et al., 2002) and sMMN (Cheng & Lin, 2013; Strömmer et al., 2014) peak amplitudes being attenuated with aging.

Along with increasing age, the level of performance in different cognitive tasks also gradually decreases (Cansino, 2009). Importantly, there is also evidence linking the age-related MMN decrement to this cognitive deterioration. It was found by Kisley et al. (2005) that MMN for an occasional stimulus onset asynchrony (SOA) shortening was much smaller in amplitude in the elderly (55–85 years) than young (18–23 years). Further, in the elderly, MMN was more attenuated in amplitude in those with a weaker performance in different cognitive performance tasks than in those with a better performance.

5.2 Temporal processing

The temporal resolution in auditory processing is decreased with aging (for a review, see Frisina et al., 2001) as indexed by gap detection paradigms. Gap detection is an important measure of the processing of rapid spectro-temporal patterns essential for speech perception. Even in healthy elderly persons, MMN to a short gap in the middle of a brief sinusoidal tone (Desjardins et al., 1999) was attenuated in amplitude, consistent with their increased difficulty in correctly perceiving rapid speech-sound patterns such as consonants (Bertoli et al., 2002). Bertoli et al. (2002) found that whereas there was no significant difference in the psychoacoustic gap-detection performance between their young (mean age 26 years) and elderly (mean age 72 years) normal healthy subjects, longer gaps were required to elicit MMN in the elderly, indicating that their temporal resolution at the pre-attentive level was reduced. The authors concluded that MMN elicited in the gap paradigm appears to be a sensitive index even for small contrasts and, further, that even though the sensitivity of the elderly at the pre-attentive level to such small gaps was considerably decreased, they could compensate this by effortful attention (as shown by psychoacoustic results). Consequently:

> Combining the results of electrophysiological tests, MMN in particular, with those from psychoacoustic tests, could allow a better delineation of the deficits that underlie the speech understanding problems of elderly persons. Perhaps these deficits could, at least in part, be located within the early stages of central auditory processing at the borderline between automatic processing and the higher levels where attentional mechanisms become increasingly important. (p. 405)

Consistent with this, Alain et al. (2004) concluded that aging affects the ability to automatically register small changes in a stream of homogenous stimuli but that this age-related decline can be compensated for by top-down controlled processes. However, Schiff et al. (2008) found that N1 and MMN were less affected by aging than were the attention-related N2b and P3, concluding that higher cognitive functions are more damaged by aging than are the perceptual and pre-attentive ones.

Whereas gap detection becomes weaker by aging, the temporal window of integration appears not to be influenced. The MMN data pattern obtained by Horváth et al. (2007) in the elderly (mean age 68.3 years) and young (mean age 21.7 years) suggested that TWI is not prolonged with aging, with both groups showing a TWI duration of 200–250 ms. Hence, in contrast to expectations based on the notion of a general slowing with aging (for a review, see Frisina et al., 2001), TWI was not longer in the elderly than that in the young.

5.3 Processing of sequential stimulus contingencies

Gaeta et al. (2002) used ascending tone pairs (with the second tone being one step higher on the musical scale than the first tone) randomly varying across 10 different frequency levels as their standards, whereas deviants were descending tone pairs. In their monaural (left-ear) condition, MMN elicited by rule violations was very similar for both their elderly (mean age 73.7 years) and young (mean age 22.3 years) subjects. When the paradigm was made even more demanding by delivering the first tone of each tone pair to the left ear and the second tone to the right ear, MMN was elicited in the younger participants but not in the elderly. This absence of MMN in the elderly under the more demanding condition was regarded as supporting the notion that the efficacy of central auditory processing declines in the elderly. However, the MMN elicitation under the easier monaural condition with ten different frequency levels demonstrates that the elderly were able to pre-attentively form neural representations of rule-based auditory features of input originating from a single source. Age-related differences in neural-trace formation must therefore lie in differences between the integration of afferent input originating from two different sources rather than from the same source. Consistent with this, Gaeta et al. (2002) concluded that the neural processes associated with the generation of abstract neural representations are intact in both the young and elderly but that there is an age-related decrease in the efficacy of neural integration processes under binaural conditions.

Previously, Alain and Woods (1999) found that infrequent stimulus repetitions in a tone sequence consisting of tones delivered at a very short constant SOA (300 ms), alternating between two frequencies (500 and 2000 Hz), elicited MMN (cf. Nordby et al., 1988) which was considerably lower in peak amplitude in the old (mean age 65.7 years) than that in the young (23.3 years). Importantly, pattern processing, as judged from MMN data, was very similar in the middle-aged (mean 43.3 years) and elderly subjects. This finding contrasts with the remarkable age-related decrease of the MMN peak amplitude for sounds deviating from standards along simple physical dimensions such as frequency, showing a linear decrement with age (Pekkonen et al., 1993; Gaeta et al., 1998; Alain & Woods, 1999).

5.4 Sensory-memory duration in audition

MMN depends on the presence of the sensory-memory trace representing the preceding stimuli at the moment of the delivery of a deviant stimulus (*Chapter 2*). By gradually prolonging SOA, MMN eventually vanishes, which enables one to assess the sensory-memory duration in audition, a potential general index of brain plasticity and hence that of brain aging (Näätänen & Kreegipuu, 2011). In young healthy adults, the trace duration, as determined in this manner, approximates 10 s (Böttcher-Gandor & Ullsperger, 1992; Sams et al., 1993; for a review of related behavioural studies, see Cowan, 1984), but is gradually shortened with aging. Pekkonen et al. (1996b) found that with an SOA of 0.5 s, the MMN amplitude for frequency change was very similar in the elderly (mean 59 years) and young (mean 22 years), suggesting that the memory-trace formation for sounds and, thus, sound perception (see Näätänen & Winkler, 1999) were not affected by aging. In contrast, with an SOA of 4.5 s, the MMN amplitude of the elderly was substantially attenuated relative to the young (Fig. 5.1), indicating that the auditory sensory-memory duration is shortened with aging. Moreover, corresponding MMN data for frequency change in patients with chronic alcoholism suggest an accelerated age-related shortening of sensory memory-trace duration, and hence a faster decrement of brain plasticity, in these patients (Polo et al., 1999; see also Grau et al., 2001).

An important paradigm improvement for determining the sensory-memory duration was introduced by Grau et al. (1998). Grau and colleagues found that in relatively older

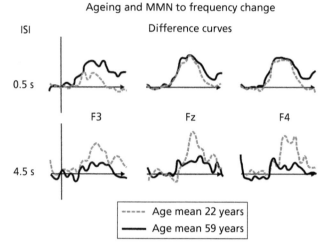

Fig. 5.1 MMN to a frequency change in young (mean 22 years) and elderly (mean 59 years) subjects when the stimuli were presented with a short (0.5 s) and long (4.5 s) constant inter-stimulus interval. Note the MMN attenuation with 4.5 s inter-stimulus interval in the older group.
Data from Pekkonen, E., Rinne, T., Reinikainen, K., Kujala, T., Alho, K., & Näätänen, R., Aging effects on auditory processing: an event-related potential study, Experimental Aging Research, 22 (2), 171–184, doi:10.1080/03610739608254005, 1996.

adults (mean age 48.1 years), MMN for tone-duration decrement was elicited in the short (0.4 s) but not long (4 s) inter-train interval (ITI) condition by deviant stimuli in the first stimulus position of a three-stimulus train (with SOA being 300 ms). In contrast, their younger subjects (mean age 21.0 years) showed very similar MMNs obtained with the two different ITIs. Consequently, this study also showed that the sensory-memory trace is shortened in duration with aging. The new and more time-effective Grau paradigm was subsequently employed by Ruzzoli et al. (2012) in three different age groups: young (mean age 33.6 years), middle-aged (mean age 50.8 years), and old (mean age 68.1 years). The standard stimuli were three consecutive sinusoidal tones of 75 ms (with SOA being 300 ms) whereas the deviant stimuli were similar tones of 25 ms in duration occasionally replacing the first tone of the three-tone sequence. It was found that MMN in the short-ITI condition (0.4 s) was very similar for all the three different age groups whereas when ITI was prolonged to 4 s, then MMN for deviants in the first stimulus position was observed for the young and middle-aged only, indexing the shortening of the sensory-memory duration with aging, particularly in the older age cohort. Importantly, the MMN amplitude over the frontal area in the 4-s ITI condition strongly correlated with the Wechsler Memory Scale (WMS) score across all subjects, highlighting the MMN amplitude as a function of ITI as an index of age-dependent brain plasticity (Ruzzoli et al., 2012). Hence, aging does not affect the precision of sound encoding whereas the retention of this sensory information is deteriorated in aging and correlates with age-related cognitive decline.

5.5 **Change detection in other sensory modalities**

Tales et al. (2002) instructed their older (mean age 77 years) and younger (mean age 30.5 years) subjects to fixate their gaze on a small blue frame at the centre of a computer monitor screen. Periodically, the centre of the blue frame filled with red (the target stimulus) and the subject had to respond to it by pressing a button. It was found that the young subjects displayed a prominent vMMN, whereas in the older ones, this vMMN was considerably reduced in amplitude. In contrast, Stothart et al. (2013) found no vMMN-amplitude decrement in their old (mean 76.8 years) relative to their young subjects (mean 20.8 years).

Lorenzo-López et al. (2004) studied vMMNs for downward-drifting gratings (deviants) occasionally replacing standards (repetitive upward-drifting gratings) in three different groups of subjects: old (mean age 62 years), middle-aged (49 years), and young (32 years), instructed to fixate their gaze on the central cross, to pay attention to the nine possible digits presented above the central cross, and to press a button as fast as possible in response to numbers lower than five of any colour. It was found that whereas behavioural reaction time was not affected by age, corresponding vMMN amplitude displayed a significant and progressive age-related decrease. The authors suggested that older adults might have difficulties in automatically detecting changes in motion direction which may lead to an inefficient perception and interpretation of the visual environment. Consequently, the decreased ability to pre-attentively detect an unattended moving object in the peripheral visual field might increase difficulties and dangers in daily activities such as driving a car (Näätänen & Summala, 1976). In the somatosensory modality, Strömmer et al. (2014) found that the somatosensory mismatch response of positive polarity to location change was attenuated in amplitude and prolonged in peak latency in their aged (mean 75 years) compared with that in their young (mean 25 years) subjects.

Hence, with aging, there is a systematic decrease of MMN amplitude and the prolongation of its peak latency in the auditory, visual, and somatosensory modalities, In audition, these changes involve multiple auditory stimulus attributes and can be observed even in middle-aged cohorts (i.e. the fourth decade of life). Furthermore, this aging effect on the MMN amplitude is considerably more robust for sound duration than frequency change, consistent with the notion of an aging-related vulnerability of temporal processing relative to that of the other stimulus features. These age-related changes occur in pre-attentive processing which attenuate, deteriorate, and delay sensory input to higher processing levels and may in particular contribute to speech-perception difficulties of the aged and delay their responses to different environmental changes.

The fact that speech-perception problems may originate even at the pre-attentive level, as shown via the study of MMN (Foster et al., 2013; Pichora-Fuller, 2003), suggests that remediation strategies which specifically target improving the accuracy and fidelity of low level pre-attentive processing may show particular promise for improving 'upstream' higher-order cognitive functions (Kujala et al., 2001; for reviews, see Ylinen & Kujala, 2015; Näätänen et al., 2007). Of particular interest are studies that demonstrate the presence of MMN in the absence of a corresponding detectable ability for behavioural discrimination (Paavilainen, 2013; Paavilainen, Arajärvi, & Tagegata, 2007; van Zuijen et al., 2006). These results locate the behavioural discrimination problem to the loss of the change-detection signal developed by the auditory-cortex MMN generator on its way to higher-level cognitive systems. That is, these higher mechanisms cannot read the impinging lower-level signal, possibly because of increased internal noise. Such findings might open new strategies for remediation, for example, by targeting the age-related increase in internal neural noise by certain types of music stimulation. Alain et al. (2014) concluded, in their review, that musical training may offer potential benefits to complex listening and might delay or even attenuate the decline in auditory perception and cognition that often emerge later in life. Moreover, it was found by Lövden et al. (2012) that cognitive training (spatial navigation) was equally effective in the old and young, with this training protecting the hippocampus against age-related volume changes during the early and late adulthood. Essential for the understanding of the speech-perception problems of the aged are MMN results indexing their decreased temporal resolution. MMN to an occasional gap in a brief sinusoidal tone showed a graded age-related decrement in amplitude, and hence a decreased temporal resolution (Pichora-Fuller, 2003).

Aging also shortened the duration of auditory sensory-memory trace, a potential objective index of decreased brain plasticity (see Cheng et al. (2013) for a proposal involving MMN as a marker of physiological aging). Consistent with this view, MMN findings suggest that the deterioration of central auditory processing may also index an age-related cognitive decline (Näätänen et al., 2012, 2014; see also De Pascalis & Varriale, 2012; Lindin et al., 2013). Firstly, performance decrement in cognitive tasks in the aged may, to some extent, be based on the higher processing levels receiving qualitatively deteriorated or delayed input from the lower levels (Pichora-Fuller, 2003), reflected by decreased and delayed MMNs. Secondly, MMN deficit in aging might also be due to the fact that impaired central auditory processing, to a great extent, results from a deficient functioning of the NMDA-receptor system (Magnusson et al., 2010) that is of crucial significance for the formation of memory traces at the different hierarchically organized levels of auditory memory (Cotman et al., 1989; Javitt et al., 1996; Magnusson, 1998; Näätänen et al., 2014; Thomas et al., 2017), for several other cognitive functions, and for the release of other neurotransmitters, hence, for general brain plasticity. This hierarchical information processing cascade model was empirically confirmed by Thomas and colleagues (2017) and is reviewed in *Chapter 7*.

5.6 **Conclusions**

(1) With aging, there is a systematic decrease of the MMN amplitude and the prolongation of its peak latency in the auditory, visual, and somatosensory modalities. In audition, these changes involve all the different auditory stimulus attributes and can be observed even in the early middle-aged cohorts. Further, this aging effect on the auditory MMN amplitude is considerably more robust for duration than frequency

change, consistent with the notion of an aging-related vulnerability of temporal processing relative to that of the other stimulus features.

(2) Age-related changes occur in pre-attentive processing which attenuate, deteriorate, and delay sensory input to higher processing levels. This may in particular contribute to speech-perception difficulties of the aged and delay their responses to different environmental changes.

(3) Most importantly, aging also shortens the duration of auditory sensory memory, an index of brain plasticity.

(4) Certain types of music stimulation could reduce age-related increase in internal neural noise, detrimental for forming and maintaining accurate neural representations. Thus, musical training may offer potential benefits to complex listening and might be utilized as a means to delay or even attenuate declines in auditory perception and cognition that often emerge later in life. Moreover, cognitive training (spatial navigation) was equally effective in old and young subjects, with this training protecting the hippocampus against age-related volume changes during the early and late adulthood.

(5) MMN data suggest that the deterioration of central auditory processing may also index age-related cognitive decline. Firstly, performance decrement in cognitive tasks in the aged may in part result from the fact that the higher processing levels receive qualitatively deteriorated or delayed input from the lower processing levels, reflected by decreased and delayed MMNs. Secondly, MMN deficit in aging might also be due to the fact that impaired central auditory processing mainly results from a deficient functioning of the NMDA-receptor system that is of crucial significance for the formation of memory traces at the different hierarchically organized levels of auditory memory.

(6) Consistent with the aforementioned, measures of auditory sensitivity and visual accuracy are strongly correlated with age-related variations in intelligence, even more strongly than are the cognitive measures of speed of processing, already accepted as robust indicators of the cognitive aging status. Consequently, age-related changes in sensory processing and cognition may have a shared pathophysiological basis.

(7) The age-related decrement of vMMN to peripheral changes in the visual field is a particularly important observation as the decreased ability to pre-attentively detect an unattended moving object in the peripheral visual field might contribute to difficulties and dangers in daily activities such as driving a car.

Chapter 6

Neurological disorders

6.1. Neurodegenerative diseases

Mild cognitive impairment

As reviewed in *Chapter 5* the MMN amplitude is gradually decreased and peak latency prolonged with aging. This effect is observed as early as middle-age and may reflect a slow age-related decline of central auditory processing and cognition. Cognitive decline can, however, be much more dramatic. Such a rapid cognitive decline may occur in individuals at risk for dementia, in particular Alzheimer's Disease (AD). The syndrome of mild cognitive impairment (MCI) is therefore an area of intensive investigation as this may reflect a possible transitory state between healthy aging and dementia. The search for biomarkers that would facilitate the early identification of MCI and/or the prediction of which MCI patients actually progress to dementia (Mowszowski et al., 2012) would be of substantial value for informing interventions. MCI is a heterogeneous clinical concept characterized by evidence for cognitive decline, without any major impairment in the performance of daily activities. Among the different subtypes of MCI, the amnestic MCI (aMCI) is the most likely one to progress to AD (Winblad et al., 2004) and is the prevalent form of dementia in the elderly (for a review, see Lindín et al., 2013). Therefore the identification of aMCI biomarkers would be of major benefit to clinicians, for such biomarkers could be used as objective diagnostic tools permitting an early, even pre-symptomatic, identification of the presence of prodromal AD. Such biomarkers would also aid treatment decisions and enable the monitoring of the progress of the disease. (See also Baldeweg & Hirsch, 2015).

A promising candidate measure for this purpose is MMN. Mowszowski et al. (2012) found that the MMN amplitude for occasional tone-duration increment recorded over fronto-temporal scalp areas (using a nose reference, revealing a polarity-reversed MMN, i.e. the mismatch positivity, MMP) was smaller in amplitude in patients with MCI than that in healthy age-matched controls. Importantly, the right temporal MMN-amplitude decrement was associated with a poorer performance in a verbal-learning task and the left-temporal MMN amplitude decrement with an increased self-rated disability. The authors concluded that these findings suggest that:

> [T]he attenuation of the early information processing mechanisms may underpin aspects of higher-order cognitive and psycho-social functioning in MCI. As such, MMN may be a viable biomarker of this transitory state between healthy aging and dementia, thus representing a practical, time-efficient and non-invasive tool for early identification of 'at risk' individuals. Given its cognitive

implications, MMN may also have utility as an outcome measure of individually tailored cognitive interventions (e.g., cognitive training programs). (Mowszowski et al., 2012, p. 216.)

In subjects performing a visual task, Lindín et al. (2013) subsequently found that the MMN amplitude was considerably attenuated in their middle-aged (between 50 and 64 years of age) amnestic MCI patients in the first evaluation. Moreover, this amplitude was further decreased at the second evaluation 18–24 months later, which was not observed in normal healthy controls. The authors suggested that this may indicate a progressive deterioration of the neural mechanisms involved in the maintenance of sensory trace and/or the pre-attentive mechanisms of the automatic detection of change in the acoustic environment. Consequently, the MMN-amplitude attenuation for tone-duration decrement provides an early biomarker, or warning signal, which is practical, time-effective, and non-invasive, of a latent initiation of brain changes leading to the cognitive deterioration known as MCI. MMN hence indexes sensory-level deterioration which is repeated at higher levels of cognitive brain functioning using outcomes of the processing carried out at lower levels (Baldeweg & Hirsch, 2015; see also Thomas et al., 2017).

In the visual modality, Tales et al. (2008) reported a significant abnormality in pre-attentive visual processing both in MCI and AD compared with healthy aging, concluding that this result shows that abnormalities in brain function in aMCI are not confined to high-level processes but rather that 'basic functions associated with the automatic detection of stimulus change within the visual environment, an important initiator of deployment of attention, are abnormal in MCI. Further, therefore, some of the high-level, cognitive, and perceptual-related deficits observed in MCI are the result, at least in part, of significant deficits in pre-cursor information processing systems.' (Tales et al., 2008, p. 1230).

Alzheimer's disease and other dementias

As described in 'Mild cognitive impairment', there is an elevated risk of AD among patients with a MCI (Winblad et al., 2004). AD is the major cause of clinical dementia in the elderly (Zamrini et al., 2011). The prevalence of AD begins to rise as people reach the age of 65 years; by the time people reach their eighties and nineties, the risk of clinical dementia amounts is nearly 50%. Consequently, Zamrini et al. concluded that treatment strategies aimed at disease modification will be the most efficacious if they can be started during the period when the pathological changes in the brain are already occurring but have not yet resulted in clinical signs and symptoms. Therefore, there has been a recent upsurge of interest in studying individuals who are in the transitional state between normal cognition and MCI in order to identify biomarkers to inform clinicians of disease-risk onset and progression. According to these authors, it seems necessary to have a biomarker that: (1) measures neuronal activity directly; (2) has good temporal and spatial resolution; and (3) is able to evaluate functional networks and the associated neuronal code. Such biomarkers could reveal the early, latent or prodromal stage of the disease before irreversible pathological changes have occurred in the brain:

Consequently, these measures may provide the best index of the earliest functional changes that may occur secondary to neuropathological processes, but prior to the onset of the clinical dementia syndrome. In order to be most effective, however, these markers must have predictive validity relative to the neuropathology of AD, as well as a modest intra- and inter-subject variability. And, they must be stable over reasonable time course (i.e., 3–6 months) in order to be useful to track change in disease, or response to medication. (Zamrini et al., 2011, p. 2.)

These biomarker prerequisites are met by MMN for AD and other neurological disorders (Light & Näätänen, 2013; Light et al., 2012, 2015). Pekkonen et al. (1994) found, in an early study, that MMN amplitude for a frequency change was only slightly smaller in patients with AD than in age-matched controls when stimulus onset asynchrony (SOA) was 0.5 s. However, when it was prolonged to 3 s, then the MMN amplitude was dramatically attenuated in patients, suggesting a pathologically shortened sensory memory duration in AD reflective of reduced neuroplasticity (Fig. 6.1; see also Pekkonen et al., 1996a; Teter & Ashford, 2002).

Subsequently, Gaeta et al. (1999) recorded MMNs of eight patients with mild to moderate AD of a mean age of 72.5 years to tone-frequency changes and novel sounds of four different categories. The SOA was constant at 1 s. It was found that both patients and controls displayed MMNs that increased in amplitude with an increasing magnitude of stimulus change. Further, these MMNs were smaller in amplitude in patients with AD than those in controls. Significant P3a responses of a small size were elicited in patients by novel sounds as a sign of involuntary attention switch to stimulus change. Gaeta et al. proposed that these results reflect 'reduced efficacy of the auditory sensory memory system,

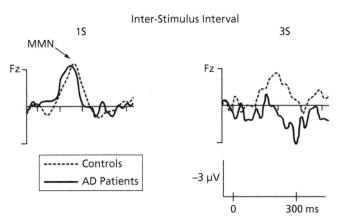

Fig. 6.1 Auditory MMN waveforms at Fz electrode with inter-stimulus intervals of 1 s and 3 s. Auditory ERPs were recorded from 9 patients with AD and 10 age-matched healthy controls. When the inter-stimulus interval increased, the MMN amplitude decreased more in the AD group than in the control group.

Data from Pekkonen, E., Jousmäki, V., Könönen, M., Reinikainen, K., & Partanen, J., *Auditory sensory memory impairment in Alzheimer's disease: An event-related potential study*, Neuroreport: An International Journal for the Rapid Communication of Research in Neuroscience, 5 (18), 2537–2540, http://dx.doi.org/10.1097/00001756-199412000-00033, 1994.

decreased sensitivity of the deviance detection mechanism, or a higher trigger threshold for involuntary attentional capture. However, because of the independent nature of these three factors, it is most likely that they all contribute' (p. 286).

Kazmerski et al. (1997) recorded MMNs to deviant tones and different environmental sounds during passive and active oddball sequences in patients with a probable AD, using a constant SOA of 1 s. It was found that MMNs were smaller in amplitude in patients compared with those in controls in both conditions. The authors suggested that even at an SOA of 1 s, either the neural representation of the standard stimulus of patients with AD is not as accurate as that of healthy controls, or the comparator mechanism is deficient in patients. Further, the fact that even patients showed significant MMNs at least in some instances suggests that these patients with a probable AD at an early stage of the disease do have a relatively normal MMN, albeit reduced in amplitude relative to healthy comparison subjects. This result implicates that the neural tissue giving rise to the primary auditory cortex component of MMN was relatively intact in the early stages of the disease process, consistent with neuropathological findings (Bouras et al., 1994). Moreover, as the authors also note, in contrast to the tonal deviants, the non-tonal deviants were able to capture attention involuntarily (as indicated by the elicitation of the N2b and P3a components).

More recently, Cheng et al. (2012) investigated P1m and MMNm in response to occasional decrements of the duration of a 1000-Hz tone in patients with a mild AD (mean age of 78 years). It was found that the P1 amplitude of the patients was larger than that of the elderly controls, suggesting, according to the authors, the presence of a deficit in inhibition for redundant auditory inputs as a sign of an early stage of cortical degeneration. In addition, the MMNm peak latency was longer in patients than that in controls. The authors proposed that the pre-attentive P1m and MMNm represent complementary brain functions in that a more efficient inhibition at the early pre-attentive stage would help the subsequent processing such as change detection. In addition, equivalent current dipole (ECD) modelling showed that the MMNm source was located anteriorly and medially to the P1m source. Therefore, as the authors concluded, distinct neural populations generate P1m and MMNm in the temporal cortex.

Subsequently, Stothart et al. (2015), in the visual modality, found no significant vMMN amplitude difference between AD patients and the age-matched healthy controls instructed to fixate and attend exclusively to a small blue frame at the centre of a monitor screen and to respond to a red target stimulus by pressing a button. Importantly, the vMMN and P1 amplitudes for the deviant stimuli emerged as a significant predictor of the Mini-Mental State Examination (MMSE) score.

In studying patients with fronto-temporal dementia and progressive supranuclear palsy, Hughes et al. (2013; see also Hughes & Rowe, 2013), using the multi-deviant MMN paradigm of Näätänen et al. (1994), observed MMNm with an attenuated amplitude to different kinds of deviant stimuli in these two different patient groups. Dynamic Causal Modelling (DCM) showed that MMNm changes in these patients were accompanied by abnormally extensive and inefficient cerebral networks. According to the authors, neurodegeneration in these two different clinical syndromes with overlapping profiles of prefrontal atrophy causes a similar pattern of reorganization of large-scale networks in the brain. In contrast, in healthy age-matched controls, the most likely pattern of connectivity was a sparse network in which there were bidirectional intra-hemispheric connections between the temporal and parietal areas and between the frontal and temporal areas, but no inter-hemispheric connections, or fronto-parietal connectivity.

The patients with fronto-temporal dementia had a delayed MMNm especially to gap deviants. This deviant-stimulus type relates to integrating information across time since the gap deviant had a brief silent pause of 25 ms in the middle of a tone of 75 ms, compared to the continuous standard tone of 75 ms. Poor time estimation, or a slow internal clock, has been observed in patients with neurodegenerative diseases such as Parkinson's disease (PD) and in those with focal prefrontal lesions, and appears to be related to abnormalities in prefrontal functions. This may explain the delayed MMNm in patients with fronto-temporal dementia to this specific deviant-stimulus type, taking into account their greater extent of frontal atrophy (for a review, see Hughes et al., 2013). It was concluded by Hughes et al. (2013) that there was a systematic change in effective connectivity in both diseases. Compared with healthy age-matched controls, who had a focal modulation of the intra-hemispheric fronto-temporal connections, the two patient groups showed abnormally extensive and inefficient networks. These changes in connectivity were accompanied by reduced MMNm responses to deviant sounds, reflecting impaired responses of the auditory cortex to deviant stimuli, despite normal responses to standard stimuli, suggesting the presence of 'a global dysfunction of change detection'.

Parkinson's disease

Parkinson's disease, a common progressive neurological disorder affecting about 3% of the population over 65 years in age (Seidl & Potashkin, 2011), is manifested by motor dysfunction such as tremor, rigidity, and bradykinesia. The primary pathology of the disease is the degeneration of the nigrostriatal brain system, which results in the loss of the dopaminergic neurons and the depletion of striatal dopamine. As the disease progresses, a variety of non-motor symptoms also emerges, most notably a gradual cognitive deterioration. Parkinson's disease dementia (PDD) ultimately develops in about 80% of the patients with PD (Rongve & Aarsland, 2006). The key brain changes in PD and PDD are abnormal microscopic deposits of a protein, alpha-synuclein. The presence of these deposits, 'Lewy bodies,' in limbic and cortical areas seems to be the main pathological feature associated with these dementias. Clinically, neuro-chemically, and pathologically, dementia with Lewy bodies (DLB) and PDD are rather similar; therefore the managements of these two forms of dementia do not markedly differ from each other (Rongve & Aarsland, 2006).

Even in the early stages of PD, impairments in various cognitive domains are observed. Foltynie et al. (2004) found that 42% of patients were cognitively impaired. In particular, executive functions may be affected. In general, cognitive deficits may initially be evident on detailed neuropsychological testing; however, in some patients, the deficits may become more severe or widespread and begin to impact on non-routine daily activities. At this point, the deficits may fulfil the criteria of MCI, which may be a precursor of a more severe cognitive syndrome, i.e. PDD.

An excellent biomarker for this cognitive decline is MMN. The first study demonstrating a PD-related MMN decline was conducted by Pekkonen et al. (1995a) who studied 13 non-demented patients with PD with a mean age of 64 years. In all patients, the PD symptoms had begun slowly. None were either demented or seriously impaired in their daily activities. It was found that MMN for a tone-frequency change was considerably smaller in amplitude in patients than that in controls. According to the authors, the MMN deficit in PD might reflect a dopamine depletion in the striatum, resulting in a decrease in the flow of sensory information through the thalamus to the cortex and hence in an impaired auditory change detection compared with that in healthy controls, and possibly in some cognitive decline (Rongve & Aarsland, 2006; Pekkonen et al., 1998).

More recently, Brönnick et al. (2010) compared MMN to tone-duration decrement of patients with PD without dementia, patients with PDD, patients with DLB, patients with AD, and normal healthy controls. MMSE scores were very similar in the different patient groups except for the PDD and DLB groups that scored somewhat lower than the PD group. The main result of the study was that the MMN amplitude was smaller in patients with PDD than that in patients with PD with no dementia. Consequently, the authors concluded that the MMN-amplitude attenuation in PD is probably associated with the pathological process leading to PDD.

Multiple sclerosis

Multiple sclerosis (MS) is a chronic demyelinating, inflammatory disease often regarded as the physically most disabling non-traumatic neurological disorder in young adults. Cognitive disorders have been reported in as many as 40–60% of the patients with MS (Beatty, 1993). For instance, MS patients exhibit attentional difficulties with a prolonged reaction time (RT) in various tasks (Foong et al., 1999). MMN provides an excellent index for these cognitive disturbances. Jung et al. (2006) recorded MMN for tone-duration decrement in 46 patients with MS (mean age 43.7 years) and 46 age-matched controls. It was found that MMN of patients was significantly smaller in amplitude than that of controls. Very importantly, MMN and P3a were considerably smaller in amplitude in patients with cognitive impairment (as assessed with a battery of neuropsychological tests) than in those with intact cognition.

The authors concluded that in MS patients with global cognitive impairment, MMN measurements may provide an indirect index of the neuropsychological deterioration gradually occurring in these patients. Subsequently, it was stressed by Guimãraes and Sá (2012) that the detection of cognitive impairment in these patients at its earliest stage has recently become increasingly important as many patients may benefit from attempts at early intervention in view of the recent advent of effective disease-modifying drugs. The decline of the MMN amplitude might reveal the early presence of the disease process before the appearance of distinct symptoms by revealing the latent onset of brain changes leading to cognitive decline. Consistent with this, Santos et al. (2006) found that the absence of MMN to duration and frequency deviants was related to cognitive impairment in these patients (see also Gil et al., 1993). For rehabilitative perspectives of patients with MS, see Flachenecker (2015).

Amyotrophic lateral sclerosis

Amyotrophic lateral sclerosis (ALS) is a neurodegenerative disease exclusively affecting upper and lower motor neurons, giving rise to progressive muscular weakness and atrophy (Mitsumoto, 2000). This decline of motor functions is rather linear, with only 8–16% of patients with ALS surviving beyond 10 years. The aetiology of the disease remains unknown but it appears that glutamate excitotoxicity is associated with the destruction of the motor neurons (Rowland & Shneider, 2001). Moreover, patients with ALS also have abnormalities in cognitive function (Hanagasi et al., 2002). Pekkonen et al. (2004), recording MEG in 12 non-demented patients with ALS and bulbar signs, found that patients had larger-amplitude P1m and N1m responses with shorter peak latencies to standard tones in both hemispheres, compared with these responses in controls. Moreover, MMNm for tone-duration decrement was also larger in amplitude in patients than controls, implicating, according to the authors, that automatic memory-based auditory discrimination is enhanced in ALS at the level of auditory cortex, which might be due to cortical overactivity of excitatory neurotransmitter glutamate.

Huntington's disease

Huntington's disease (HD) is an autosomal dominant neuropsychiatric disorder, caused by an abnormality in chromosome 4, accompanied by severe motor disturbances. The pathological process in HD is associated with a severe neuronal loss in the striatum but neocortical brain areas are also affected, albeit to a lesser extent. One of the pathological mechanisms suggested is excitotoxicity (Beal & Ferrante, 2004) associated with cell death resulting from the activation of excitatory amino-acid receptors. In HD, voltage-dependent NMDA receptors probably are abnormally receptive to endogenous levels of glutamate (Beal & Ferrante, 2004), increasing glutamatergic neurotransmission and thereby leading to excitotoxic cell death. Given the selective sensitivity of MMN to the NMDA receptor system, one might expect that MMN and hence sensory memory are enhanced in HD. According to Beste et al. (2008), this would sharply contrast with other cognitive functions which decline in HD. Studying symptomatic and pre-symptomatic HD patients, these authors found that the symptomatic HD group had larger MMN amplitudes for a tone-frequency change, shorter behavioural response latencies, and more accurate performance than those of controls and pre-symptomatic HD patients. According to the authors, their results showed that specific cognitive functions, namely, auditory sensory memory, as indexed by MMN (and reorientation of attention, as indexed by reorienting negativity (RON)), do not deteriorate and may even be enhanced in late stages of HD, where a pathogenic increase in the responsiveness of a transmitter system occurs. Based on their study, the authors concluded that the assumption of a general cognitive decline taking place in the course of neurodegeneration in HD has to be modified. 'Thus, highly circumscribed elevations of cognitive functions can be embedded within a pattern of more general decline' (p. 11700).

Conclusions

(1) The attenuation of the MMN amplitude for tone-duration decrement provides the earliest biomarker, or warning signal, which is practical, time-effective, and non-invasive, for the latent initiation of brain processes leading to the cognitive deterioration known as MCI.

(2) MMN indexes sensory-level deterioration which is repeated at higher levels of cognitive functioning using outcomes of the processing carried out at lower levels. Consequently, MMN may predict which patients with MCI are in the greatest danger of transition to AD and provide a biomarker of this gradual deterioration and conversion from MCI to AD.

(3) The MMN provides an objective biomarker for the gradual cognitive deterioration of patients from MCI to AD.

(4) The rapid decrease of the MMN amplitude as a function of the increase of SOA indexes the accelerated time course of the decay of the auditory sensory-memory trace and hence that of the general plasticity of the brain, dramatically affected in patients with AD.

(5) The MMN deficit for tone-frequency change provides an excellent biomarker for cognitive decline occurring in patients with PD.

(6) This MMN deficit is probably associated with the pathological brain processes leading to PDD.

(7) In MS patients with a global cognitive impairment, the MMN attenuation may reveal the presence of the disease process before permanent damage occurs, which is particularly useful because of the recent development of effective disease-modifying drugs.

(8) In ALS, the MMNm amplitude may be pathologically enhanced due to the over-activity of excitatory neurotransmitter glutamate.

(9) The results on HD showing enhanced cognitive performance and increased MMN and RON challenge the view that a late stage of neurodegeneration is necessarily associated with a global decline in cognitive abilities.

6.2. **Epilepsy**

Epilepsy is one of the most common neurological disorders, affecting more than 1% of the population and 65 million people world-wide (England et al., 2012). The most common form of acquired epilepsy is temporal-lobe epilepsy (TLE). Epilepsy is characterized by the repeated occurrence of spontaneous bursts of neuronal over-activity, i.e. seizures which usually arise in restricted regions of the brain and may remain confined to these areas or may spread to both cerebral hemispheres. Temporal-lobe structures including the hippocampus, amygdala, and piriform cortex are among the most epileptogenic regions of the brain (Pitkänen & Sutula, 2002). The behavioural manifestations of the seizures, as well as the severity of the epileptic condition, are related to the brain regions where neuronal over-activity occurs. Recent studies showed that several developmental factors such as congenital brain malformations and defects in postnatal maturation of neuronal networks contribute to the epileptogenesis, resulting in the view that epilepsy is, in fact, a neurodevelopmental disorder (for a review, see Bozzi et al., 2012). Unfortunately, intellectual impairment such as memory problems usually accompany epilepsy, and this is particularly true for mesial temporal-lobe epilepsy (MTLE). The cognitive decline is increased with the duration of epilepsy and with the younger age of onset (for a review, see Kaaden & Helmstaedter, 2009).

More recently, Liasis et al. (2006) studied children suffering from Benign Focal Epilepsy with Centro-Temporal Spikes (BECTS), a common form of childhood epilepsy, to determine whether nocturnal epileptic spike discharges are associated with long-term effects on their central auditory processing which could underlie their language deficits. In all five patients with unilateral spikes present in sleep, there was an absence of the auditory P85-120 contralaterally to the epileptic activity, in contrast to the normal symmetrical vertex distribution in controls. Most importantly, no MMN was detected. The authors concluded that the P85-120 abnormality and the absence of MMN in wake recordings may arise because of the long-term effects of spikes occurring during sleep, resulting in the disruption of the evolution and maintenance of echoic memory traces. The absence of MMN in these children was a 'striking' finding, since MMN is almost always recorded, even in patients with unilateral structural lesions (see Alho et al., 1994b). Moreover, the absence of MMN even over the non-affected side may suggest 'a more global disruption of the maintenance of the echoic memory trace' (pp. 947–8) and partly explain the language difficulties described in children with BECTS. Further studies are needed to determine whether these ERP abnormalities are, like epilepsy, age-related phenomena, or a permanent marker of dysfunction in the auditory/language cortex (Liasis et al., 2006).

Subsequently, Boatman et al. (2008) also studied cortical auditory dysfunction in BECTS in children of 7.5–11 years of age. Based on parental reports, all children had experienced decreased academic performance with the onset of their seizures, including distractibility, increased reading-comprehension difficulties, and difficulty in following classroom instructions, but these changes were not sufficiently severe to require special-education services or the diagnosis of a learning disability. In ERP recordings, with children watching a video, standard stimuli were tones of 1000 Hz while the deviant stimuli were tones of 1200 Hz, presented at 1 s intervals to the child's right ear. In further stimulus blocks, speech stimuli were delivered: digitized syllables /ba/ (standard) and /da/ (deviant). It was found that three children showed no measurable speech MMN and, consistent with this, they also exhibited the most severe speech recognition impairments. In contrast, MMN was present in all the seven normally developing control children. For tone changes, MMN was present in all but one of these patients which suggests, according to the authors, that the abnormality may be specific to speech or similarly complex sounds. It was therefore concluded that longitudinal studies are needed to determine whether these speech-recognition impairments are transiently associated with EEG spiking or resolve with clinical remission, which occurs usually by age 16.

Comprehensive testing of auditory functions using behavioural and electrophysiological methods is important to identify children who could benefit from early interventions (Boatman et al., 2008). Consistent with this, Tomé et al. (2014) found a decrease or absence of MMN in children with BECTS with a mean age of 10 years, concluding that this might indicate a disruption of the evolution and maintenance of echoic memory traces, possibly leading to an impairment in speech recognition and a consequent risk for reading difficulties (Boatman et al., 2008).

Korostenskaja et al. (2010) recorded MMNm by employing the multi-feature 'Optimum-1' MMN paradigm of Näätänen et al. (2004) in children of 13 years (mean age) with intractable epilepsy. The MMNm amplitude was attenuated in patients in comparison with that of the age-matched controls for all five different deviants used. In addition, the afferent M100, M150, and M200 components (corresponding to the N1-P2-N2 complex recorded with the EEG; Näätänen & Picton, 1987) were also smaller in amplitude in patients than those in controls. These results were interpreted as indexing a general dysfunction of cortical auditory processing in patients with intractable epilepsy. Importantly, there was a strong negative correlation between the right-hemispheric MMN peak latency for a gap deviant and the age at epilepsy onset. Furthermore, the authors also found a strong positive correlation between the left- and right-hemispheric MMNm peak latencies for gap deviant and epilepsy duration. They concluded that the deficiencies in both N1m and MMNm indicate that both the early and late stages of auditory processing such as the encoding of the stimulus features, the sensory-memory trace formation, and discrimination are abnormal in patients with intractable seizures. In support of this conclusion, an fMRI study of Zhang et al. (2009) demonstrated the presence of a decreased functional connectivity within the regions of the auditory network in patients with MTLE.

Consistent with Zhang et al. (2009), Nearing et al. (2007) found that drug-resistant TLE can be a progressive disorder leading over time to both neuroanatomical and metabolic changes and cognitive decline. Moreover, Lin et al. (2007) observed, in patients with mesial TLE, that their MMNm-peak latency for tone-duration decrement was longer than that in healthy age-matched controls. Also, the right-hemispheric predominance of MMN for non-linguistic stimulus changes (Paavilainen et al., 1991) was not consistently observed in patients with a right-sided temporal epileptic focus, suggesting that 'the epileptic abnormality in the right mesial temporal area may affect the interhemispheric balance of auditory memory processing' (pp. 2520–1).

Importantly, Lin et al. (2007), evaluating the phase-locking consistency across the trials of the responses elicited by standards and deviants (see also Sinkkonen et al. 1995), found that neural activations were strongly phase locked in the bilateral temporal regions to the onset of deviant sounds. The main difference in phase locking between the responses to deviants and standards was observed at around 150–250 ms from stimulus onset, which overlaps in time with MMN obtained by using the conventional subtraction procedure. Consequently, the phase-locking characteristics of cortical signals in this time frame may also reflect 'the differentiation between cerebral activity to standard and deviant sound stimuli' (p. 2521). Very importantly, an increase in this phase-locking response to deviant sounds was observed in those patients who became free of seizures after surgery. The phase-locking enhancement for the theta and alpha oscillations occurred over the bilateral temporal and frontal regions (corresponding to MMN generation loci), which suggests, according to the authors, the occurrence of a plastic change following the removal of a mesial temporal lobe seizure focus.

MMN for speech sounds in adult patients with TLE and focal epilepsy was studied by Hara et al. (2012). The standard stimuli consisted of a sequence of Japanese vowel speech sounds presented at an SOA of 500 ms whereas the deviant stimuli were occasional exemplars of another Japanese vowel. It was found that MMN recorded at the mastoids (with a nose reference, i.e., the mismatch positivity, MMP, indexing auditory cortex activation), was smaller in amplitude in patients with TLE than that in their age-matched controls, whereas the MMN amplitude in the frontal and vertex recordings showed no significant difference between the two groups. Importantly, the frontal MMN amplitude was smaller in patients with more frequent seizures than that in those with less frequent seizures, thereby indexing the degree of severity of the patient's condition.

Miyajima et al. (2011) investigated MMN in adult patients with TLE for frequency and duration changes using pure tones. Their most important result was the considerably larger fronto-central MMN amplitude in patients than that in controls, explained by the authors in terms of frontal-lobe hyperexcitability to compensate for the temporal lobe dysfunction: 'a larger number of synchronously activated frontal neurons may be required for successful automatic attention-switching in TLE patients than controls, due to impairment of an initial sensory memory mechanism in the temporal lobe' (p. 155).

More recently, Hirose et al. (2014) recorded MMNs of adult patients with TLE to frequency and duration changes of the standard stimulus of 1000 Hz with a duration of 100 ms. The patients were watching silent cartoon movies under an instruction to ignore sounds. It was found that the MMP of the patients for tone-duration change was smaller in amplitude than that in the healthy age-matched controls. In contrast, for frequency change, no significant difference was observed between the two groups. The authors concluded that TLE may produce specific deficits in the processing of temporal sound information and, further, that MMN elicited by duration change may be a sensitive index of impaired auditory pre-attentive memory function in TLE.

Gene-Cos et al. (2005) investigated MMN in adults with epilepsy and those with non-epileptic seizures (NES) by employing standard tones of 1000 Hz and deviant tones of 922 Hz. It was found that both patient groups had larger MMN amplitudes when compared with those of controls, which, according to the authors, might be in part related to impaired sensory/sensorimotor gating and the subsequent increased intrusiveness of novel stimuli, associated with a state of hypervigilance (Lang et al., 1995). In further support of this suggestion, the authors mention that an increase in the startle response with a loss of its normal inhibitory modulation has been shown in patients suffering from the post-traumatic stress syndrome (PTSD). Consistent with this, Morgan and Grillon (1999) observed a larger MMN amplitude in female rape victims when compared with normal healthy controls; a significant correlation between the MMN amplitude and the Mississippi PTSD Symptoms Scale Scores was also observed. A connection between PTSD and NES in the clinical setting has already been proposed (Betts, 1997). Gene-Cos and her colleagues concluded that the MMN changes observed in NES may play a significant role in the clinical picture of the condition: 'Patients with NES, at times of stress, may become overloaded with irrelevant stimuli, surpassing their coping abilities. These responses to such a situation may then be externalized as seizure-like activity' (p. 371).

Landau-Kleffner Syndrome (LKS) is a rare form of childhood epilepsy accompanied by acquired aphasia. The first cases of LKS were described by Landau and Kleffner (1957) who reported on five children with a gradual regression of language abilities associated with paroxysmal unilateral or bilateral spike-and-wave discharges usually localized in the temporo-parietal brain regions. One of the main features of LKS is language regression which is primarily related to auditory comprehension, and thought to be specific to phonological processing (see Korkman et al., 1998). Furthermore, a specific EEG pattern, i.e. an almost continuous spike-and-wave activity, is always present in children with LKS which usually starts between the ages of 3 and 8 years (for a review, see Honbolygo et al., 2006). Fortunately, the outcome of the syndrome is rather benign: a complete spontaneous recovery is likely to occur by the beginning of the adolescence which is, however, not the case with the acquired language deficit. In contrast to LKS, in children with an acquired language deficit, a severe residual language deficit may remain; the younger the child is at onset, the worse is the chance of recovery (Bishop, 1985).

The abnormal EEG pattern in LKS is also characterized by another syndrome: i.e. one involving continuous spikes and waves during slow-wave sleep (CSWS). The two syndromes share several common features. Both are childhood disorders characterized by a specific EEG disturbance but with no structural lesions. However, in CSWS, the cognitive deficit associated with epileptic activity involves not only language but other cognitive functions as well (for a review, see Honbolygo et al., 2006). In their review of neuropsychological findings in Rolandic epilepsy and LKS, Metz-Lutz and Philippini (2006) concluded that MMN might help one determine at an early stage whether interictal discharges were affecting the auditory cortex and its development and, consequently, the ability to discriminate different speech sounds.

As for the treatment of epilepsy, a number of patients with epilepsy do not respond to conventional treatments despite multiple combinations of antiepileptic drugs; these patients are therefore considered drug-resistant. The management of seizures in patients with epilepsy by conventional and newer antiepileptic agents is successful in most cases but up to 30% of the patients do not respond to treatment even when drugs are given at maximal tolerated doses and in various combinations (Borghetti et al., 2007). In this population of drug-resistant patients, vagal nerve stimulation (VNS) provides a valid therapeutic option (for a review, see Ben-Menachem 2000). Importantly, recent studies suggest that the beneficial effects of VNS may even extend to mood and cognition (Schachter, 2004). Borghetti et al. (2007) recorded MMN to tone-frequency change (standards of 1000 Hz, deviants of 1200 Hz) in patients (mean age 40.3 years) with remote symptomatic epilepsy before the VNS implantation and twice post-implantation. It was found that the implantation of VNS successfully decreased the baseline seizure frequency by 15–25% in most patients but did not significantly change the MMN amplitude or peak latency for a tone-frequency change. However, in two patients with a severely impaired MMN baseline parameters, who did not experience a significant reduction in seizure frequency, the MMN peak latency was shortened and amplitude increased after 1 year of VNS stimulation. According to the authors, this improvement, even though limited in size, is consistent with findings of improvement in specific memory tasks as a result of VNS stimulation using selected stimulation intensities.

As for the mechanisms accounting for VNS effects, Borghetti et al. (2007) regarded as the most attractive a hypothesis that involves the role of the locus coeruleus (LC) in the antiepileptic effect of VNS. Seizure suppression by VNS may therefore depend on the release of norepinephrine (NE), a neuromodulator with anticonvulsant effects (Borghetti et al., 2007). The positive effect on seizures could hence be explained by the LC-NE system, whose activation is also reflected in pre-attentive auditory discrimination, sensory memory, and involuntary attention. 'The final effect is either the lack of deterioration or enhancement of MMN response, with an increase in the absolute peak values and a decrease in mean latency. This response is not impaired in those subjects with normal values at baseline, thus confirming the absence of cognitive negative effects of VNS' (p. 84).

Hence, it appears that intracranially recorded MMN enables one to locate the epileptogenic zones in child patients in preparation for surgical epilepsy operation. In addition, in children with BECTS, an absence of MMN might index a long-term consequence of spikes occurring during sleep, resulting in the disruption of the evolution and maintenance of sensory memory and therefore in the deterioration of higher-level cognitive processing. The MMN decline in these patients therefore appears to index brain changes predicting their decreased academic performance including increased distractibility, reading comprehension difficulties, and difficulty in following classroom instructions. The multi-feature MMN paradigm (Näätänen et al., 2004; Pakarinen et al., 2007, 2009; Vuust et al., 2011; see also Lovio et al., 2009, 2010), enabling one to determine the individual auditory discrimination profiles in patients with intractable epilepsy across the various different stimulus-feature dimensions, shows that in these patients, there is an overall decrease of automatic discrimination accuracy in audition, suggesting the presence of a general dysfunction in their cortical auditory processing system. Importantly, an increase in the phase-locking response, paralleling and overlapping MMN to deviant stimuli, was observed in the five patients who became seizure free after the removal of the right temporal epileptic focus, predicting which patients will become free of epileptic seizures after surgery. In addition, MMN might index the effectiveness of VNS in epilepsy (Borghetti et al., 2007).

Conclusions

(1) Intra-cranially recorded MMN may enable one to locate the epileptogenic zones of the brain in child patients in preparation for surgical epilepsy operation.

(2) In children with BECTS, the absence of MMN appears to be a long-term consequence of spikes occurring during sleep resulting in the disruption of the evolution and maintenance of sensory memory which is in turn reflected in the deterioration of higher-level cognitive processing.

(3) In these patients, the MMN data pattern suggests that the abnormality may be specific to speech and similarly complex stimuli. An important implication of these results therefore is the possibility of identifying children who could benefit from early interventions.

(4) The MMN amplitude is smaller in patients with more frequent seizures, suggesting that this MMN deficit might index the long-term cumulative effects of epilepsy.

6.3. Altered states of consciousness: coma, persistent vegetative state, and anaesthesia

Coma and persistent vegetative state

One of the most important clinical applications of MMN involves coma-outcome prediction. This is of major significance because clinical assessment cannot establish the prognosis, for instance, in traumatic brain injury, with confidence. The first study demonstrating that MMN can predict the recovery of consciousness in comatose patients was conducted by Kane et al. (1993) who studied 18 adult patients with coma after blunt head trauma. The standard stimuli were tones of 800 Hz while the deviant stimuli were those of 1600 Hz. All the healthy volunteers of the age-matched control group exhibited an MMN response whereas of the 18 patients, 14 had no detectable MMN while 4 patients showed MMN. Consciousness returned in all the latter four patients within 48 hours from the recording whereas of the remaining patients, five died soon after without regaining consciousness. A sixth patient developed an MMN on a subsequent testing one week post-injury and within 48 hours from that started to open his eyes to speech but 1 week later lapsed into unconsciousness, MMN could no longer be elicited, and he soon died from septicaemia. The remaining eight patients with no detectable MMN in initial recordings developed MMN in subsequent serial recordings while still unconscious, preceding the return of comprehension of simple commands by 48–72 hours. Kane et al. (1993) concluded that MMN is the earliest available indicator of awakening from coma and may reflect 'the recovery of neurochemical mechanisms for information processing in the cerebral cortex associated to cognition' (p. 688).

Kane et al. (1996) confirmed and extended these pioneering findings in their subsequent study including 54 comatose traumatic brain injury patients. The main outcome measure was the Glasgow Coma Scale (GCS) assessed 3 months after coma onset. ERP recordings were repeatedly carried out. The best response obtained while the patient still was in coma was retained. The presence of MMN predicted the return to consciousness (89.7% sensitivity and 100% specificity) and preceded changes in GCS. Subsequently, Kane et al. (2000) found that the MMN peak latency measured at hospitalization of survivors of coma caused by severe head injury predicted their expressive language ability and visuospatial performance at 1 year from injury. Moreover, Kotchoubey et al. (2003) demonstrated that in using MMN to objectively assess the remaining cognitive capacity, it is better to use complex rather than simple sound stimuli that may result in a severe underestimation of the remaining capacity. For an exhaustive review of the available neuropsychological assessment techniques for use in severely brain-damaged patients even without residual motor function, see Neumann and Kotchoubey (2004). Subsequently, it was found by Qin et al. (2008) that MMN elicited by the patient's own name as a deviant stimulus predicted the recovery of the patient in a chronic disorder of consciousness to MCI. The authors concluded that the patient's own name is effective in eliciting MMN in patients with chronic disorder of consciousness and, further, that this MMN has a potential prognostic value in predicting the recovery of consciousness. For corroborating results, see Holeckova et al. (2008). Moreover, Fischer et al. (2008) showed that P3 increases the prognostic value of MMN in response to the patient's own name in predicting awakening from coma.

Pioneering work in the field of coma outcome prediction was also conducted by Fischer et al. (1999). Their sample consisted of 128 patients aged between 15 and 93 years who were in intensive care in hospital and were in a comatose state, with GCS lower than 8 at the time of ERP recording at 12 days from coma onset. The causes of the coma were head injury, cardiac or respiratory failure, ischaemia or haemorrhagic stroke syndrome, complications of neurosurgery, or encephalitis. In the ERP recordings, the standard stimuli were pure tones with a duration of 75 ms whereas the deviant tones were of 30 ms in duration. MMN was observed in 33 out of the 128 patients. N1 was observed in 84 out of the 128 patients. The N1 and MMN amplitudes were considerably smaller in patients than those in controls (see Fig. 6.2). Also, the N1 peak latency was prolonged in patients compared with that in controls. Importantly, out of the 33 patients with MMN, 30 patients returned to consciousness (the positive predictive value 90.9%). Further, out of the 84 patients showing N1, 70 returned to consciousness, yielding a positive predictive value of 83.3%. It was concluded that in particular the presence of the MMN in a comatose patient is 'a strong predictor of the return of consciousness' (p. 1609). Thus, the use of MMN and related ERP parameters such as N1 offers tremendous promise for improving the prediction of coma outcomes.

In their subsequent study of 346 coma patients with various different aetiologies tested approximately 10 days from coma onset, Fischer et al. (2004a, 2004b) confirmed that the presence of MMN in these patients is associated with a high percentage of awakening and, importantly, excludes the progression to the persistent vegetative state (PVS). Moreover, according to Fischer and Luauté (2005), none of the 88 patients who showed MMN at an early state of coma progressed to PVS: 'Hence, our study showed—for the first time—that

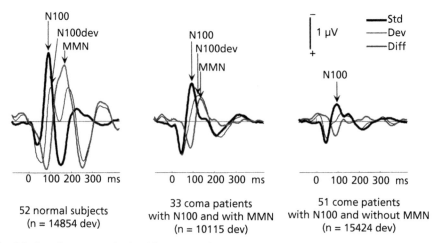

Fig. 6.2 Grand averages obtained from normal subjects, coma patients with N100 and MMN, and coma patients with N100 and without MMN. In patients in a comatose state, the N1 and MMN amplitudes for a tone-frequency change are considerably smaller than those in healthy controls.

Reprinted from Clinical Neurophysiology, 110(9), Fischer, C., Morlet, D., Bouchet, P., Luaute, J., Jourdan, C. & Salord, F., *Mismatch negativity and late auditory evoked potentials in comatose patients*, 1601–1610, Copyright (1999), with permission from Elsevier.

the presence of an ERP at the early stage of coma, precisely the MMN, precludes coma patients from progressing to a PVS' (p. 378).

Luauté et al. (2005), using a large number of consecutively sampled comatose patients with different aetiologies, found that MMN for tone-duration decrement showed, among a variety of different measures used, the highest positive predictive value for a good outcome, concluding that particularly MMN and N1 provide strong prognostic factors for a good functional outcome. The estimated probability to achieve a good functional outcome was around 70% when MMN was detected at an early phase of coma, regardless of the aetiology. In addition, N1 also was significantly associated with a good outcome. The authors developed a tree-based classification analysis for the prognosis of awakening from severe anoxic coma (for an improved version, see Fischer et al., 2006a, b). Luauté et al. (2005) concluded that their study, using a large sample and comprehensive statistical analysis, demonstrated that late auditory ERPs are strong individual prognostic factors for a good functional outcome: 'Hence, with a few clinical and electrophysiological variables, which are easy to collect at the early stage of coma, it is possible to be more confident about what is likely to happen, to give more reliable information to relatives and, it is hoped, to enhance caregivers strategies' (p. 922). (See also Morlet & Fischer, 2014.) Naccache et al. (2005) confirmed the Fischer et al. (1999) results, also proposing some useful methodological improvements:

The simple and automatized EEG signal processing adopted here offers a result within a few minutes. In spite of this simplicity, this methodology enables the recording of sufficient trials to obtain individual statistically significant results. Therefore, we think that this reliable procedure might be adopted by a large set of Intensive Care units in order to flexibly evaluate current level of cognitive integration of comatose patients, to evaluate their dynamic impact of sedative drugs, and to predict their clinical outcome. (Naccache et al. 2005, p. 988.)

A novel, ingenious stimulus paradigm for the objective assessment of the degree of consciousness in patients with disorders of consciousness by using MMN and other re-lated responses was introduced by Bekinschtein et al. (2009a; see also Bekinschtein et al., 2009b, 2009c). In this 'ERP Local-Global Paradigm', on each trial, a sequence of five brief complex tones are presented over a total period of 650 ms. The first four sounds are always identical, either high or low tones, whereas the fifth tone could be identical to ('locally standard trials') or different from ('locally deviant trials') the preceding ones. The global regularity, in turn, was defined according to the relative frequency of the two types of five-tone sequences. Globally standard sequences were pseudo-randomly delivered on 80% of the sequences, whereas globally deviant sequences were delivered at a probability of 20%. Importantly, the local and global regularities could be manipulated orthogonally; hence, there were four types of trials: local standard, local deviant, global standard, and global deviant. In healthy controls, the violation of local regularity (local deviant) elicited a vertex-centred MMN after the onset of the fifth tone. When subjects were instructed to relax the local ERP effect was essentially identical to that observed in an active counting task. In sharp contrast, the global effect was dramatically decreased. This disappearance of the global effect coincided with the absence of the subjective awareness of the global stimulus structure. It was concluded that an ERP signature of global violations ('a late P300b response') was observed only when subjects were consciously aware of the global regularity structure and of its violation. These pioneering results were confirmed by Faugeras et al. (2011) using a larger sample of patients in the vegetative state (VS). In add-ition, the results of Bekinschtein et al. (2009a) were confirmed and extended by King et al. (2013a, b) who demonstrated that the multivariate pattern classifiers can extract subject-specific EEG patterns and predict single-trial global (P300b) or local (MMN) 'novelty re-sponses'. Moreover, the study confirmed, in controls, that the local responses are robust to distraction whereas the global responses depend on attention and are easily distractible.

MMN can also track and predict the recovery from PVS. Wijnen et al. (2007), in a pioneering study, repeatedly examined (every 2 weeks) these patients over a period of 3–4 months. A 'striking result' was the dramatic MMN amplitude increase, up to the level of controls, during the period leading to the recovery of consciousness (Fig. 6.3). Moreover, their results on the predictive value of MMN extend the previous results of Fischer et al. (2004a, 2004b) from the acute phase showing that MMN predicted the awakening from coma and excluded a regression to VS. In addition, very importantly, the MMN ampli-tude measured at 9 days from hospitalization strongly predicted the level of consciousness at discharge, which was not predicted by the level of consciousness at admission. Wijnen et al. (2007) concluded that MMN is a powerful tool in predicting the recovery from VS, stressing the fact that a sudden increase in the MMN amplitude within minimally con-scious state (MCS) strongly predicts the recovery of consciousness. Consistent with this,

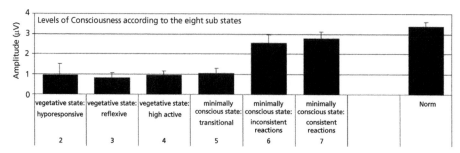

Fig. 6.3 The MMN amplitude at different levels of consciousness in comatose patients from vegetative state to minimally conscious state and in normal state.
Reprinted from Clinical Neurophysiology, 118(3), Wijnen, V.J., van Boxtel, G.J., Eilander, H.J. & de Gelder, B., *Mismatch negativity predicts recovery from the vegetative state*, 597–605, Copyright 2007, with permission from Elsevier.

van der Stelt and Boxtel (2008) proposed that MMN may have utility in differentiating VS from MCS. (See also de Tommaso et al., 2013.)

Boly et al. (2011) recently provided a seminal contribution to our understanding of brain functional abnormality in VS by demonstrating that feed-forward processes are preserved whereas top-down processes are severely impaired in these patients. The effective connectivity was assessed by using MMN in response to tones delivered in the roving paradigm (Baldeweg et al., 2004) in which each deviant stimulus immediately becomes a new standard stimulus; hence, the development of the memory trace for the standard stimulus started anew again after each deviant stimulus, i.e. a new standard stimulus. Boly and her associates found that the only difference between patients in VS and controls was an impairment of backward connectivity from frontal to temporal cortices in patients, suggesting that a selective disruption of the top-down processes from high levels of cortical hierarchy can lead to loss of consciousness in brain-damaged patients, and can clearly differentiate VS from MCS. Boly et al. proposed that their MMN-based approach could constitute a new diagnostic tool to quantify the level of consciousness at the patient's bedside. Vanhaudenhuyse et al. (2008), in their review, concluded that data on MMN in comatose patients converge on the conclusion that MMN is 'a very good predictor of recovery, notably so in anoxic coma'. Consistent with this, in their meta-analysis of ERP studies of coma-outcome prediction in patients with different aetiologies, Daltrozzo et al. (2007) concluded that MMN and P300 appear to be reliable predictors of awakening from coma.

Tzovara et al. (2013) conducted, using an MMN paradigm, two EEG recordings: the first within 24 hours after coma onset and under mild therapeutic hypothermia, and the second 1 day later but this time under normo-thermic conditions. The EEG responses were analysed using a multivariate decoding algorithm that automatically quantifies neural discrimination at a single-patient level. Importantly, the progression of auditory discrimination between the first and second recordings was informative of the patient's chance of survival: all patients with an MMN amplitude enhancement between the two recordings survived. In contrast, an MMN amplitude decrease was observed in all non-survivors and therefore yielded a 100% predictive value outcome for MMN-amplitude change in the second vs first recording. The authors concluded that this method is able to identify those patients who will awaken in an automatic and quantifiable fashion, providing an early automatic outcome prediction within 48 hours after coma onset.

More recently, Sculthorpe-Petley et al. (2015) aimed at validating the Halifax Consciousness Scanner (HCS) which essentially is a rapid, automated ERP evaluation of brain functional status. ERP results, obtained by using repetition and intensity deviants in a tone paradigm (lasting 2.5 min) and in a separate speech-sound paradigm (lasting 2.5 min) in 100 healthy subjects, showed that the HCS stimulus sequence successfully evoked all the ERP responses of interest, among them N1, MMN, and P300 in a 5-min recording time only. The authors concluded that the ability to probe a spectrum of ERPs in a short period of time is critical in view of clinical applications, such as the evaluation of the functional status of a patient following brain injury. Short testing times are also essential in a clinical context due to the logistical constraints. Additionally, short testing times avoid fluctuations in vigilance, attention, and fatigue, which present a significant challenge in the clinical applications of the ERPs (Neumann & Kotchoubey, 2004). In order to meet these requirements, a rapid methodology for the examination of multiple ERP components is needed such as that of Sculthorpe-Petley et al. (2015).

Anaesthesia

It was long believed that there is no cognitive processing during anaesthesia. However, early MMN studies radically changed this view. The first MMN studies in anaesthesia were conducted by Yppärilä et al. (2002) and Simpson et al. (2002). Yppärilä et al. monitored auditory ERPs before and after cardiac surgery in 29 patients. It was found that deep and moderate levels of propofol sedation delayed and diminished N1 and MMN responses which suggests, according to the authors, that there is a deficit in sensory memory function during sedation. Simpson et al. (2002), also investigating the effects of propofol anaesthesia, found that both the duration- and frequency-change MMNs were abolished before consciousness was lost whereas N1 could identify the transition from consciousness to unconsciousness:

> It is possible that the concentration of propofol at which MMN disappears is that at which the ability to lay down explicit or implicit auditory memory is lost, as opposed to that at which consciousness is lost ... the disappearance of the MMN before loss of consciousness would be in accord with the dissociation between awareness and the ability to establish memories. (Simpson et al., 2002, p. 387.)

Subsequently, Heinke et al. (2004) recorded MMN, together with P1, and ERAN (early right anterior negativity elicited by music-syntactic violations) pre-operatively as a function of a gradually increasing propofol sedation in 18 non-musician patients. In the MMN blocks, the standards were 440 Hz while the deviants were 496 Hz. In the ERAN blocks, music-syntactically regular chords served as standards, whereas music-syntactically irregular chords served as deviants (which elicit ERAN in normal healthy listeners familiar with the major–minor tonal system). It was found that P1 elicited by standard tones and in-key chords could be observed at all levels of sedation but was markedly reduced in amplitude during unconsciousness. Furthermore, both MMN and ERAN were elicited, even during both light and deep sedation, but decreased in amplitude with increasing propofol sedation, vanishing in unconsciousness. In addition, during wakefulness and light sedation, MMN was accompanied by P3a which vanished during deep sedation. The authors concluded that the mechanisms underlying physical and music-synthetic auditory irregularity detection function even under deep sedation and, further, that these processes are uniformly affected by an increasing propofol sedation. In contrast, P1 may discriminate drug-induced sedation from adequate anaesthesia, which is consistent with previous intra-cranial recordings, with electrodes implanted in the Heschl's gyrus, that demonstrated only weak effects of even deep anaesthesia on early cortical responses to auditory stimuli. Consequently, the results indicate differential effects of propofol sedation on cognitive functions that mainly involve the auditory cortices and those that involve the frontal cortices. In other words, sedative concentrations first affect auditory change-detection processes (reflected by MMN) that involve the frontal cortices, whereas the processes merely involving the primary auditory cortex are only affected by propofol dose causing unconsciousness. The findings strongly suggested that the cerebral cortex is not uniformly affected by propofol which rather has differential effects on the different cortical areas and hence functions associated with these areas. For a review of the effects of anaesthetics on different indices of cognitive brain function, see Heinke and Koelsch (2005).

In their subsequent study, Koelsch et al. (2006) again recorded MMN and ERAN under sedation. After the sedation phase, the propofol anaesthesia was increased over a period of 8 min to produce unconsciousness in 19 healthy volunteers. It was found that in deep sedation, the MMN amplitude was markedly reduced but still was significant whereas no ERAN was observed. In addition, a P3a was elicited in deep sedation by those deviants that were task-relevant in the discrimination task performed before sedation. As soon as subjects again regained consciousness, a normal MMN was elicited, suggesting that the auditory sensory-memory operations become normal as soon as consciousness is recovered.

Conclusions

(1) MMN is the earliest available indicator of awakening from coma.

(2) MMN recorded in a comatose patient predicts the recovery of consciousness in the near future and precludes the progression of the patient to PVS.

(3) MMN can also track and predict the recovery from PVS, with the MMN amplitude dramatically increasing before the recovery of consciousness.

(4) The MMN-based approach developed by Boly et al. constitutes a new diagnostic tool to quantify the level of consciousness at the patient's bedside.

(5) Deep and moderate levels of sedation delay and diminish the N1 and MMN responses, reflecting the absence of auditory memory-trace formation and, apparently, a greatly reduced brain plasticity, with these ERP responses disappearing before consciousness is lost.

(6) During wakefulness and light sedation, MMN is accompanied by P3a which is no longer elicited when the sedation becomes deeper, indicating the loss of the automatic attention-switch function, except perhaps for deviant stimuli which have some meaning to the patient.

(7) Importantly, MMN recovery during the wake-up period reflects the return of consciousness and memory-trace formation.

6.4. **Brain lesions**

Aphasia

In patients with stroke, a focal cerebral infarction in the affected core territory is often accompanied by damage in cerebral regions that can be quite remote, including even contralateral regions, from the locus of infarction. This wide-reaching damage explains, at least in part, the widespread cognitive and other neurological defects in these patients (Dhawan et al., 2010). As such, MMN amplitude for different kinds of stimulus changes in stroke patients usually is considerably attenuated, correlating with the nature and magnitude of the perceptual and cognitive loss. Importantly, MMN permits the objective monitoring of the latent post-stroke recovery process when reliable behavioural measurements are not yet possible. This was demonstrated by Ilvonen et al. (2003), who found that at 4 and 10 days after left-hemispheric stroke onset, the sound discrimination of patients was impaired in their left hemisphere, as suggested by attenuated MMN amplitudes for duration and frequency change in a repetitively presented harmonically rich tone, especially when stimuli were presented to the right ear (Fig. 6.4). However, at 3 months post-stroke onset, MMN for right-ear stimuli was considerably increased in amplitude, and was again of a normal size. Moreover, a remarkable increase in the left-ear frequency-MMN amplitude was observed between 3 and 6 months post-stroke onset. In addition, during the follow-up period, a progressive improvement in speech-comprehension test scores was also found, there being a close relationship between the duration-MMN amplitude increase and an improvement in Boston Diagnostic Aphasia Examination speech-comprehension test score from 10 days to 3 months post-stroke. (For an Editorial in *Stroke*, see Cramer, 2003).

In their study of stroke patients, Särkämö et al. (2010), divided 60 middle cerebral artery stroke patients into music-listening, audiobook-listening, or control groups and recorded MMNm to frequency and duration changes in a binaural complex tone. In addition, all patients received normal hospital treatment and rehabilitation treatment for stroke. As expected, MMNm amplitudes were generally smaller in the lesioned than in the opposite hemisphere. Importantly, the frequency-MMNm amplitude increased more in both

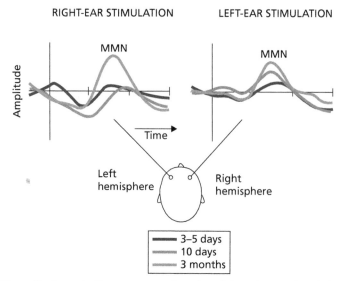

Fig. 6.4 MMN amplitude gradually recovers as a function of time elapsing from left-hemispheric stroke. Ilvonen et al. measured MMN from aphasic, left-hemisphere-stroke patients 3-5 days, 10 days, and 3 months after stroke. At 3 months after stroke, MMN had significantly increased and during the follow up period, progressive improvement was also observed in speech-comprehension tests.

Data from Ilvonen, T. M., Kujala, T., Kiesilainen, A., Salonen, O., Kozou, H., Pekkonen, E., Roine, R.O., Kaste, M. and Näätänen, R., *Auditory discrimination after left-hemisphere stroke: a mismatch negativity follow-up study*, Stroke, 34 (7), 1746–1751, doi:10.1161/01.STR.0000078836.26328.3B, 2003.

music and audiobook groups than that in the control group during the 6-month post-stroke period. In addition, the amplitude of the duration MMNm increased more in the audiobook group than that in the other two groups. Furthermore, the frequency-MMNm amplitude increase correlated with the behavioural improvement in verbal memory and focused attention induced by music listening. These results demonstrate that merely listening to music or speech starting early in the post-stroke period can induce long-term plastic changes in sensory processing, as reflected by the MMNm-amplitude enhancement, which may, in turn, facilitate the recovery of the higher cognitive functions. These remarkable results strongly suggest the use of music and speech stimulation in the early post-stroke period. Music stimulation has been successfully used in other clinical contexts, too. (See Raglio et al., 2014, who found positive effects of music stimulation in patients with dementia.)

In another related study, Särkämö et al. (2010; also see Särkämö et al., 2009a, 2009b) addressed amusia caused by left or right middle cerebral artery stroke. They found that amusia caused by right-hemisphere damage, especially that involving temporal and frontal areas, was more severe than that caused by left-hemisphere damage. Moreover, the severity of amusia correlated with a lower amplitude of the frequency MMNm in amusic right-hemispheric patients. Within the right-hemisphere damage group, the amusic patients who had damage in the auditory cortex showed worse recovery from amusia and weaker MMNm responses throughout the 6-months follow-up period than did non-amusic patients or amusic patients with no auditory cortex damage. Further, amusic patients performed worse than did non-amusic patients on a number of tests measuring different aspects of cognitive performance (including working memory, attention, and cognitive flexibility). These findings implicated, according to the authors, domain-general cognitive deficits as the primary factor underlying amusia with no auditory cortex damage, whereas amusia with auditory cortex damage was associated with both auditory and cognitive deficits. In a previous study, Kohlmetz et al. (2001) observed a major amplitude attenuation in the frequency MMN in left-hemispheric stroke patients with amusia whereas left-hemispheric stroke patients with no amusia showed normal-size MMN.

Consistent with this, Auther et al. (2000) found that the presence of MMN for speech-sound change in patients with aphasia better predicted auditory comprehension than did the absence of MMN. In addition, MMN absence and poor comprehension were associated with temporal-lobe lesions. Moreover, it was found by Wertz et al. (1998) that MMN for speech-sound change occurred in only 54% of aphasic patients. In addition, among patients showing this MMN response, the duration of the MMN response was considerably shorter with more severe aphasia as revealed by the Western Aphasia Battery, the Porch Index of Communicative Ability, and the Token Test. In another study on patients suffering from aphasia, Peach et al. (1992) found that their MMN peak latency for a tone-frequency change in ignore conditions was similar to that in healthy controls but that in the active target-detection task using the same stimuli, patients showed slower behavioural responses than did controls. The authors concluded that in these patients, the attentional processes for detecting changes in auditory stimuli are initiated within a normal time frame but that an abnormally long time may be required to make decisions regarding discrimination of the deviant stimuli. Subsequently, Peach & Newhoff (1994) obtained corroborating MMN results which they interpreted as being consistent with the presence of attentional deficits at the earliest, 'preconscious' levels of attention. More recently, Pettigrew et al. (2005) reported that patients with aphasia showed MMN responses with attenuated amplitudes to deviations in complex-tone duration and in speech sounds. Importantly, the amplitudes of these MMNs strongly correlated with performance on auditory comprehension as measured by using the Western Aphasia Battery. The authors concluded that MMNs for such complex changes better separate patients from controls than do simple tone-frequency changes, as previously suggested by Aaltonen et al. (1993), Csepe et al. (2001), and Neumann and Kotchoubey (2004). (See also Tome et al., 2015.)

Csepe et al. (2001) used MMN to determine the neurophysiological abnormalities underlying impaired speech perception in patients with aphasia. Their principal finding was that MMN elicited by pitch deviations is not sensitive enough to distinguish between patients and age-matched controls (see also Aaltonen et al., 1993); therefore one should employ speech-sound contrasts. Their finding showed that MMN elicited by consonant contrasts was the most vulnerable response in patients with aphasia. In addition, MMNs elicited by contrasts in voicing and place of articulation were either totally lacking or distorted, or their scalp distribution was abnormally limited. Moreover, these MMN deficits correlated with deficits found in a behavioural phoneme-discrimination task.

Pure word deafness

MMN in Pure Word Deafness (PWD) was studied by Jacobs and Schneider (2003) in a patient with a lesion in his left fronto-parietal area. As expected, a significant MMN was elicited by tone-frequency but not by phonetic changes. Speech perception testing indicated that he had difficulty with spectral and spectro-temporal discrimination and in combining phonological and semantic information. Consistent with this result, Sun et al. (2015), studying patients with traumatic brain injury, found that their MMN amplitude for a tone-frequency change was smaller than that of controls and was highly significantly correlated with daily living function and 'extremely positively' with Social Disability Screening Schedule scores. The authors concluded that MMN might accurately reflect functional outcomes in patients after traumatic brain injury.

Unilateral neglect

MMN has also provided important information on unilateral neglect, often accompanying a right-hemispheric damage. These patients are often unaware of visual, auditory, or tactile stimuli occurring on the left side. Deouell et al. (2000a) proposed that MMN may be used to probe the integrity of the pre-attentive processes playing a role in triggering the switching of involuntary attention: 'a capacity which is apparently malfunctioning in neglect' (p. 354). To this end, the authors examined MMNs elicited by pitch, duration, and location changes occurring on the left and right sides of patients with right-hemispheric lesions and left-side neglect. They found that for these three dimensions of stimulus change, MMN was elicited 'quite consistently' when the deviant stimulus occurred on the right side of the patient whereas when the deviant stimulus occurred on the left side then MMN for pitch, and in particular for location change, was reduced in amplitude (or was even absent in some of the patients). This pattern of MMN deficits suggests, according to the authors:

> [T]he existence of a rather early, albeit selective, deficit in the stream of auditory processing in right hemisphere -damaged patients with neglect. ... The difficulty in eliciting an adequate contra-lesional mismatch detection process in our patients may be related directly to the essential feature of unilateral neglect, the fact that significant events fail to attract attention reflexively when they occur on the contra-lesional side. ... The present MMN results suggest that neglect patients may suffer from a deficient bottom-up process (signalled by MMN) that normally serves to 'call' for attention resources to be disengaged and relocated to an event whose perception has been accomplished by the sensory system (signalled by early evoked potentials such as N1). This deficit may contribute to and aggravate concomitant higher order deficits in these patients, leading to different manifestations of the lateralization bias characteristic of neglect ... This hypothesis was supported by the robustness of the side of stimulus effect on the MMN elicited by deviance in spatial location (across patients) compared with that elicited by deviance in pitch or location. ... The present MMN results provide strong evidence that spatial attributes (more than other attributes) corresponding to events on the contra-lesional side are either not encoded, or at least that their encoding is not useful, and that the deficit is probably independent of attention. This particular deficiency may

provide a clue for understanding the lack of awareness of the left hemisphere in neglect. (Deouell et al., 2000, pp. 360–361.)

More recently, Tarkka et al. (2011) assessed the evolution of changes in sensory processing and neglect symptoms over a 6-months post-stroke follow-up period. Consistent with the results of the previous studies (for a review, see Deouell et al. 2000b), their data suggested that automatic orientation and deviance detection are impaired in the right hemisphere. 'This deficit contributes to the neglect syndrome and demonstrates in part the subject's failure to link a perceived event in the surroundings to the attentional system in the brain. The hyperexcitability of the left hemisphere and the deficits in N1 and MMN functioning in the right hemisphere both may have important and complementary roles in neglect' (p. 278). Fortunately, as stated by the authors, the neglect syndrome mostly fades away by about 9 months from stroke onset along with the reduction of the severity of the neglect.

Closed-head injury

Closed-Head Injury (CHI) occurs as a consequence of sudden movements and stretching of the brain tissue within the skull by external acceleration–deceleration forces commonly resulting in a predictable focal injury in the frontal poles and in a diffuse axonal injury (DAI). DAI essentially reduces connections between the frontal and other brain areas. However, the pathological consequences of CHI, for instance DAI in its whole extent, are not necessarily detected by structural brain-imaging techniques such as MRI. The typical symptoms accompanying CHI include, among other things, disorders of planning, initiation of motor or cognitive actions, as well as forgetfulness, fatigue, slowness of information processing, and increased distractibility and attentional deficits (Kaipio et al., 1999). Kaipio et al. (1999) aimed to determine whether ERPs could be used for evaluating attentional problems in CHI patients, who are very easily distracted and frequently complain about such attentional problems. The authors presented their subjects, instructed to ignore sounds and to perform a visual-motor tracking task, with auditory stimulus sequences consisting of 600 Hz standard tones, 660 Hz deviant tones, and complex novel sounds. The only ERP difference found between the patients and controls was in the larger amplitude of the late portion of P3a to novel sounds which, according to the authors, could indicate 'stronger involuntary switching of attention in the patient group because of their measured difficulties in suppressing of irrelevant stimuli' (p. 2128).

In their subsequent study on CHI, Kaipio et al. (2001) used frequency and duration deviants in sequences of tone stimuli, and observed that the MMN amplitude for frequency deviants decreased in the patient group considerably faster than that of the control group during the session. This result suggested to the authors a faster vigilance decrease in these patients, consistent with clinical observations. In keeping with this, Polo et al. (2002) also found MMN evidence for a faster vigilance decrement in CHI patients than that in controls. These patients showed MMN for tone-frequency changes in irrelevant background stimulation which attenuated in amplitude more rapidly than that of the controls. The strongly attenuated MMN amplitude for auditory deviants was interpreted as signifying that CHI leads to an impairment in the automatic stimulus-change detector mechanism reflected by MMN.

The effects of lesions of the frontal cortex were also studied by Alho et al. (1994b), who found that dorsolateral prefrontal cortex lesions attenuated the MMN amplitude for tone-frequency change in subjects performing a visual RT task. This finding confirmed the previous results (Giard et al., 1990), showing that the frontal cortex plays a central role in the neural circuitry underlying MMN. In addition, P1 to standard and deviant sounds was enhanced in amplitude in patients, reflecting a reduced frontally mediated gating of sensory input to auditory cortex. (See also Knight et al., 1989; Knight, 1991.)

MMN has also been studied in patients with cerebellar lesions. These studies significantly contributed to our current understanding of the functional role of cerebellum. In a study on patients with cerebellar cortical atrophy, Moberget et al. (2008) provided evidence for a cerebellar contribution to the automatic processing and anticipation of auditory stimuli. While patients were watching a silent movie, a stream of task-irrelevant sounds was presented in the background, composed of standards and four different types of deviants differing from standards in one of four dimensions: duration, intensity, pitch, or location. Patients exhibited a delayed MMN peak latency for duration deviants and a similar trend for intensity deviants, whereas the pitch and location MMNs did not differ from those of the controls. According to the authors, their results are at odds with a view suggesting a role of cerebellum in sensory prediction but instead provide partial support to the timing hypothesis, which holds that the cerebellum is critical in generating precisely timed expectancies. It was concluded that 'the auditory mismatch paradigm can reveal important and meaningful data clarifying the functional role of the cerebellum. Our results provide support for a cerebellar contribution to the automatic processing and anticipation of auditory stimuli' (p. 2577).

Interestingly, Restuccia et al. (2007) demonstrated that cerebellar damage in patients with unilateral cerebral lesions was associated with a clearly abnormal somatosensory MMN (sMMN) to stimulation of the affected hand (ipsilateral to the affected cerebellar hemisphere), suggesting that cerebellar processing is involved in the pre-attentive detection of somatosensory input changes and, further, that patients with cerebellar damage may be impaired in the cortical processing of somatosensory input.

Thalamic infarctions

The effect of thalamic infarctions on MMNm and brain rhythmic activity was investigated by Mäkelä et al. (1998b), who found that lesions of non-specific thalamic nuclei may disturb brain rhythms in widespread cortical areas. Moreover, MMNm to pitch-deviant tones was absent in two patients, markedly decreased in amplitude in three patients, and normal in two patients, implicating that pathways passing through the anteromedial thalamus contribute to the MMNm modulation. The authors concluded that local unilateral lesions in the anteromedial thalamus may cause extensive, bilateral alterations in the electric brain activity and impair the patient's sensory memory.

Herpes simplex encephalitis

In another study of MMNm, Mäkelä et al. (1998b) addressed the functional brain changes caused by left-hemisphere dominant herpes simplex encephalitis (HSE) and the associated memory disorders. Four patients (mean age 52 years) with left-sided brain lesions caused by HSE were investigated at 24–36 months after the acute encephalitis. It was found that the N1m response actually was enhanced in amplitude in patients in comparison with that in controls. According to the authors, it is possible that diminished inhibition from anterior temporal areas or from the frontal cortex contributed to this enhancement. Furthermore, MMNm was smaller in amplitude in patients than that in controls, especially over the left, more affected hemisphere, implying, according to the authors, that the formation of sensory memory traces is affected by HSE lesions.

Conclusions

(1) In patients with stroke, the attenuated MMN for different kinds of stimulus changes correlates with the nature and magnitude of perceptual and cognitive loss.

(2) MMN permits the objective monitoring of the latent post-stroke recovery process when no informative behavioural measures can yet be used.

(3) The frequency- and duration-MMN recovery reflects the post-stroke recovery of brain mechanisms of speech comprehension.

(4) The improved post-stroke recovery caused by music and audio-book stimulation is indexed by the faster increase in the strength of the MMNm responses to frequency and duration changes in a binaural complex tone.

(5) The enhancement of the MMNm response to frequency change in these patients correlated with improvement in verbal memory and focused attention.

(6) In patients with aphasia, the presence of the MMN for speech-sound change predicts better auditory comprehension than does the absence of MMN, which rather indexes the presence of temporal-lobe lesions.

(7) In patients with aphasia, the duration of the MMN response was considerably shorter for those with more severe aphasia, hence serving as an index for the severity of aphasia.

(8) In patients with aphasia, MMN amplitude for complex-tone duration decrement and consonant-vowel syllable change correlated with auditory comprehension.

(9) MMN may be used to probe the integrity of the pre-attentive processes playing a role in triggering involuntary attention, a function apparently malfunctioning in neglect.

(10) In closed-head injury patients, MMN can be used for assessing their attentional problems such as their increased distractibility and, in particular, their abnormally fast vigilance decrease.

(11) MMN studies have also contributed to our current understanding of the role of, for example, the cerebellum in information processing, in particular its role in

automatic anticipation of auditory stimuli and in the processing of somatosensory stimuli.

6.5. **Cochlear lesions and implants**

For profoundly deaf individuals, the sensation of hearing can often be restored by means of cochlear implants (CI). CIs currently are the most successful and widely used sensory neuroprosthetics. In a large percentage of individuals fitted with CI, a remarkable degree of language communication via the auditory domain is restored. Nevertheless, objective, non-behavioural measures of auditory discrimination such as MMN remain a potentially powerful, but as yet under-utilized, application for this patient population (for a review, see Näätänen et al., 2017). Kraus et al. (1993) conducted their pioneering study of MMN in CI users, employing syllable contrasts. They found that MMN elicited in CI users was remarkably similar to that recorded from a group of age-matched normal-hearing (NH) controls. These results therefore suggested that despite the major differences in peripheral input, the brain of the CI user was processing basic speech units similarly to controls. Kraus et al. therefore concluded that MMN shows promise as a measure for the objective evaluation of CI function.

Consistent with these results, Ponton et al. (2000; see also Ponton & Don, 1995, 2003), recorded MMN elicited by a single contrast in stimulus duration from adult CI users and from age-matched NH adults, and also found that MMNs of the two groups were rather similar to each other. In a more detailed investigation with patients separated into two groups based on the benefit gained by using CI, Groenen et al. (1996) reported that patients who benefitted from the CI showed a MMN response, while those who did not failed to generate a comparable response. The authors concluded that 'there seems to be a relation between speech perception ability and MMN quality. To fundamentally understand the effects of electrical stimulation of the inner ear and to clinically adjust rehabilitation, diverse data are needed on different aspects of auditory processing. Optimizing the procedure to elicit MMN is therefore of great value' (p. 112). Furthermore, Kelly et al. (2005) reported a similar failure to record MMN from CI users defined as poor performers on the basis of their speech scores. Consistent with this, Zhang et al. (2011) found that good CI performers displayed MMNs with a large amplitude whereas moderate-to-poor performers showed small or absent MMNs.

An analogous data pattern can also be observed in children with CIs. Kileny et al. (1997) found that in children with CIs between ages of 4 and 12 years, the MMN and P3 amplitudes for a tone-frequency change significantly correlated with results of tests evaluating speech recognition skills. They concluded that the clinical use of cognitive evoked potentials in children with CI is 'feasible and informative'. Further:

> Given the strong relationship between some of the measures of the cognitive evoked potentials and traditional speech recognition scores, this procedure holds promise as a clinically useful technique for evaluating young children with cochlear implants. In particular, this measurement allows us to evaluate central auditory processing skills of young children in whom behavioral measurement

may be difficult or unreliable. In addition, this technique has the potential of providing insight into auditory learning and auditory memory in this patient population. (Kileny et al., 1997, p. 168.)

Lonka et al. (2004), in longitudinally tracking the changes in language function after a group of deaf adults had received their CIs, found that while MMN was absent for approximately 12 months post-surgery, it subsequently emerged first for a large vowel contrast, and then later for a more subtle vowel difference. A corresponding behavioural performance improvement was also observed during the follow-up period. According to Lonka et al., their results suggested that plastic changes occurred in the auditory cortex while the discrimination of speech sounds improved. The most important of these plastic changes might be the re-activation of cortical phoneme traces (Näätänen et al., 1997) that were formed before the deafness occurred. Consistent with this hypothesis, the results of Salo et al. (2002) suggest that the neural memory traces once developed for the mother tongue speech sounds remain quite stable even in total deprivation from supportive stimulation. The stability of these memory traces probably explains the fact that the post-lingually deafened patients benefit from CI soon after the operation: their language abilities have remained accessible. The information delivered through the implant seems to activate neural phonetic memory traces underlying the generation of MMN. Consistent with this, Perkell et al. (1992), who studied speech of post-lingually deafened patients before and after CI activation, suggested that 'production gains are governed at least as much by prior linguistic experience as by perceptual gains' and, further, that there exist somewhat degraded internal models of the relation between the production routines and the resulting acoustics which needs auditory feedback for recalibration.

The improvement of vowel discrimination in the early post-implant period was also investigated by Kraus et al. (1993). They found that MMN for a syllable change of a patient with a CI was small in amplitude at 2 months post-implant but was considerably enhanced at 8 months post-implant. Consistent with this result, the behavioural speech-sound discrimination ability of the patient was much better at 8 than 2 months post-implant. The authors concluded that MMN shows promise as a measure of objective evaluation of CI function. Moreover, the ability to measure MMN in CI recipients indicates that the response might be used to evaluate the success of implantation in a more objective manner than is practiced currently: 'Because of its involuntary nature, the MMN might be particularly useful as a tool for evaluating cochlear implant function in young deaf children. In addition, because the MMN appears to be an effective neurophysiologic index of fine acoustic stimulus processing, it may provide a neurophysiologic basis for the design of cochlear implant rehabilitation programs and signal-processing strategies' (pp. 123–4).

More recently, Liang et al. (2014) conducted a longitudinal study of the auditory cortex functional development using MMN in pre-lingual severely-to-profoundly hearing-impaired children of 1–6 years old post-implantation. The standard was a 1000 Hz tone while the deviant was of 1500 Hz. The MMN incidence in individual ERP averages gradually increased during the follow-up period of 6 months. Moreover, the MMN peak latency decrement from month 3 to month 6 correlated with the increment of scores assessing auditory-ability development in children. The authors concluded that 'MMN incidence increment and latency decrement are likely to be the objective and noninvasive indicators for evaluating auditory central development at the early stage in children after CI power-up.' Moreover, the MMN peak latency decrement from month 3 to month 6 significantly correlated with the increment in the scores assessing auditory ability development, 'indicating a fast maturation period, which might be a key period for auditory rehabilitation.'

In their long-term study of patients with CIs, Singh et al. (2004a, 2004b) and Liasis, Rajput, and Luxon (2004) observed that initially there were MMN responses in 80–85% of good performers in speech perception but only in 15–20% of poor performers. When the subjects were reassessed after 2 years, 50% of the poor performers with MMN had become good performers, whereas only 25% of poor performers with no MMN had become good performers. It was concluded that the presence of MMN could be a good indicator for evaluating cortical status after CI implantation. Consistent with this, Turgeon et al. (2014) found that MMN elicited by speech-sound contrasts distinguished between the adult CI users with a good behavioural performance in a speech-recognition task and those with a poorer performance. The amplitude of MMN in good performers, in fact, resembled that of the normal healthy controls. Moreover, a bivariate binomial correlation analysis showed a positive correlation between the MMN amplitude and the speech-recognition score. The authors concluded that MMN can distinguish between CI users who have good vs poor speech recognition ability as assessed with conventional tests. Further, MMN can assess speech recognition proficiency even in CI users who cannot be tested with regular speech recognition tasks, like infants and other non-verbal populations, suggesting that MMN could be used 'to evaluate speech recognition and to assess improvement following implantation and intervention in infants and non-verbal adults' (p. 834). Consequently, these results indicate, according to the authors, that the clinical use of MMN is 'feasible and informative'. This conclusion was supported by Kelly et al. (2005) who observed that MMN for tone-frequency change was absent or degraded in CI patients with poor speech scores, concluding that MMN is a useful tool for objectively assessing auditory discrimination in patients with CI: 'Since auditory evoked potentials relate to CI performance, they may be a useful tool for objectively evaluating the efficacy of speech processing strategies and/or auditory training approaches in both adults and children with cochlear implants' (p. 1235).

Subsequently, Ortmann et al. (2013) aimed to determine the central factors accounting for developing satisfactory speech performance in pre-lingually deafened children and adolescents. Two groups of CI users, one with a 'very good' and the other with a 'very bad' speech perception, were matched according to the hearing age and the age at implantation to determine whether these two CI groups differed from each other with regard to their phoneme discrimination ability and auditory sensory memory capacity. These functions were measured behaviourally and by using MMN. It was found that the behaviourally measured phoneme discrimination ability was comparable in the CI group of good performers to that in matched healthy controls and was better in both groups than that in the bad performers. Furthermore, source analyses revealed a larger-amplitude MMN in good than bad performers, which was generated in the frontal cortex and positively correlated with behavioural measures of working memory. These results indicate, according to the authors, that the two CI groups developed different auditory speech processing strategies and stress the role of phonological functions of auditory sensory memory and the prefrontal cortex in positively developing speech perception and production.

Trautwein et al. (1998) and Ponton et al. (2000), assessed patients with CI by using non-speech stimuli and obtained results that relate back both to speech performance and training. Trautwein et al. found that while the psychophysical thresholds were superior to MMN-estimated discrimination thresholds for duration contrasts in the control group, the opposite was true for a group of adult CI users. Thus, in a number of patients, there was neurophysiological evidence for discrimination based on MMN, without the patient being able to behaviourally discriminate the difference. Based on the apparent separation of discrimination at the level of sensation vs perception, Ponton et al. (2009) developed a protocol based on a pre-training MMN evaluation to determine whether there was neurophysiological evidence for discrimination in the absence of behavioural discrimination. This knowledge was then used to develop a training protocol which resulted in a significant improvement in behavioural frequency discrimination as well as in combined consonant and vowel discrimination in a single profoundly trained adult CI user.

In addition, Nager et al. (2007) found that CI users are impaired in the pre-attentive registration, indexed by a greatly attenuated P3a response to novel sounds in the passive oddball condition, an index of automatic orienting of attention. In contrast, in the active condition, the patients and controls did not differ from one another in hit rates and RTs. Furthermore, the ERPs elicited by novel stimuli were characterized by enhanced N2b and P3b components that did not differ in amplitude between the two groups. The authors concluded that the finding involving a clearly diminished P3a response in an unattended stimulus stream is of note because it provides the first direct evidence demonstrating that auditory novel events outside the attentional focus fail to automatically capture attention in cochlear implantees: 'This has implications for the ability of such patients to operate and navigate in the acoustic environment, as this clearly involves the movement and re-orientation of the attentional focus triggered by novel or deviant events in the auditory scene' (p. 395). This might also have important, even fatal, implications for traffic safety (see Näätänen & Summala, 1976).

As noted by Roman et al. (2005), there is a clear application of MMN in clinical testing and training of CI populations. However, refinements are needed in methods and recording technique to optimize protocols for these purposes. These authors studied postlingually implanted adult patients and found that a frequency discrimination ability (between tones of 1000 and 1500 Hz) could be demonstrated in all but one of their patients with CI by using MMN. A commendable methodological aspect of their investigation was to average MMN from eight fronto-central electrodes together, covering the scalp area with the highest MMN amplitudes, which revealed, according to the authors, MMN 'more precisely'. A further major refinement of the methodology was introduced by Ponton et al. (1997) who developed a statistic named MMNi, or the MMN-integrated, in which the averaged evoked potentials for the standard and deviant stimuli are integrated and compared to the individual's own variability for the standard stimulus across randomized, multiple trials. Based on their findings, Ponton et al. (2000) promoted use of MMNi as a clinical tool for examining individual differences in speech perception and discrimination, and in auditory short-term memory (for a review, see Johnson, 2009).

Previously, an important methodological contribution was provided by Wable et al. (2000), who analysed MMN in patients with CI to assess electrode discrimination in these patients, following the example given by Ponton and Don (1995). The latter authors compared MMN responses in an electrode-pair stimulation paradigm of patients with CI to tone-burst stimulation in NH subjects, finding shorter-latency MMN responses with electrical stimulation. This result may be explained, according to the authors, by a more synchronized activation of neurons in response to electrical stimulation. Consistent with this, Wable et al. found that MMN can be elicited when stimulating two different electrodes, with one for standards and the other for deviants. In order to avoid the overlap of MMN by ERP components related to the physical attributes of the two stimuli, two stimulus blocks were administered for each electrode pair: the first with Stimulus 1 as the repetitive standard and Stimulus 2 as the randomly interspersed deviant stimulus, and the contra protocol with the two stimuli being reversed (Ponton & Don, 1995).

Koelsch et al. (2004) studied music perception of CI users and found that CI users can perceive timbre, judging from MMN elicited by timbre deviants (for the timbre MMN, see Tervaniemi et al., 1997; Toiviainen et al., 1998). Moreover, music-syntactic violations elicited an ERAN, which again was considerably smaller in amplitude than that elicited in controls but nevertheless demonstrated that the central neural mechanisms underlying music perception are activated by musical stimulation even through CI (even though these patients reported difficulty in discriminating musical information and that they were in general frustrated by their inability to accurately perceive music). The finding that MMN and ERAN were smaller in amplitude in CI users reflects, according to the authors, the fact that the amount of sensory information received through a CI is smaller compared to that received through a natural cochlea. Consistent with this result, Zhang et al. (2013) reported that most post-lingually deafened adult CI users describe music as a noise-like and unpleasant stream of sounds. Zhang et al. (2013) found that MMN was present in all control group individuals but only in approximately half of the CI listeners studied. Moreover, in the CI users with MMN present, the MMN peak amplitude was smaller and peak latency longer than those of the controls. The authors concluded that MMN in CI users may be a useful objective tool to indicate the extent of sound registration in the auditory cortex in future efforts to improve CI design and speech strategy. Supporting these results, Sandmann et al. (2010) found, by using the multi-feature MMN paradigm with six different levels of magnitude of deviation for each feature that CI users had difficulties in discriminating small changes in the acoustic properties of musical sounds, judging from the small MMN amplitudes elicited. The authors concluded that an impaired discrimination ability in different acoustic dimensions may, at least partially, account for poor musical sound perception in CI users. Furthermore, according to Sandmann and colleagues, this type of paradigm could be of substantial clinical value by providing a comprehensive profile of the extent of the restored hearing in CI users.

Moreover, an inverse relationship was found between the MMN amplitude and the duration of profound deafness, indexing the adverse effect of this period. However, very importantly, there was also evidence for experience-related plastic cortical changes associated with CI use (Sandmann et al., 2010). According to these authors, MMN responses could be used as an objective marker for assessing auditory rehabilitation in different acoustic dimensions following cochlear implantation. An objective marker would be particularly helpful for young children who receive implants before language acquisition by indicating whether CI provides sufficient stimulation to allow the normal development of the central auditory functions (Sharma & Dorman, 2006). Importantly, Sandmann et al. (2010) also found a relationship between speech intelligibility (tested by the Oldenburg Sentences Test) and the MMN amplitudes for frequency and intensity deviations.

Timm et al. (2012) studied temporal and feature perception in post-lingually deafened CI users employing musical stimuli. They manipulated the first 60 ms of a cornet sound to determine whether these differences in the temporal envelope of the sounds, in particular the attack time, are detected by CI users. They found that, in an oddball paradigm with one of the stimuli at a time as standard and the others as deviants, MMN was only elicited in normal controls. Consequently, the authors concluded that small acoustic differences are difficult for CI users to perceive and encouraged musical training in CI users since it strongly affects ERPs (for a review, see Näätänen et al., 2017).

In their subsequent study on the residual neural processing of musical sound features in adult CI users, Timm et al. (2014) used the musical multi-feature MMN paradigm of Vuust et al. (2011, see also Vuust et al., 2012a, 2012b) which enables one to determine automatic auditory discrimination of six different types of sound-feature changes inserted within a musically enriched stimulus setting lasting for 20 min only. The musical multi-feature paradigm is an extension of the 'optimal paradigm' of Näätänen et al. (2004) but with a rich musical context and higher complexity obtained by presenting standards and deviants within an 'Alberti bass' configuration which is commonly used in the Western musical culture in both classical and improvisational music genres. In this paradigm, deviant sound features (such as pitch, timber, intensity, and rhythm changes) are embedded in the 'Alberti bass' where three different pitches alternate in a four-note pattern changing over the twelve keys. The stimuli therefore provide a more musical context than the original multi-feature paradigm. Indeed, the musical multi-feature paradigm has shown MMN differences between different kinds of musicians, which were closely related to the style-specific aspects of the music practiced (Vuust et al., 2011).

In their study employing this paradigm, Timm et al. (2014) found significant MMNs in the CI users for five deviant-stimulus categories, while obtaining significant MMNs for all six different deviant-stimulus categories in controls. MMNs in the CI users were lower in amplitude and their peak latencies were longer than those of the controls for deviations of pitch and guitar timbre, whereas no differences were found for intensity and saxophone timbre. Furthermore, MMNs in the CI users reflected their behavioural scores. These results indicate, according to the authors, that even though the CI users are not performing on the same level as the controls they have potential processing abilities for music listening. However, MMNs in CI users for rhythm were absent, indicating their diminished perception of rhythm within a melodic pattern.

Timm et al. results extend the view of the neural abilities for musical feature processing in adult CI users who were implanted after their childhood. Importantly, in a music-like stimulation paradigm, the brains of CI users are able to extract much more information from sound than previously reported, as indexed by the distinct MMNs for several musical features. This indicates the existence of residual encoding abilities in the brains of adult CI users which provide a ground for possible effective rehabilitation programmes. The authors further proposed that the musical multi-feature MMN paradigm implemented in their study may be adopted for routine clinical use as it may yield objective data on the capability of the current implants in an everyday listening situation. However, future research in the ERP method needs to reach sensitivity at the single-subject level 'to enhance reliability of individual multi-attribute profiles of sound discrimination abilities'.

Torppa et al. (2012) studied cortical processing of musical sounds in 22 early implanted children (mean age 6 years 10 months) who had had their implants for at least 22 months prior to the ERP recording, and 22 NH children. The standard stimulus was a piano tone D4 in the Western musical scale (295 Hz) with a duration of 200 ms. The deviants differed from the standards either in fundamental frequency (with all harmonics changing with the fundamental frequency), duration, intensity, gap (a short gap in the middle of the tone), or musical-instrument sound (representing a change in timbre). Each deviant randomly occurred at three different magnitudes of stimulus change. The standards and deviants alternated with each other, with the deviants being presented in a random order in every other stimulus position (see Näätänen et al., 2004). They found that this multi-feature MMN paradigm, with a recording time of 36 min, yielded significant P1, MMN, and P3a responses. Typically, the medium magnitudes of change elicited significant MMNs in both child groups, showing that they are optimal deviant-stimulus types for children. The authors concluded that with natural sounds presented in the multi-feature paradigm, it is possible to obtain novel information about the development and plasticity of cortical processing of musical stimuli. Further, in these early implanted CI children, MMN indicated less accurate change detection than that in NH age-matched children which probably reduced involuntary attention shifts to changes of musical instruments. Importantly, the authors proposed that these difficulties might be alleviated or abolished with appropriate auditory rehabilitation. In addition, their results suggest that despite the different sensory information provided by a CI, early and unilaterally implanted CI users process the acoustic properties of piano tones with natural harmonics and a fast presentation rate with the same neurocognitive mechanisms as do NH control children, as indexed by MMN and P3a. This is intriguing, the authors note, because adults with CI have great difficulties in perceiving F0 changes of piano tones in particular.

According to Torppa et al., these results are in line with the findings of Koelsch et al. (2004) who reported the occurrence of fast and fairly automatic music-syntactic processing in adults with CI using piano-like stimuli. Further:

> The apparent similarities in neurocognitive mechanism in the present study may begin to explain how CI children are able to process the auditory events that make up music. Even if cortical processing of auditory discrimination is less accurate and the perceptual cues to acoustical differences are different in CI than in NH children, there seem to be reliable and similar to NH children neurocognitive responses to changes in most of the key acoustic features of musical sounds. This may allow the development of higher-order musical perceptual and cognitive processes that allow the attribution of musical meaning to auditory events in a way that is analogous to the way that NH children adapt to music from different musical cultures. … This in turn may allow CI children to derive from music the same self-regulatory, emotional and arousing effects as the NH population … which is an extremely important factor in attracting them into the world of music and sound - and explain why early-implanted children enjoy music. … Moreover, our results on similar processing indicate that like in NH children, multisensory musical experiences could be an effective way to enhance auditory cortical functioning, discrimination accuracy and auditory skills in general. (Torppa et al., 2012, p. 1978.)

Recently, Petersen et al. (2015) wanted to determine the behavioural and neural correlates of music perception in the new generation of pre-lingually deaf adolescents who grew up with CIs. MMN was recorded to changes in musical features in adolescent CI users and in NH peers. Significant MMNs were found in CI users for deviations in timbre, intensity, and rhythm, indicating the presence of residual neural prerequisites for musical feature processing. By contrast, only the larger one of the two pitch changes used elicited MMN in the CI users. This pitch discrimination deficit was supported by behavioural measures in which the CI users scored significantly below the level of the NH controls. Overall, the MMN amplitudes were smaller in the CI users than those in the controls, suggesting a poorer music discrimination ability. According to the authors, this is the first study to show significant brain responses to musical feature changes in pre-lingually deaf adolescent CI users, implying the presence of neural predispositions for at least some aspects of music processing.

Conclusions

(1) MMN enables the objective assessment of the functioning of the CI in different patient groups, for it provides a quantitative measure for CI functioning strongly correlating with speech perception and hence pinpointing the potential problem areas for attempts at remediation.

(2) MMN enables the objective monitoring of the gradual improvement of auditory, in particular speech discrimination, after CI implantation.

(3) Importantly, MMN can be used to evaluate the effectiveness of different training and rehabilitation programmes intended for the improvement of the CI function of a patient.

6.6. **Tinnitus**

Tinnitus is a phantom auditory perception in the absence of any corresponding acoustic stimulus (Mahmoudian et al., 2013). It was estimated that 4–15% of the population experience tinnitus (Hoffman & Reed, 2004). By using the multi-feature MMN paradigm of Näätänen et al. (2004), Mahmoudian et al. (2013) found that the MMN topographic maps for different types of sound changes (frequency, duration, gap) of tinnitus sufferers differed from those of the control subjects. According to the authors, these findings suggested that there was possibly a deficit in pre-attentive change detection in patients with tinnitus. Further, tinnitus can cause a reduction in the duration of sensory memory in the auditory cortex of these patients, which might lead to decreased MMN amplitudes. The authors concluded that their study 'provides electrophysiological evidence supporting the theory that the pre-attentive and automatic central auditory processing is impaired in individuals with chronic tinnitus. Considering the advantages offered by the MMN paradigm used here, these data might be a useful reference point for the assessment of sensory memory in tinnitus patients which can reliably assess success in treatment monitoring' (pp. 161–2). Previously, Weisz et al. (2004) interpreted MMN results as suggesting that hearing loss is the basis of the development of tinnitus: 'It is likely that some central reorganization follows a damage to hearing receptors.' They concluded that 'so far diagnosis of tinnitus has solely relied on reports made by the subject. If the measures found here prove to be replicable, this could implicate first steps in the direction of an objectification of tinnitus and its related distress. They could serve e.g. as dependent variables in evaluation of therapies that currently lack objective markers' (p. 7).

Conclusion

(1) MMN data recorded from patients with tinnitus suggest a possible deficit in automatic central auditory processing mechanisms and the shortening of their auditory sensory-memory duration.

6.7. **Persistent developmental stuttering**

Persons with developmental stuttering suffer from speech disfluency. In a study of adults with persistent developmental stuttering, Corbera et al. (2005) reported normal MMNs for simple tone contrasts whereas the supra-temporal left-lateralized MMN-amplitude was enhanced for phoneme contrasts. Furthermore and very importantly, this MMN-amplitude enhancement correlated positively with speech disfluency as self-rated by the subjects. The authors concluded that individuals with persistent developmental stuttering have abnormal permanent memory traces for speech sounds in their auditory cortex (see also Salmelin et al., 1998, 2000a, 2000b). In addition, these abnormal speech-sound memory traces serve as a reference for producing the respective speech-sound utterances (Näätänen, 1999), probably underlying their speech disorder. Furthermore, it was also found that MMNs for prototypical and non-prototypical phonetic contrasts were very similar with each other, indicating that adults with developmental stuttering 'have difficulties in discriminating non-native from native sounds properly, suggesting abnormal auditory processing of all kind of speech-like signals' (Corbera et al., 2005, p. 1250). Subsequently, Jansson-Verkasalo et al. (2014) found no P1 and N1 amplitude differences between children with stuttering and age-matched controls, whereas MMN for only the very salient vowel-duration change was significant in children with stuttering, in contrast to the control children in whom significant MMNs were elicited by all the different types of stimulus change used (consonant, vowel, vowel duration, frequency, intensity). Furthermore, the MMN amplitudes were overall diminished in the children with stuttering and there was a significant correlation between the stuttering severity and the MMN amplitude. The authors concluded that in children with stuttering, central auditory speech-sound processing was normal at the level of sound encoding whereas speech-sound discrimination was atypical.

Conclusions

(1) The abnormally enhanced MMN response recorded in adults with stuttering suggest that there might be pathological excitation in their auditory cortex encoding the different speech-sound representations.

(2) Diminished MMNs, in turn, were reported in children with stuttering, whose MMN was significantly elicited only by the most salient change in the syllable stimuli. It remains to be investigated which issues influence the MMN in stuttering (stimulus type and magnitude, age).

6.8. **Migraine**

Migraine is one of the most common headache disorders affecting about 11% of the adult population (Stovner et al., 2007). In a study of 22 female migraine patients suffering from menstrually related migraine, Morlet et al., (2014a) found that MMN to a tone-duration decrement was normal across different phases of the menstrual cycle, and that the migraine patients showed no impairment compared with age- and cycle-matched control females. In contrast, the normal MMN was succeeded by a late and prolonged N2b in the migraine patients. The authors concluded that their study showed normal auditory sensory processing in patients with migraine but that automatic attention orienting processes to auditory changes (and more generally to any auditory stimulus) were enhanced: 'The pathophysiologic basis of such heightened attentional response recorded in migraineurs is still unknown, but could, at least partially, be linked to the close relationship observed between environmental stimuli and migraine. Understanding the links between photo/phonofobia and an increased automatic attention orienting in migraine is a challenge for future studies' (p. 510). Previously, De Tommaso et al. (2004) reported that the MMN peak latency correlated positively with duration of illness in patients with migraines, suggesting that 'the hypofunctioning state of cortical automatic processing of acoustic stimuli may also develop in the course of the disease' (p. 666).

Conclusion

(1) In patients with migraine, automatic sound discrimination as reflected by the MMN peak amplitude is not affected whereas MMN peak latency is increased with the duration of the illness.

6.9. **Chronic pain and fibromyalgia**

Fibromyalgia (FM) is a common chronic pain disorder characterized by widespread pain and tenderness, often accompanied by affective and cognitive symptoms. A large number of patients with FM exhibit cognitive deficits in attention, executive functioning, and working memory (for a review, see Choi et al., 2015). Dick et al. (2003) studied 12 patients with a diagnosis of chronic pain for at least 6 months but with no history of psychiatric problems or head trauma. The mean length of time since the onset of chronic pain was 13.75 years (mean age 52.8 years). It was found that in these patients, the MMN amplitude for tone-frequency change was attenuated when the patient experienced chronic pain compared to when he/she did not experience it. The authors, stating that this is the first result demonstrating an effect of pain at such an early level of cognitive processing, explained this effect by referring to the model of Eccleston and Crombez (1999), maintaining that 'as a stimulus, chronic pain is distracting and disruptive'. This MMN effect mainly occurred when the frequency change was small in magnitude. The authors concluded that their results provide an electrophysiological correlate to previous findings that high levels of pain disrupt cognition during the performance of demanding tasks (see also de Tommaso et al., 2013).

Choi et al. (2015) recently aimed at determining whether patients with FM exhibit any abnormality in preattentive auditory processing as assessed by using the auditory MMNm. It was found that the MMNm amplitude in the right hemisphere was smaller and showed left-ward asymmetry in patients with FM compared with that in healthy controls. Furthermore, the right-hemisphere MMNm source in the FM group differed from that in healthy controls. Choi and colleagues concluded that the functional and structural abnormalities, as potential signatures of the cortical reorganization of chronic pain in FM, could have caused alterations in the MMNm source location. Moreover, the authors also point to the accumulating evidence that FM might be related to a global sensory disturbance rather than abnormalities restricted to pain processing.

Conclusion

(1) Chronic pain attenuates the MMN amplitude, presumably indexing the distracting effect of chronic pain.

6.10. **Essential tremor**

Essential tremor, which is clinically characterized by an 8–12 Hz kinetic tremor of the arms, often accompanied by head and voice tremors, represents the most common pathological tremor in humans (Louis, 2009). These patients also suffer from cognitive deficits which are typically mild but progressive. Pauletti et al. (2014) recorded MMN to deviant sounds (1100 Hz) in a sequence of standard sounds (1000 Hz) while the patient was watching a video. These MMNs did not differ in amplitude from those recorded in healthy age- and sex-matched controls. However, there was a strong positive correlation between the MMN peak latency and the age at disorder onset. The authors suggested that the deficit in pre-attentive auditory discrimination in elderly onset patients may be due to a possible impairment in locus-coeruleus functioning.

Conclusion

(1) The MMN peak amplitude is not affected by essential tremor whereas its latency strongly correlated with the patient's age at disorder onset.

Chapter 7

Psychiatric disorders

7.1. Schizophrenia

Schizophrenia (SZ) is a severe, chronic, and often debilitating psychiatric disorder affecting approximately 1% of the population worldwide (Jablensky, 1997). It is primarily characterized by 'positive' (e.g. hallucinations and delusions) and 'negative' (e.g. affective flattening, anhedonia, and alogia) psychotic symptoms. Cognitive impairments affect approximately 75% of people diagnosed with SZ (Palmer et al., 2009) and constitute a primary barrier to optimal functioning (Green, 1996; Green et al., 2000). While conventional treatments for the disorder have primarily aimed to reduce psychotic symptoms with antipsychotic medications, recent years have shifted the focus of treatment to include the restoration of the disabling cognitive deficits. Despite widespread consensus about the need for effective cognitive remediation in SZ, however, cognitive impairments remain one of the most intractable aspects of the illness, with both pharmacological and behavioural interventions often failing to produce statistically or clinically significant improvements (McGurk et al., 2007; Wykes et al. 2011). Neuroscience-derived biomarkers like MMN have ushered in a revolution in cognitive treatment for SZ, due to their suitability for probing the earliest stages of sensory-perceptual processing and linking cognitive deficits to specific neural systems (Braff & Light, 2004, 2005; Javitt et al., 2008; Light & Makeig, 2015; Rissling et al., 2014).

The first evidence of MMN abnormality in SZ was reported nearly three decades ago (Shelley et al., 1991). To date, a Medline search for 'mismatch negativity' and 'schizophrenia' yields over 400 results. In the time since Shelley et al.'s initial study, robust MMN amplitude reductions (effect sizes ≈ 1.00) in SZ have been firmly established in this population via independent studies, meta-analyses and large-scale multi-centre studies (Erickson et al., 2016; Light et al., 2015; Thomas et al., 2017; Umbricht & Krljesb, 2005). Fig. 7.1 shows individual MMN data (amplitude colour coded) for each of n=877 SZ patients and n=753 healthy comparison subjects as well as group grand averages adapted from Light et al., 2015.

Reduced MMN amplitude is evident even in the absence of psychotropic medication (Catts et al., 1995; Kasai et al. 2002b; Korostenskaja et al., 2005; Light et al., 2015; Rissling et al., 2012; Umbricht et al., 1998, 1999), suggesting that the underlying neural dysfunction may result from the illness process itself, rather than a consequence of antipsychotic medications. MMN reductions in SZ have been associated with impairments across several cognitive domains (e.g. Baldeweg et al., 2004; Kawakubo et al., 2006; Kiang et al.,

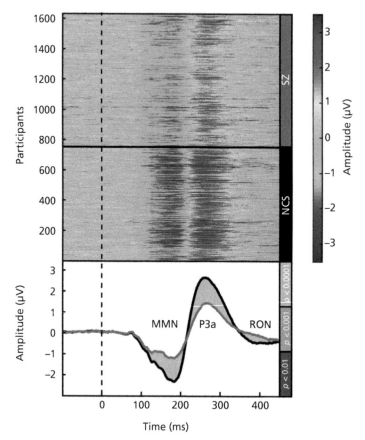

Fig. 7.1 Individual subject and group averaged waveforms: Individual subject Deviant–Standard difference wave averages (color coded by amplitude) are shown in the upper portion of the figure for healthy comparison subjects (n=753) and schizophrenia patients (n=877). Group averaged waveforms are shown in the lower portion of the figure (negativity downwards).

Data from Light, G. A., Swerdlow, N. R., Thomas, M. L., Calkins, M. E., Green, M. F., Greenwood, T. A., … Turetsky, B. I., *Validation of mismatch negativity and P3a for use in multi-site studies of schizophrenia: Characterization of demographic, clinical, cognitive, and functional correlates in COGS-2,* Schizophrenia Research, 163 (1), 63–72, doi:https://doi.org/10.1016/j.schres.2014.09.042, 2015.

2007; Lee et al., 2014; Rissling et al., 2014), including processing speed and attention (Hermens et al., 2010), verbal and working memory (Baldeweg et al., 2004; Kawakubo et al., 2006; Todd et al., 2010), verbal fluency (Baldeweg et al., 2004), and social cognition (Jahshan et al., 2013; Wynn et al., 2010). Deficits in MMN are highly associated with SZ patients' impairments in identifying real-world environmental sounds (Joshi et al., 2018). MMN has further been correlated with clinician ratings of global psychosocial functioning (Kawakubo & Kasai 2006; Koshiyama et al., 2017; Lee et al., 2014; Light & Braff 2005a, 2005b; Light et al., 2015; Rissling et al., 2014; Thomas et al., 2017) and self-reported quality of life (Hermens et al., 2010). Moreover, MMN deficits are a stronger predictor of functional impairments than neuropsychological tests (Lee et al., 2014).

Several studies have investigated whether MMN abnormalities represent state-vs trait-markers of SZ. MMN deficits appear to be independent of fluctuations in clinical state and symptoms (Light et al., 2012; Shinozaki et al., 2002). Cohorts of individuals at high clinical risk for developing psychosis as well as patients in the early stages of illness (i.e. within five years of onset) have consistently shown reductions in duration-MMN (dMMN); studies of frequency-MMN (fMMN) in early stages of illness have yielded mixed findings of deficits (Bodatsch et al., 2011; Erickson et al., 2016; Haigh, Coffman & Salisbury, 2017; Hay et al., 2015; Hermens et al., 2010; Koshiyama et al., 2017b; Nagai et al., 2013a, 2013b; Perez et al., 2014b; Salisbury et al., 2002; Salisbury et al., 2007; Salisbury et al., 2017; Salisbury et al., 2018; Shaikh et al., 2012; Todd et al., 2008; Umbricht et al., 2006). This dissociation of dMMN and fMMN has contributed to the suggestion that dMMN impairments may constitute a vulnerability marker for psychosis, while reductions in fMMN may instead provide an index of illness progression (e.g. Nagai et al., 2013b). Consistent with this view, fMMN deficits have further been associated with illness duration (Umbricht & Krljesb 2005), and progressive fMMN reduction across the first 1.5 years of illness has been correlated with progressive reduction in left temporal lobe gray matter (Salisbury et al., 2007). In another longitudinal study, patients were assessed during periods of acute illness and symptom remission. While there was no difference in fMMN measured at Fz during the two stages of illness, mastoid fMMN was significantly reduced during the acute phase (Shinozaki et al., 2002).

Several studies have attempted to determine whether problems with sensory memory, sensory encoding, or predictive estimation may be the primary contributor to MMN deficits in SZ. More pronounced MMN deficits are not evident at longer inter-stimulus intervals, suggesting that reduced MMN is not solely a consequence of impairments in sensory memory (Javitt et al., 1998; Shelley et al., 1999). Sensory encoding, however, does appear to be problematic. Using standard and deviant stimuli with frequency differences derived from individualized pitch discrimination thresholds, Leitman et al. (2010) showed that SZ patients no longer demonstrated reduced MMN compared to nonpsychiatric controls. In a similar study controlling for temporal discrimination thresholds, however, Todd et al. (2003) found that dMMN was reduced even in patients whose temporal discrimination abilities were equivalent to that of controls; bottom-up encoding imprecision therefore does not appear to be the sole contributor to reduced MMN, as demonstrated by Javitt et al. (1998). They reported that patients with SZ actually demonstrate the greatest MMN impairments when the magnitude of difference between standard and deviant stimuli is large, as opposed to small. In both patients and nonpsychiatric controls, the degree to which MMN amplitude increases with progressively larger frequency differences appears to reach a plateau (at 100% frequency difference in (Javitt et al., 1998); cf. Horton et al. (2011) for SZ vs control group differences at 5% deviants). In patients, the plateau was significantly lower than it was for controls, suggesting that the maximum amplitude of MMN that can be evoked may be reduced in SZ patients.

With regard to top-down influences, MMN generation can be elicited in the absence of directed attention. When participants are engaged in highly demanding foreground tasks (e.g. continuous performance task), MMN to task irrelevant auditory stimuli can be suppressed. Interestingly, the amount of MMN amplitude from low- to high-demand conditions correlates with concurrent attentional functioning (Rissling et al., 2013). Since MMN relies on the ability to abstract expectations about one's auditory environment, MMN is thus thought to result when a deviant stimulus violates one's expectations formed as a result of exposure to standard stimuli. Evidence of MMN generation in SZ is itself reflective of the ability to generate expectations about the environment. Furthermore, in patients, MMN amplitude is sensitive to the same factors to which it is responsive in controls, namely deviant probability and magnitude of change in the deviant stimulus. Some MMN paradigms specifically assess higher order abilities, e.g. pattern violation detection (Salisbury & McCathern 2016; Todd et al., 2014, 2018) or speech syllable category changes (Kasai et al., 2002a), and SZ patients tend to show deficits in those paradigms as well (Green et al., 2000).

Estimating the degree of stimulus error, however, may be problematic. In a study by Baldeweg and colleagues (2004), the authors utilized an ingenious 'roving' stimulus paradigm and varied the number of standards that preceded deviant tones in both SZ patients and nonpsychiatric control subjects. They found that, in controls, not only did MMN amplitude increase with a higher number of standards between deviants, but that a 'repetition positivity' that became larger with a higher number of standard repetitions was observed. The authors argued that this positivity might reflect the encoding of the regularity of the standard stimulus. Patients did not show this positivity, nor did they generate larger MMN to less frequent deviant stimuli, suggesting that patients may have difficulty encoding environmental regularities and thus lack the expected adaptability of MMN to stimulus likelihood. As noted by Todd et al. (2012), 'a failure to distinguish between probabilities could mean that the brain signal for something that sometimes occurs is indistinguishable from that produced to something that almost never occurs. Likewise, a failure to represent different magnitudes of change could mean that an event that is somewhat unusual is coded the same way as an event that is grossly different.' The authors go on to postulate that perhaps it is not the *absolute* MMN amplitude that holds functional implications, but rather the *relative* changes in amplitude that may be problematic in schizophrenia. A restriction in representational range may mean that, in fact, auditory changes are more likely to 'max out' the MMN response, and that patients may be more likely to orient attention toward stimuli that may not be particularly novel or salient. Nonetheless, the use of conventional and novel paradigms that can probe the capacity for neuroplasticity is an intensive emerging area of research (Perez et al., 2017; Rissling et al., 2013; Swerdlow et al., 2016).

Links to neural circuits/mechanisms

The neural sources of MMN in healthy subjects have been extensively characterized using a variety of methods with consistent evidence of contributions from temporal and frontal brain regions. Takahashi et al. (2013) utilized distributed EEG tomography (Exact Low Resolution Electromagnetic Tomography; eLORETA) to characterize the neural sources of MMN and P3a in schizophrenia in large samples of patients and healthy controls. With regard to MMN current density, the authors found a *group difference* that was relatively circumscribed to medial frontal regions, with maximal group differences in right medial frontal gyrus (Fig. 7.2). Other significant SZ abnormalities were identified in the right cingulate gyrus and right paracentral lobule. In contrast to the relatively circumscribed areas of MMN deficits in SZ patients, group differences in P3a current density were broadly distributed across frontal, temporal, and parietal lobes, including bilateral anterior cingulate, cingulate gyrus, parahippocampal gyrus, posterior cingulate, paracentral lobule, medial frontal gyrus, superior frontal gyrus, postcentral gyrus, inferior parietal lobule, precuneus, and sub-gyral, with maximum deficits in schizophrenia patients at the right post central gyrus (Takahashi et al., 2013). Similarly, Rissling et al. (2014) used a novel

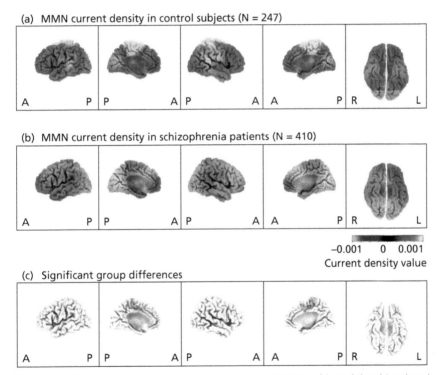

Fig. 7.2 Current density of mismatch negativity in nonpsychiatric subjects (A), schizophrenia patients (B), and group differences (C). Blue color shows the location where patients had smaller current density compared to controls (p<0.001). Abbreviations: A, anterior; P, posterior; R, right; L, left.

Data from Takahashi, H., Rissling, A. J., Pascual-Marqui, R., Kirihara, K., Pela, M., Sprock, J., … Light, G. A., *Neural substrates of normal and impaired preattentive sensory discrimination in large cohorts of nonpsychiatric subjects and schizophrenia patients as indexed by MMN and P3a change detection responses*, NeuroImage, 66, 594–603, doi:10.1016/j.neuroimage.2012.09.074, 2013.

approach to deconstruct cortical sources using independent component analysis. This approach identified generators centered in superior temporal, inferior frontal, ventral mid-cingulate, anterior cingulate, medial orbitofrontal, and dorsal mid-cingulate cortical source areas. The independent component analysis derived source analyses substantially improved the sensitivity for detecting group differences and relationships to many important domains of clinical, cognitive, and psychosocial functioning in schizophrenia patients. The collective pattern of source findings suggest that the distributed neural architecture supporting initial auditory sensory discrimination (i.e. MMN) is similar in schizophrenia patients and healthy controls but that these impairments in medial frontal regions conceivably cascade forward and result in generalized neurocognitive deficits (Braff & Light 2004; Javitt et al., 1995; Rissling et al., 2014; Tiitinen et al., 1994).

Such a hierarchical information processing cascade model was recently tested and expanded by Thomas et al.'s (2017) large-scale structural equation modeling study in over 800 schizophrenia patients. Thomas et al. found that impairments in the MMN-P3a-RON 'auditory deviant response complex' (Rissling et al., 2014; Fig. 7.3), reflecting early auditory information processing, are causally related to generalized impairments in both cognitive and psychosocial functioning. Importantly, the model predicts that if the auditory deviant response complex could be increased collectively by 1 microvolt, cognition would be expected to increase by an effect size of at least d=0.78. It is notable that while single-doses of both pharmacological (e.g. Swerdlow et al., 2016) and nonpharmacological (e.g. Perez et al., 2017) treatments can 'move' MMN, single exposure to any treatment is obviously not expected to produce enduring improvements in cognition (e.g. Bhakta et al., 2016). Thus, further research is needed to clarify the time course and requirements for promoting cognitive enhancement. In this regard, pharmacological augmentation of cognitive training (PACT; Swerdlow 2012; Light & Swerdlow 2015) represents a promising new approach for treatment development. This collection of findings provide compelling support for the use of MMN in the development of pharmacological and/or nonpharmacological treatments.

Examination of the neurochemical contributions to MMN has provided evidence of the widespread neural dysfunction in schizophrenia, even challenging the conventional beliefs of the time of schizophrenia as a disorder characterized predominantly by hyperactivity within the dopamine (DA) system. The DA model of schizophrenia was historically based on observations of decreased hallucinations and delusions in response to chlorpromazine and other DA antagonists, as well as induction of psychotic symptoms by DA agonists (Javitt et al., 2012). However, DA hyperactivity appears to be specifically associated with positive symptoms, while having little to no effect on negative symptoms or cognitive functioning (Kantrowitz & Javitt 2010), or MMN amplitude (Leung et al., 2007, 2010; Oranje et al., 2017). In addition, even positive symptoms persist in the absence of DA hyperactivity, suggesting an altogether limited role for DA in the disorder's pathology (Kantrowitz & Javitt, 2010).

Glutamatergic dysfunction has become increasingly accepted as an aetiopathological model of schizophrenia based on observations that phencyclidine, ketamine, and similar

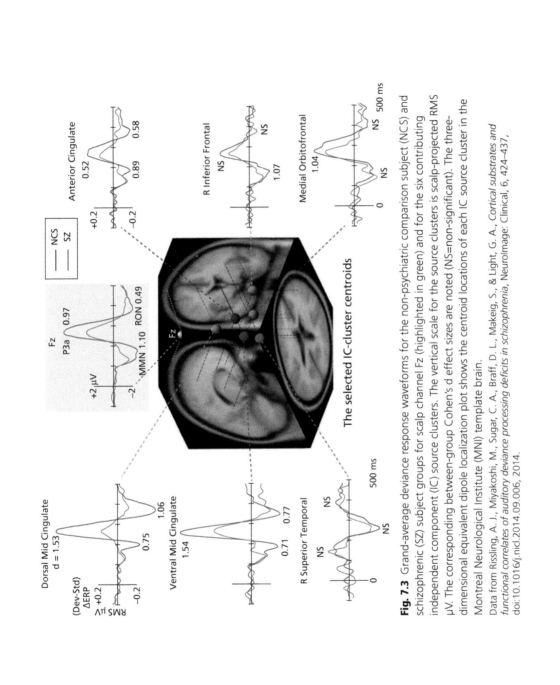

Fig. 7.3 Grand-average deviance response waveforms for the non-psychiatric comparison subject (NCS) and schizophrenic (SZ) subject groups for scalp channel Fz (highlighted in green) and for the six contributing independent component (IC) source clusters. The vertical scale for the source clusters is scalp-projected RMS µV. The corresponding between-group Cohen's d effect sizes are noted (NS=non-significant). The three-dimensional equivalent dipole localization plot shows the centroid locations of each IC source cluster in the Montreal Neurological Institute (MNI) template brain.

Data from Rissling, A. J., Miyakoshi, M., Sugar, C. A., Braff, D. L., Makeig, S., & Light, G. A., *Cortical substrates and functional correlates of auditory deviance processing deficits in schizophrenia*, NeuroImage: Clinical, 6, 424–437, doi:10.1016/j.nicl.2014.09.006, 2014.

psychomimetic compounds induce a schizophrenia-like psychosis in nonpsychiatric controls by blocking neurotransmission at N-methyl-D-aspartate glutamate receptors (NMDAR; Goff & Coyle 2001; Javitt & Zukin 1991; Krystal et al., 1994). NMDAR are widely distributed throughout the brain, both cortically and subcortically, implicating NMDAR in the generalized sensory and cognitive deficits of schizophrenia (Kantrowitz & Javitt 2012). Indeed, in addition to inducing positive symptoms of psychosis, like hallucinations and delusions, NMDAR blockade also mimics negative symptoms and cognitive deficits common in schizophrenia. Support for the role of NMDAR in schizophrenia has also been shown at the neurophysiological level, with studies demonstrating MMN sensitivity in healthy subjects administered drugs that engage the NMDAR (Avissar & Javitt 2018; Greenwood et al., 2018; Hamilton et al., 2018; Javitt et al., 2012; Mathalon et al., 2014; Swerdlow et al., 2016).

Animal model studies have also confirmed a major role of glutamate in regulating MMN (Ahnaou et al., 2017; Amann et al., 2010; Featherstone et al., 2017; Harms 2016; Javitt et al., 1996; Lee et al., 2017; Sivarao et al., 2014). Gil-da-Costa et al. (2013) further extended a substantial and rapidly evolving knowledge base of the neural substrates of MMN by demonstrating cross-species homology of electrophysiological responses to subanesthetic doses of the NMDA receptor antagonist ketamine, further establishing MMN and the closely linked P3a component as translational biomarkers that can model some of the core cognitive impairments of schizophrenia and related psychotic disorders.

Although the cause of temporal grey matter reductions in schizophrenia is not yet known, two primary hypotheses have garnered empirical support. The first involves the NMDAR system and its purported influence on dendritic spine density. Through facilitation of long-term potentiation (LTP), NMDAR play a key role in learning and memory and, more generally, experience-dependent synaptic plasticity. Neurotrophic factors produced through LTP result in the proliferation of dendritic spines and subsequent strengthening of synaptic connections. Conversely, long-term depression at NMDAR is associated with scarcity of dendritic spines (Mattson 2008; Singer 1995). Grey matter reductions and related MMN deficits may therefore occur at least partially as a result of dysfunction within the NMDAR glutamate system.

MMN as a genetic endophenotype of schizophrenia

Endophenotypes are measures reflective of genes predisposing one to developing a particular disorder (Braff & Light 2005; Light et al., 2014). They are measured by laboratory tests, are not discernable by the naked eye, and provide a more direct 'link' to genes than do observable behaviours. Endophenotypic abnormalities may be present in the absence of behavioural pathology and thus may serve as indicators of increased genetic risk for development of a disorder, making the identification of endophenotypes essential for early detection and intervention. Endophenotypes may also be useful for identifying subtypes of more complex psychiatric phenotypes. Endophenotypes are a special class of biomarkers that are: 1) associated with a disorder and represent stable, reproducible impairments in an individual patient, 2) highly heritable, 3) evident in unaffected family members, 4) rapidly and easily measured, and 5) reflect the functional status of neurobiological mechanisms related to pathophysiology of disorder and action of limited number of genes (Turetsky et al., 2007). MMN fulfills all of these criteria, as described below.

MMN deficits are associated with SZ (d~1.0) with high test-retest reliability coefficients (ICCs=0.90) over both short and 1-year retest intervals in healthy subjects and SZ patients (Light et al., 2012). The effect size of deficits and stability coefficients are comparable to or even exceed concurrently measured neuropsychological test performances (Light et al., 2012). In addition, MMN deficits are present in some people at genetic risk for psychosis (Atkinson et al., 2017; Baker et al., 2005; Jahshan et al., 2012; Jessen et al., 2001; Michie et al., 2002; Schreiber et al., 1992) and appear to be heritable; family members of schizophrenia patients often show either amplitude reduction (Jessen et al., 2001; Michie et al., 2002) or values that fall between healthy controls and schizophrenia probands (Price et al., 2006). MMN heritability estimates range from 0.56 to 0.68 (Hall et al., 2006; Hong et al., 2012). While not all studies have supported the contribution of genetics to MMN (Bramon et al., 2004; Hong et al., 2012; Kim et al., 2014), the MET allele of the VAL108/158MET COMT polymorphism gene has been implicated in MMN deficits (Baker et al., 2005; Cheour et al., 1997). Rodent studies have demonstrated a role of NRG1 gene. NRG1 (+/-) mice showed selective deficits in MMN, but not obligatory ERPs, like P20 and N40 or evoked gamma power (Featherstone et al., 2015). Large-scale human studies are underway to identify genes associated with MMN and related neurophysiological measures (Light et al., 2015; Turetsky et al., 2015).

Utility of MMN as a biomarker to guide diagnosis and treatments of neuropsychiatric disorders

There has been a recent surge of interest in improving the prediction of psychosis onset in individuals at high risk for developing schizophrenia (e.g. Light & Näätänen 2013; Nagai et al., 2013a, 2013b; 2017). Evidence suggests that people with longer periods of time between symptom onset and initiation of adequate treatment (i.e. longer durations of untreated psychosis; DUP) tend to have worse clinical and functional outcomes, with mortality rates more than six times higher than of patients with short DUPs within the decade following illness onset (Farooq et al., 2009; Marshall et al., 2005; Perkins et al., 2005). Several of the structural brain changes that have been detected in SZ patients also appear to occur early in the course of illness, including decreased frontal white matter volume, increased frontal lobe CSF volume, and increased ventricular volume (DeLisi et al., 1997; Ho et al., 2003a, 2003b; Lieberman et al., 2001). In clinical high-risk (CHR) samples, which include subjects with both a genetic risk for developing a psychotic disorder in addition to demonstrating sub-threshold psychotic symptoms, specific preventive treatment (including pharmacological and/or psychosocial interventions) has been found to delay or prevent onset of psychotic disorders, or reduce severity of psychotic symptoms (Amminger et al., 2010; McGorry et al., 2002; Morrison et al., 2007; Morrison et al., 2012; Stafford et al., 2013). Early detection and intervention is therefore crucial.

In the past decade, several groups have developed clinical criteria to identify individuals at CHR for psychosis. Under the Criteria of Prodromal Syndromes (COPS; Miller et al., 2002) or the comparable At-Risk Mental States criteria (ARMS; Yung & McGorry 1996), 18–36% of the individuals identified as CHR for psychosis subsequently developed a psychotic disorder within a 2–3 year follow-up period (Cannon et al., 2008; Fusar-Poli & Borgwardt 2012). This means that approximately 65–80% of individuals identified as being at high risk do not convert to psychosis. This low 'hit rate' is a major barrier for attempting prophylactic pharmacological interventions, particularly with antipsychotic medications, which cause metabolic or motor side effects. Ultimately, this lack of predictive power when relying on clinical information alone has raised doubt about the utility of the CHR syndrome (Yang et al., 2010).

Although the vast majority of MMN studies in schizophrenia have consisted of cross-sectional characterizations of patient deficits, longitudinal studies have recently shown that the prediction of psychosis in CHR can be considerably improved by means of simple MMN recordings. In the first of these studies, Bodatsch et al. (2011, 2015) compared CHR participants who did vs did not convert to psychosis during follow-up. At baseline, converters had significantly smaller MMN amplitude, one comparable to that in early illness patients, whereas MMN in nonconverters was comparable to that of healthy age-matched controls. Perez et al. (2014b) extended these findings to show that severity of MMN amplitude deficits also 'forecasts' the time lag to psychosis onset in CHR individuals; those with more severe MMN reductions had shorter times to psychosis. MMN may therefore be useful in predicting the development of psychosis and enhancing individualized risk-estimation/prevention strategies.

MMN may also be useful for treatment development, as well as guiding individualized assignment to interventions and subsequently monitoring response to those interventions. Translational neurophysiological biomarkers are powerful tools for accelerating the pace of development of new treatments (Braff & Light 2004; Javitt 2015; Light & Näätänen 2013; Light & Swerdlow 2015). MMN and related measures have been instrumental in demonstrating that an experimental treatment engages its intended target; biomarkers can also facilitate dose selection, and serve as surrogate end points. Ultimately, the hope is that neurophysiological biomarkers can be used to assign patients to receive treatments where there is a likelihood of success (Light & Swerdlow 2015; Perez et al., 2014a).

EEG biomarkers, such as MMN, may provide a functional probe of the frontotemporal brain network underlying a number of functionally relevant abilities and may therefore lead to more precise 'neuroscience-informed' diagnoses. In addition, the potential for MMN to probe functionally relevant neural activity may have further implications for estimating the likelihood of patient response to a new generation of neuroscience-informed interventions.

MMN also shows great potential to guide treatment and inform outcome studies, based on evidence that amplitude is: 1) extremely reliable in both healthy individuals and schizophrenia patients tested over a 1-year interval (Light et al., 2012); 2) insensitive to order or practice effects unlike some behavioural tests (Kathmann et al., 1999; Light et al.,

2012; Pekkonen et al., 1995); 3) robustly related to level of everyday functioning in schizo-phrenia patients (Friedman et al., 2012; Kawakubo et al., 2007; Kiang et al., 2007; Light & Braff 2005a, 2005b; Rasser et al., 2011; Wynn et al., 2010); 4) responsive to pharma-cological models of schizophrenia (Javitt et al., 1996; Lavoie et al., 2008; Swerdlow et al., 2016; Umbricht et al., 2000, 2002); and (5) easily assessed in patients with a broad range of function given the low effort associated with task demands.

Despite the many available antipsychotic agents that reduce the dramatic and defining positive psychotic symptoms of SZ, there has been little progress in the way of using pharmacological interventions to ameliorate the disabling cognitive features of the ill-ness. Yet, there is reason to be hopeful about our ability to produce lasting improve-ments in the cognitive functioning of people with schizophrenia. Emerging findings indicate that the impaired neural systems of psychiatric illnesses are not fixed, but may be modified by carefully designed training interventions that harness neuroplasticity-based learning mechanisms (Fisher et al., 2009). One promising intervention, Targeted Cognitive Training (TCT), is designed to sharpen the accuracy and fidelity of audi-tory information processing in psychosis via daily, computer-based cognitive exercises (Fisher et al., 2009; Vinogradov et al., 2012). Plastic changes within the neural sys-tems that subserve early perceptual processing are thought to feed forward to enhance higher-order cognition. Studies in schizophrenia patients who completed 50 hours (1 hour/day, 5 days/week) of TCT demonstrated large effect size gains that generalized to auditory-dependent cognitive domains (verbal learning and memory, d=0.86–0.89) as well as global cognition (d=0.86) and quality of life (Fisher et al., 2009). Although TCT is efficacious at the group level, individual participant responses vary consider-ably; some patients show little or no benefit after even a full course of training (Fisher et al., 2009). As such, there is a need to identify predictive biomarkers of response to this daily, resource-intensive intervention. Given that MMN is regarded as a robust, reliable, and sensitive index of central auditory system plasticity (Näätänen 2008), it is a promising candidate biomarker for indexing treatment-related changes in physi-ology, as well as predicting treatment response. These investigations have demonstrated that MMN predicts response to intensive computerized cognitive training (Kujala et al., 2001; Lovio et al., 2012) and psychosocial skills training (Kawakubo et al., 2007) in clin-ical populations.

Menning, Roberts and Pantev (2000) demonstrated that 3 weeks of intensive (~1hr/day) auditory frequency discrimination training produced significant increases in MMN amplitude that persisted for several weeks after the cessation of training in healthy volun-teers. Other studies have shown that MMN both predicts and corresponds to changes in language acquisition, musical training, and other auditory-dependent cognitive tasks in nonpsychiatric individuals. Likewise, MMN exhibits malleability after just 3 h of audi-tory training in dyslexic children, which was associated with a significant amelioration of cognitive impairment in phonological processing, reading, and writing (Lovio et al., 2012). Thus, changes in MMN are detectable in the early stages of cognitive training, predict generalized improvements in non-trained higher-order cognitive domains, and correspond to measurable changes of cortical plasticity in intact and impaired neuro-psychiatric populations.

Since MMN improves the prediction of psychosis in CHR individuals, and it reflects the neural systems targeted by TCT, it may prove useful in future treatment stratification algorithms. Current symptom-based models of diagnosis and treatment employ clinical assessment for symptom stabilization using medication, hospitalization, and psychotherapy as treatment methods. Biomarker profiles could indicate neural circuitry patterns subserving/predicting: 1) disruption of auditory processing centres calling for neuroplasticity-based cognitive enhancing treatment such as TCT; 2) neuropsychological impairment to be addressed with compensatory cognitive remediation strategies (e.g Twamley et al., 2012b); 3) maladaptive thoughts and social skills targeted by cognitive behavioural and social skills treatment for psychosis (e.g. Granholm et al., 2005); or 4) impaired role development requiring vocational training and rehabilitation services (e.g. Twamley et al., 2012a, 2013). If successful, biomarker-informed treatment stratification could delineate subgroups of individuals for better responses to even currently available treatments and contribute to future diagnostic classifications validated by predictive therapeutic utility (McGorry et al., 2013).

Consistent with the model of using MMN to predict and monitor response to interventions, Perez and colleagues (2017) conducted a proof of concept study of SZ patients who underwent MMN testing immediately before and after completing 1 h of a speeded time-order judgment task of two successive frequency-modulated sweeps (Posit Science 'Sound Sweeps' exercise that is an essential component of TCT; Tarasenko et al 2016). Perez et al. found that all SZ patients exhibited the expected improvements in auditory perceptual learning over the 1 h training period (p<0.001), consistent with previous results (Tarasenko et al., 2016). Larger MMN amplitudes recorded both before and after the training exercises were associated with greater gains in auditory perceptual learning (r=-0.5 and r=-0.67, respectively, p <0.01 for both). Significant pre- vs post-training MMN amplitude reduction was also observed (p<0.02). These findings support the view of MMN as a sensitive index of the neural systems engaged by auditory-based TCT in SZ and encourage future trials of MMN as a biomarker for individual assignment, prediction, and/or monitoring of patient response to pro-cognitive interventions, including auditory cognitive training in SZ.

Conclusions

(1) Individuals at high risk for developing psychosis as well as patients in the early stages of illness have consistently shown MMN reduction to duration changes; studies of MMNs to frequency changes in early stages of illness have yielded mixed findings.

(2) MMN studies suggest that patients with SZ have an impaired sensory memory encoding rather than sensory memory duration; furthermore, they may have a difficulty encoding environmental regularities, lacking the expected adaptability of MMN to stimulus likelihood.

(3) MMN current density analysis in SZ indicates abnormalities in multiple brain regions with marked impairments in medial frontal lobe sources.

(4) MMN reductions in SZ have been associated with impairments across several cognitive domains, including processing speed and attention, verbal and working memory, verbal fluency, and social cognition.

(5) MMN shows high test-retest reliability coefficients (ICCs=0.90) and therefore is promising for predicting and monitoring response to targeted CNS interventions.

7.2. **Major depression**

Major Depressive Disorder (MDD) is a debilitating psychiatric disorder characterized by a range of emotional and behavioural symptoms, with core features including persistently depressed mood and decreased interest or pleasure in activities usually enjoyed by the individual. MDD is also highly prevalent; for instance, it has been estimated that almost 20% of the population experience at least one clinically significant episode of depression in their lifetime (Kessler et al., 2009). It has been long observed that depressed patients perform poorly on cognitive tasks, especially those involving memory and concentration, and frequently display a slowing of cognitive processes. In their review, Hammar and Ardal (2009) concluded that depression is associated with cognitive impairment in the acute phase of the disorder (for a review, see Castaneda et al., 2008), and, further, that some studies (e.g. Kennedy et al., 2007) indicate that this impairment might be long lasting despite symptom reduction and recovery. Moreover, in their study on visual ERPs, Normann et al. (2007) provided evidence in humans for a central role of decreased synaptic plasticity in the pathophysiology of depression. In addition, Thomas and Elliott (2009), in their review, concluded that it seems that impaired cognitive performance in these patients is associated with reduced cortical function while normal performance can only be achieved through enhanced cortical function.

Because the MMN amplitude is, in general, attenuated with cognitive decline, then one would expect MMN amplitude attenuation in major depression. There are only a few MMN studies on depression. Most of these studies suggest that the MMN amplitude is indeed attenuated in depression. It was found by Takei et al. (2009) that the magnetic local field power (mGFP) of the MMNm in response to duration and frequency changes of pure-tone stimuli and in response to across-category vowel changes was considerably smaller in their major depressive disorder patients than in healthy control subjects. Further, because the P1m amplitude was not affected, the authors concluded that information processing at the pre-attentive level is impaired in major depressive disorder, and that this dysfunction is not due to a dysfunction at the lower level of information processing. In addition, because there was a lack of a significant correlation between the MMNm power and clinical symptoms, the authors suggested that the MMNm power reduction in these patients may be assumed to reflect the trait for developing major depressive disorder or the morbid process of developing this disorder. Moreover, the unchanged MMNm dipole location in the major depressive disorder patients in their study suggests, according to Takei et al. (2009) that MMNm abnormalities in these patients are more functional rather than structural.

Consistent Takei et al.'s (2009) results, Lv et al. (2010) obtained data suggesting that the MMN amplitude for novel sounds was attenuated compared with that in controls, but the fact that only an active behavioural discrimination task was used makes the interpretation of their results uncertain, as far as the MMN is concerned. The authors interpreted their pattern of results as suggesting that the ERP abnormality reflected by the fronto-central waveform elicited by novelty may be highly correlated with the negative experiences in depression.

In a further study by He et al. (2010), subjects were patients with treatment-resistant depression, those with borderline personality disorder and normal controls. The authors found that the frontal MMN amplitude for tone-frequency change of the patients with treatment-resistant depression was in fact larger than that of the controls, contrary to the authors' expectations (see also Kähkönen et al., 2007). As for the patients with the borderline personality disorder, their MMN amplitude did not differ from that of the controls. He et al. (2010) suggested that the relatively larger MMN at Fz (compared to those at Cz and Pz) might imply a lack of inhibition to the irrelevant stimuli or an increased cortical neuronal excitability (or both), especially in the frontal cortex, in the patients with depression. This lack of inhibition might then impact later stimulus evaluation processes (reflected by the reduced P3 amplitude). The authors further suggested that their results are in line with Bajbouj et al.'s (2006) study which demonstrated a cortical inhibition deficit using the trans-cranial magnetic stimulation in patients with unipolar major depressive disorder. Further results consistent with those of He et al. (2010) were provided by Ogura et al. (1991, 1993) who found an increased N2b amplitude for a wide tone-frequency change in depressed subjects aged 18–22 years, which might reflect the increased distractibility in these patients. In contrast, the MMN amplitude was attenuated in comparison with that in control subjects.

In patients with late-life depression, Naismith et al. (2012) found that the amplitude of their mastoid MMN, but not that recorded from fronto-central scalp sites, for tone-duration increase was considerably reduced, suggesting depression-related decrease of the auditory-cortex generated MMN. Importantly, there was a strong relationship between the MMN-amplitude decrease and self-rated disability (for both the left and right mastoid recordings). This MMN deficit was also linked to poorer semantic fluency as assessed by a neuropsychological task considered to recruit fronto-temporal and particularly temporal-lobe neural circuits (Rascovsky et al., 2007). However, as the authors also reported, the MMN deficit was not clearly associated with other neuro-psychological functions that probe fronto-temporal circuits, namely learning and memory, nor was the MMN deficit related to depressive symptom severity. Therefore the authors further concluded that their data pattern suggests that MMN dysfunction may exist as a relatively distinct marker of underlying brain change. Moreover, stressing their finding that MMN deficit in this sample was strongly associated with higher levels of disability, they suggested that this biomarker has 'relevance for daily functioning', highlighting the utility of the MMN for understanding the neuro-biological basis of affective disorders, even in the remitted state.

Previously, Lepistö et al. (2004), studying MMN in treatment-naive children with major depression, found that their MMN to syllable change peaked considerably earlier than that of control children (whereas the MMN amplitude was not affected), which led the authors to conclude that in major depression of childhood, the neural excitability of the central auditory system might be enhanced, probably reflecting the increased irritability of these patients, consistent with the diagnostic criteria of childhood depression in DSM-IV (American Psychiatric Association, 1994). This interpretation is supported by the enhanced P3a amplitude elicited by sounds disrupting performance in visual primary tasks (Escera et al., 1998, 2000a, 2001; Gumenyuk et al., 2001; Yago et al., 2001a). Moreover, the P3a amplitude is enhanced in several patient groups characterized by increased behavioural distractibility (Kaipio et al., 1999, 2000; Kilpeläinen et al., 1999; Polo et al., 2003). Hence, as further concluded by the authors, in children with major depression, the neural hyper-excitability, as suggested by the shortened MMN peak latency, may render the threshold for triggering involuntary attention switch abnormally low.

Conclusions

(1) Attenuation of the MMN amplitude has been reported in major depression, for instance, to frequency changes of pure tones and across-category vowel changes.

(2) However, also enhanced MMNs have been reported, including those to frequency and duration changes of tones. Furthermore, an association was found between MMNs to duration changes and self-rated disability and diminished semantic fluency. In children with major depression, shortened MMN peak latencies were found for syllable changes. The amplified and speeded MMNs may reflect enhanced neural excitability, consistent with the increased irritability associated with depression.

7.3. **Bipolar disorder**

Bipolar Disorder (BD) is a highly heritable, chronic, and disabling illness which has a complex aetiology. Attempts have been made to determine endophenotypes that can reduce the phenotypic complexity of bipolar disorder, improve the power in the identification of possible gene carriers, and help in clarifying the genetic and biological basis of the disorder (Hall et al., 2007). At the end of the 19th century, it was thought that affective psychosis could be separated from dementia praecox by the fact that BD patients tended to experience natural remission without cognitive dysfunctions whereas patients with dementia praecox did not. However, later it was realized that patients with BD and other recurring mood disorders also can show cognitive impairments (Bulbena & Berrios 1993; Tham et al., 1997).

As a possible reason for this dysfunction, Tham et al. (1997) found that the patients with impaired cognitive functioning had a larger number of hospitalization episodes and their illness was longer in duration than that of the BD patients with normal cognitive functioning. Further, previous studies appeared to indicate that the cognitive dysfunctions in BD are state dependent (e.g. Coffman et al., 1990). However, cognitive impairments have also been found in euthymic BD patients, thus suggesting that these cognitive dysfunctions represent a trait marker (Sapin et al., 1987; Savard et al., 1980; Tham et al., 1997). Consistent with this idea, during a depressive episode, acute phase of illness, or remission, BD patients demonstrated neuropsychological deficits in executive function, verbal learning, immediate and delayed verbal memory, abstraction and set-shifting, sustained attention, response inhibition, and psychomotor speed (Robinson et al., 2006; Thompson et al., 2005); for a review, see Takei et al. (2010).

Nevertheless, in contrast to schizophrenia, many studies of BD patients have failed to identify attenuated MMN amplitude (Catts et al., 1995; Hall et al., 2007, 2009; Kaur et al., 2012; Salisbury et al., 2007; Takei et al., 2010; Umbricht et al., 2003) even though cognitive decline in different cognitive brain disorders is usually associated with the attenuation of the MMN amplitude (for reviews, see Näätänen et al., 2010, 2012, 2014). Takei et al. (2010), however, found that the peak latencies of the MMNm for tone-duration increment and frequency change were prolonged in the right hemisphere of patients with BD, in comparison with those of controls. There was also an equivalent current location difference in the left hemisphere between the patients and controls.

Moreover, Andersson et al., (2008), studying patients with bipolar II disorder, found that their MMN for tone-duration decrement was smaller in amplitude and longer in peak latency in comparison to those of the controls and, further, that the patients performed worse than controls in different neuropsychological tasks. Moreover, Reite et al. (2009) have described structural and functional abnormalities in the auditory cortex of BD patients which, according to the authors, may be related to the cognitive impairments observed in these patients (Bruder et al., 1975, 1981).

Conclusion

Whereas many studies failed to find attenuated MMN amplitudes in BD, some studies have shown diminished and delayed MMNs to tone-duration deviant stimuli. A delayed right-hemispheric MMN was also found in such patients.

7.4. **Post-traumatic stress disorder**

Post-Traumatic Stress Disorder (PTSD) may develop as a consequence of a traumatic event that is beyond normal human experience. Soldiers in combat, for instance, are at risk of developing PTSD, as also are victims of traffic accidents. Most individuals with PTSD continuously re-experience the traumatic event, persistently avoiding stimuli and situations associated with this event, and showing chronic hyperarousal (for a review, see Ge et al., 2011). In their pioneering study, Morgan and Grillon (1999), studying a group of sexual assault victims, found that the MMN amplitude for a tone-frequency change was significantly larger in the affected individuals than that in controls (Fig. 7.4). It was concluded that there were abnormalities in the preconscious auditory sensory memory

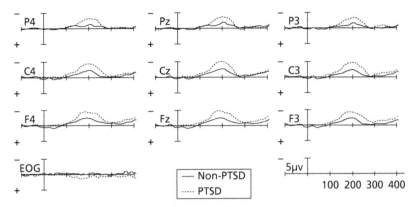

Fig. 7.4 The MMN amplitude for a tone-frequency change is enhanced in patients with post-traumatic stress disorder (PTSD) compared to that in control subjects.

Reprinted from Biological Psychiatry, 45(7), Charles A Morgan and Christian Grillon, *Abnormal mismatch negativity in women with sexual assault-related posttraumatic stress disorder*, 827–832, Copyright 1999, with permission from Elsevier.

in patients with PTSD that were manifested as increased sensitivity to stimulus changes at the automatic level. Subsequently, Ge et al. (2011) investigated survivors of a tremendous earthquake that occurred in the Sichuan Province, China, in 2008 that measured 8.0 on the Richter Scale and killed about 69,000 people. Subjects were not injured and received no psychiatric treatment or medication before the study but they exhibited significantly enhanced MMN amplitudes for a minor tone-frequency change, interpreted as suggesting the presence of an increased sensitivity of the automatic stimulus-comparator mechanism, which may reflect 'generalized chronic hyperarousal that sensitizes PTSD victims to any change in the environment' (p. 234).

Cornwell et al. (2007) aimed to determine brain regions that show potentiated responses to stimulus deviation during anticipatory anxiety, 'a key symptom of anxiety disorders such as posttraumatic stress disorder' (p. 282). Tone sequences with occasional frequency changes were presented in a passive oddball paradigm under two different conditions: during a threat of an unpleasant electric shock and a 'safe' condition. Source analyses of MMNm revealed greater right auditory-cortex and inferior parietal-cortex response to deviant stimuli under threat relative to the safe condition. It was also found that brain structures related to the evaluation of threat, the left amygdala and the right insula, showed increased activity to stimulus deviation under threat. According to the authors, these findings fit with evidence of a potentiated MMN in PTSD relative to healthy controls and 'warrant closer evaluation of how these structures might form a functional network mediating sensitization to stimulus deviance during anticipatory anxiety' (p. 282). Further, 'heightened vigilance, whether by experimentally induced anxiety or by chronic anxiety, sensitizes the individual to changes in the auditory environment, which may in turn facilitate auditory discriminative processes' (p. 286). For a meta-analytic review of the ERP studies in PTSD, see Karl et al., (2006). It can be concluded that MMN/MMNm to frequency change is enhanced in amplitude in patients suffering from PTSD, signaling their sensitization to abrupt auditory changes.

Conclusion

MMN amplitudes in PTSD victims (sexual assault victims and earthquake survivors) were found to be enhanced to tone-frequency changes. This was interpreted to reflect generalized and increased hyperarousal sensitizing individuals with PTSD to environmental changes.

7.5. **Panic disorder**

Panic Disorder is a mental disorder characterized by recurrent panic attacks and worrying about having subsequent attacks. In medication-free patients with panic disorder, it was found by Chang et al. (2015), using the multi-feature MMN paradigm of Näätänen et al. (2004), that these patients had a significantly increased MMN amplitude for sound intensity and location changes compared with those elicited in healthy controls. The correlation between the intensity-MMN amplitude and disorder severity was also significant. Tang et al. (2013) recently used vMMN to study the detection of facial emotions in patients with panic disorder. (For the expression-related MMN, see the review by Liu et al., 2016). vMMN was recorded in 12 patients to schematic facial emotions. It was found that the vMMN amplitude for both the negative and positive emotions was significantly decreased in these patients in comparison with that of age- and education-matched controls.

Conclusion

In patients with panic disorder, the MMN amplitude is enhanced in response to auditory change and, further, that the MMN amplitude for intensity change correlates with the severity of the panic disorder. However vMMN amplitude appears to be decreased in patients with panic disorder compared to controls.

7.6. **Alcohol and alcoholism**

Acute effects

MMN has provided a major contribution to our understanding of the acute and chronic effects of alcohol on cognitive processing and its brain basis (for a review, see Ahveninen et al., 2000a). Jääskeläinen et al. (1995b) used a dichotic-listening task to determine the acute effects of ethanol on different ERP components. Subjects were ten healthy young adult volunteers (social drinkers). The standards were tones of 300 Hz and deviants those of 330 Hz in the left ear while the frequencies in the right ear were 1000 Hz and 1100 Hz, respectively. Subjects performed a target-detection task in a designated ear while being instructed to ignore all input to the opposite ear. Alcohol attenuated the MMN amplitude proportionally more than that of any other ERP component measured (N1, P2, N2b, P3b, processing negativity). On these grounds, the authors concluded that automatic processes are first affected by alcohol and that this occurs at a relatively low dose of alcohol (at blood-alcohol concentration (BAC) 0.05–0.06 ‰). Moreover, the dampening of the automatic change-detection process outside of the focus of attention reduces the attentional switch triggered by the pre-attentive change-detection process (indexed by MMN), a prerequisite for the occurrence of an attentional switch to change. Consequently, the MMN attenuation indexes an increased accident risk due to a deficient orienting of attention to acoustic changes. For instance, traffic accidents in which the driver was engaged in a secondary activity when encountering a hazard might result from a decreased ability, due to alcohol intoxication, to detect unattended stimuli and stimulus changes in the environment.

These results were confirmed and extended by Jääskeläinen et al. (1995a) who found that the MMN-amplitude suppression was relatively stronger with smaller stimulus changes, implicating that the threshold for detecting acoustic deviations outside the scope of attention is elevated after ingestion of alcohol. Because the attention-related ERP components were, in contrast, not affected by alcohol it was concluded that:

> automatic high-level processing is more sensitive to low dosages of alcohol than is attention-dependent processing, at least within the auditory modality. The total reduction of the MMN amplitude caused by alcohol intoxication was proportionally high and seems to be larger than the alcohol effect on the other ERP components that we studied, at least with low BAC. In addition, MMN elicited by the smaller magnitude of frequency change was attenuated by alcohol more than MMN elicited by the larger magnitude of frequency deviation. This suggests that the effect of alcohol on MMN is pronounced when stimulus deviations are relatively small (Jääskeläinen et al., 1995a, p. 494).

Subsequently, these results were confirmed and extended by the MMNm results of Kähkönen et al. (2005).

In their next study, Jääskeläinen et al. (1996c) wished to determine alcohol effects separately on the two MMN subcomponents, the auditory- and frontal-cortex ones. It was concluded that the MMN-amplitude attenuation observed was mainly due to the effect of alcohol on the frontal MMN subcomponent only, with the supra-temporal MMN generator being relatively resistant to alcohol (Fig. 7.5). This would suggest, according to the authors, that the locus of the alcohol effects on the central auditory processing is above the level of the basic sensory processing occurring in auditory cortex. Hence, alcohol had an effect on the brain mechanisms leading to an attention switch beyond the pre-perceptual change detection occurring in auditory cortex. Consequently, in view of the role of the MMN-generator activation in passive attention in audition (Näätänen, 1990, 1992; Schröger, 1996), the frontal MMN suppression by alcohol may be related to an increased risk of traffic and other accidents. A strong effect of alcohol on the MMN amplitude was observed even at modest doses of alcohol which gives a serious warning signal to those who believe that it is fully safe to drive after the ingestion of 'only' a couple of beers (see also Grillon et al., 1995). Nevertheless, Jääskeläinen et al. (1996a) also observed some positive effects of alcohol on cognitive task performance. They used a visual choice-reaction time (RT) task in which each visual stimulus

The differential effects
of ethanol on MMN

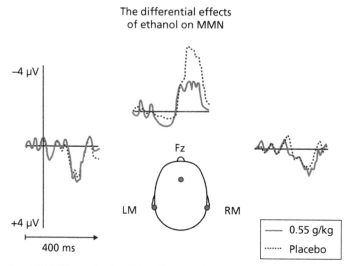

Fig. 7.5 The frontal MMN amplitude, elicited by tone duration changes, is attenuated by an acute ethanol intoxication (0.55 g/kg dose of alcohol) whereas the mastoid-recorded (with a nose reference) MMN amplitudes are not affected.

Reprinted from Biological Psychology, 43(1), Jääskeläinen, I., Pekkonen, E., Hirvonen, J., Sillanaukee, P., and Näätänen R., *Mismatch negativity subcomponents and ethyl alcohol*, 13–25, Copyright 1996, with permission from Elsevier.

was shortly preceded either by an auditory standard stimulus (a tone of 600 Hz), a deviant stimulus (a tone of 660 Hz), or a 'novel' sound (e.g. a telephone ringing). In the placebo condition, RT was prolonged by a preceding deviant or novel sound, and the hit rate was decreased by deviant sounds. During alcohol intoxication, however, the hit-rate decrease caused by deviant tones was significantly smaller than that in the placebo condition. This suggests, according to the authors, that the attention-capturing effects of disturbing sounds were suppressed by alcohol. Consequently, a small dose of alcohol may even improve cognitive performance in noisy conditions. These results were corroborated by Jääskelainen et al. (1999), who found that an RT prolongation caused by a task-irrelevant frequency change in the task stimuli was attenuated in the alcohol condition in comparison with the placebo condition. According to the authors, their findings 'demonstrate a detrimental effect of alcohol on involuntary attention shifting, evident with doses considerably smaller than previously described, and still acceptable in road traffic in most countries' (p. 16). Moreover, this data pattern was observed even at a dose (0.3 g/kg), which was far lower than those previously documented (for a review, see Jääskeläinen et al., 1996b).

Hirvonen et al. (2000) aimed to determine the possible role of the adenosine receptors in the suppression of the MMN amplitude by alcohol. It was found that caffeine, a selective antagonist of the adenosine A1 and A2a receptors, at concentrations achieved during normal consumption, blocked the effects of alcohol on the MMN peak latency at a relatively low dose. This novel finding suggests, according to the authors, that the alcohol-induced disturbance on MMN is caused by an alcohol-induced increase in extra-cellular adenosine levels acting on the A1 and A2a receptors, which are abundant in the temporal and frontal cortices involved in MMN generation. Importantly, the detrimental effects of alcohol on P3b and processing negativity were not blocked by caffeine, which suggests, according to the authors, a relatively specific role of the adenosine receptors in the generation of, and in the detrimental alcohol action on, MMN.

Naltrexone, an opioid antagonist used in the treatment of alcoholics, was employed by Jääskeläinen et al. (1998). Alcohol when ingested alone prolonged the MMN peak latency for a tone-frequency change. This effect was further increased when alcohol and nal-trexone were ingested together. It was concluded that the detrimental effects of alcohol on involuntary attention were augmented by naltrexone. In the visual modality, Kenemans et al. (2010) obtained vMMN results analogous to those in the auditory modality, con-cluding that 'a moderate amount of alcohol that is considered legally acceptable in many societies, disrupts a dedicated, rapid visual-cortex mechanism that may be crucial for the detection of unexpected events outside the focus of attention' (p. 844).

On the basis of these studies, it can be concluded that alcohol dramatically attenuates the auditory MMN amplitude and that this effect can be observed even at low alcohol dos-ages, resulting in elevated thresholds of detecting acoustic deviations outside the scope of attention and therefore an increased risk of traffic and other types of accidents even at low doses of alcohol. Importantly, effects of alcohol on pre-attentive processing, as reflected by MMN and P3a, may sometimes be even greater than those on higher-level processing, judging from the fact that alcohol effects on MMN were relatively stronger than those on longer-latency ERP components reflecting higher-level processing. Consistent with this, alcohol effects on the frontal MMN subcomponent are stronger than those on the auditory-cortex MMN subcomponent, accounting for the detrimental effects of alcohol on the brain mechanisms of involuntary attention switching and thereby the elevated acci-dent risk. In the visual modality, analogous MMN results were obtained by using vMMN. The dampening effect of even small amounts of alcohol on the attention-switching mech-anism for unattended peripheral changes may even have life-threatening effects.

Chronic alcoholism

In chronic alcoholism, MMN shows a delay in stimulus discrimination, an increased distractibility by task-irrelevant changes, and a shortened sensory-memory duration, an index of decreased brain plasticity (Näätänen & Kreegipuu, 2010). Kathmann et al. (1995) found a delayed MMN peak latency for a wide frequency change in detoxified chronic alcoholics performing a visual tracking task, consistent with the previous 'N2' results of Realmuto et al. (1993). Some studies, however, showed that soon after the onset of abstin-ence from chronic alcohol abuse, there is a period lasting for some weeks when ERP/MEG responses, at least in the hemisphere ipsilateral to the ear stimulated, are accelerated, such as MMNm (Pekkonen et al., 1998) which can be attributed to the hyperexcitation of the brain related to alcohol withdrawal. MMN studies also showed that chronic alcoholism has detrimental effects on different forms of memory, at least on sensory and working memories. Ahveninen et al. (1999) found that an increased backward masking in these patients abolished MMN but not that in social drinkers. Importantly, in chronic alcoholism, the MMN-amplitude decrement correlated with an impaired performance in the ACT (auditory consonant trigrams test; Peterson & Peterson, 1959). Furthermore, the MMN-amplitude attenuation by masking significantly correlated with the patients' self-reported weekly alcohol consumption. It was concluded that MMN might provide the first index of the functional brain damage developed in the early stages of alcoholism and, further, that the MMN backward-masking paradigm may provide an objective method for the evaluation of the early-phase changes in alcohol-induced CNS disorders.

Chronic alcoholism also makes the affected individuals more easily distractible by irrelevant stimulation. Ahveninen et al. (2000b) found that occasional irrelevant changes in tone frequency elicited MMN which was larger in amplitude in individuals with alcoholism with an early than late onsets. The authors concluded that attentional deficits in the abstinent alcoholics, as indicated by MMN and RT, suggest that the MMN enhancement reflected impaired neural inhibition of involuntary attention shifting in these patients. For corroborating P3a results, see Polo et al. (2003). P3a diminished in amplitude toward normal values as the withdrawal period continued. Subsequently, Marco-Pallares et al. (2007), studying MMN for tone-duration change, found evidence indicating that the automatic discrimination of these changes was deteriorated in chronic alcoholism. An attenuated MMN was observed in the left frontal and right anterior and posterior temporal areas.

MMN results also indicate the life-long cumulative effects of alcohol abuse. Polo et al. (1999), studying MMN generation in young and middle-aged chronic alcoholics, found that in these patients (with a mean abstinence of 56 days), the MMN peak amplitude was diminished in older alcoholics, whereas no MMN-amplitude reduction was observed in younger alcoholics (Fig. 7.6). It was concluded that the automatic stimulus-change detector mechanism of the brain, reflected by MMN generation, is impaired in chronic alcoholics over the age of 40 years, suggesting that the neuro-toxic effects of chronic consumption of alcohol are more prone to appear after a critical age, consistent with numerous previous studies (e.g. Berglund et al., 1987; Pfefferbaum et al., 1997, 1998).

Chronic alcoholism also shortens the duration of sensory memory, an index of general brain plasticity. In a particularly important study, Grau et al. (2001) found that the sensory-memory trace duration, as indexed by MMN, was shortened in abstinent chronic alcoholics. These authors recorded MMN to infrequent decrements in tone duration while subjects were performing a visual task. It was found that with an ISI of 0.4 s, there was no significant difference between the chronic alcoholics and age-matched controls. However, when the ISI was prolonged to 5 s, then no significant MMN was elicited in the patients any more whereas MMN was still present in the controls. It was suggested that this shortening of the sensory-memory duration, indexed by MMN, may functionally reflect grey-matter volume loss in the auditory cortex previously found by using MRI in patients with chronic alcoholism (Pfefferbaum et al.,

Difference wave

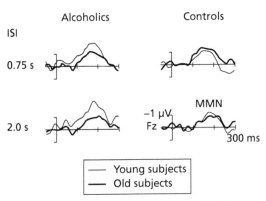

Fig. 7.6 MMN in abstinent chronic alcoholics and healthy control subjects with inter-stimulus intervals of 0.75 s and 2.0 s, after dividing the groups according to age into young and old subjects, cutoff point being 40 years of age. MMN was attenuated in chronic alcoholics, who were older than 40 years of age.

Reproduced from Polo, D., Escera, C., Gual, A., and Grau. C., *Mismatch Negativity and Auditory Sensory Memory in Chronic Alcoholics*, Alcoholism: Clinical and Experimental Research, 23(11), 1744–1750, Figure 2, DOI: 10.1111/j.1530-0277.1999.tb04069.x, Copyright © 1999, Research Society on Alcoholism.

1997, 1998) and decreased brain plasticity in these patients. Consistent with this, MMN in chronic alcoholism is a state rather than trait marker (Fein et al., 2004; Cloninger et al., 1986). However, it was found by Zhang et al. (2001) that high-risk individuals (with fathers diagnosed as alcohol dependent and hospitalized for chronic alcoholism) have a larger-amplitude MMN for a change in tone frequency than that in controls. The authors proposed that their results offer the possibility that, as measured by MMN, high-risk individuals may be characterized by a deficit in cortical inhibition (excessive neural excitation) and, further, that this pre-existing CNS excitatory state may lead to ethanol use for self-medication. As already mentioned, a CNS hyper-excitability in chronic alcoholism was demonstrated by accelerated MMN (Ahveninen et al., 2000b) and MMNm responses (Pekkonen et al., 1998a).

The effects of chronic alcoholism on MMN may be summarized as follows: the MMN peak-latency prolongation and amplitude attenuation observed in chronic alcoholism reflect delayed and less sensitive auditory stimulus discrimination in these patients and provide the first index of functional brain damage in the early stages of chronic alcoholism, demonstrating an accelerated age-related decrease of general brain plasticity in these patients.

Conclusions

(1) Even a small dose of alcohol diminishes the amplitude of the MMN, particularly its frontal component. This is associated with diminished distractibility and may lead to insufficient sensitivity to react to potentially important environmental events.

(2) Soon after the abstinence from chronic alcohol abuse the MMN/MMNm is enhanced, presumably reflecting neural hyperexcitation and elevated distractibility.

(3) Backward masking abolishes the MMN in alcoholics but not in social drinkers, suggesting vulnerability to memory-trace disruption. MMN is also abnormally diminished by stimulus interval prolongation in alcoholics, which suggests shortened duration of the memory trace. These atypical MMN findings may contribute to the memory dysfunctions observed in alcoholics.

Chapter 8

Concluding discussion

This book has shown that the MMN/MMNm has had a profound impact on cognitive neuroscience with several promising applications for improving the understanding and treatment of different clinical conditions. One might therefore wonder what potential common underlying factors could link MMN/MMNm deficiency to such a broad range of heterogeneous clinical conditions. In the past four decades since the initial description of the MMN component, a common factor that has emerged across the different conditions appears to be acquired or progressive deterioration of CNS function. In this context, MMN also offers a unique vista into the neural substrates of cognitive deficits: neuroplasticity. In patients with CNS impairments, acquired either due to injury or illness, the brain is not able to develop and maintain accurate representations or memory traces for sensory stimuli. This process is robustly reflected in the MMN response using conventional passive auditory oddball paradigms. Innovative procedures for eliciting MMN and isolating plasticity have also been developed. As proposed by Baldeweg and Hirsch (2015), the 'memory-trace effect' can be quantified to assess the capability of the brain to encode auditory stimulus events and to maintain these representations.

In other words, the MMN/MMNm is a probe of the plasticity of the central auditory system and thereby, possibly, that of the functional condition of the whole brain. This idea is supported by the close connections between the MMN and cognitive status reviewed in the foregoing: it indeed appears that the lower level, sensory representations as measured via MMN/MMNm tap into the requisite neurophysiological substrates of higher-level cognitive operations (see Thomas et al., 2017).

Consistent with this hierarchical information processing cascade model of Thomas et al. (2017; see *Chapter 7* in schizophrenia; *Chapter 8*, Verhaeghen & Salthouse, 1997; Salthouse, 1991), changes in the cognitive system are associated with 'some general and fundamental mechanism'. Moreover, Pichora-Fuller (2003) proposed that cognitive deterioration associated with aging might reflect widespread neural degeneration, including the neural mechanisms of perception. Similarly, since auditory sensitivity and visual accuracy are strongly correlated with age-related variations in intelligence, Lindenberger and Baltes (1994) argued that the age-related decrement in sensory processing and cognition has a shared pathophysiological basis, which appears to be a general decrease in brain plasticity reflected by attenuated MMN amplitudes indexing affected memory-trace formation and maintenance which, in turn, results in lower fidelity sensory representations and compromised cognitive functioning. Moreover, the mounting evidence of associations among low-level perceptual functioning with higher-order cognition underscores the importance of fully accounting for perceptual deficits when investigating cognitive decline in older age (Roberts & Allen, 2016). This general decrease of brain plasticity in aging and in different cognitive brain disorders might, besides structural age-related changes, result, to a large extent, from age-related changes in the NMDA-receptors and the other neurotransmitter systems (for a review, see Magnusson et al., 1998). There is compelling evidence for the role of a deficient NMDA-receptor action in the generation of attenuated MMNs in different animals (for a review, see Baldeweg & Hirsch 2015). Moreover, Schmidt et al. (2012) showed that in human subjects an NMDA-receptor blockage reduced the magnitude of the memory-trace effect, indexing decreased brain plasticity.

For instance, in chronic alcoholism, the brain change, exceeding that due to normal aging, illustrates a clear case of dramatically decreased brain plasticity in that the MMN is strongly attenuated in amplitude. This abnormality is further increased when the SOA is prolonged, indexing the abnormally short duration of sensory-memory traces in these patients. Such an adverse effect appears to accumulate with increased age: it was shown by Polo et al. (1999) that the MMN-amplitude attenuation (for tone-frequency change) occurred in patients in an accelerating manner after a critical age, approximately 40 years (see also Kiang et al, 2009). Consequently, in chronic alcoholism, MMN data suggest an accelerated age-related decrement of brain plasticity.

Further, in some patients in a comatose state who do not imminently regain consciousness, no MMN can be recorded, demonstrating that memory traces are not formed for sensory stimuli; that is, brain plasticity is temporarily lost or at least at a very low level. In contrast, the presence of MMN among comatose patients indicates the recovery of the ability of the brain to form sensory-memory traces, and foreshadows the recovery of consciousness in these as-yet unconscious patients. Likewise, when a patient is emerging from a persistent vegetative state, the MMN response rapidly increases in amplitude, demonstrating the functional recovery of brain plasticity permitting memory-trace formation.

In aging, the MMN gradually decreases in amplitude, with the magnitude of this attenuation correlating with the concomitant normal decline in cognition, suggesting an age-related decrease in brain plasticity. This age-related MMN-amplitude decrease is dramatically amplified by the prolongation of the SOA, indicating that reduced brain plasticity is indeed involved as sensory-memory traces can no longer be maintained for longer than 1–2 s.

Importantly, reduced brain plasticity may also be present in the early phase of life in certain developmental brain disorders. For instance, in 7–8 years old children with cleft palate, the MMN amplitude for tone-frequency change was of normal amplitude with short SOAs (350 and 700 ms), whereas the prolongation of the SOA to 1400 ms attenuated their MMN amplitude much more than it attenuated that of age-matched control children (Čeponiene et al., 1999a). An analogous pattern of results was observed in infants with cleft palate; this abnormality was even greater in magnitude in children with the CATCH-22 Syndrome (Cheour et al., 1997, 1998, 1999).

In addition, an abnormally short sensory-memory duration, as reflected by MMN data, was associated with a delayed linguistic development in children. Grossheinrich et al. (2010) showed that late talkers had a shorter sensory-memory duration, as judged from MMN data for tone-frequency change as a function of the ISI, recorded at the age of 4 years and 7 months. In addition, Barry et al. (2008) obtained MMN data for tone-frequency change as a function of the ISI that suggested a shorter sensory-memory duration in parents of children with specific language impairment than that of control parents of normally developing children.

In the case of stroke, besides the local damage, there are also widespread cortical sequelae that may also result in decreases in general brain plasticity. Särkämö et al. (2010) suggested that the improved recovery of their stroke patients caused by music and speech stimuli presented to the patients resulted from long-term plastic changes induced by the stimulation, that is, increased brain plasticity.

Consequently, it now appears that the MMN/MMNm provides a unique access to brain plasticity, which is affected in a very wide range of cognitive brain disorders and which therefore is of central importance in clinical brain research and patient work. However, before the MMN really is ready for every-day clinical patient work, some procedural improvements still have to be made, in particular in biosignal analysis and interpretation, in order to obtain reliable information even at the single-patient level. For recent considerable progress toward this end, see Schall et al. (2016), Bishop and Hardiman (2010), Ponton et al. (1997), Sinkkonen and Tervaniemi (2000), Petermann et al. (2009), McGee et al. (1997), Kalyakin et al. (2007, 2008, 2009), and Light et al. (2015).

In summary, there are several promising clinical applications of MMN/MMNm, including:

(1) The prediction of conversion to psychosis among clinically at-risk individuals.

(2) The prediction of the recovery of consciousness and cognitive capabilities in patients in a comatose or persistent vegetative state.

(3) The early identification of the presence of mild cognitive impairment (MCI), in particular that of the amnestic MCI (aMCI), the one that is the most likely to progress to Alzheimer's disease. Here the MMN provides an objective evaluation of the memory function of the patient, using in particular the sensory-memory duration indexed by the MMN as a general index of brain plasticity. This information could guide clinicians in their treatment decisions, in evaluating treatment effectiveness, and in monitoring the progress of the disorder.

(4) The objective evaluation of the cognitive and functional status of the patient and that of cognitive decline occurring in different brain disorders such as schizophrenia, epilepsy, Parkinson's disease, Alzheimer's disease, MCI, and multiple sclerosis.

(5) The prediction of cognitive recovery after the occurrence of a stroke or other brain injury and that of the effectiveness of different potential means to facilitate and expedite this recovery.

(6) The objective monitoring of age-related cognitive brain change and, possibly, testing the effectiveness of different potential countermeasures to slow down this age-related cognitive decline.

(7) The feature-specific monitoring of the early central auditory system development by means of MMN recordings conducted at different time points in infants and young children, which can be extended even to the foetal stage by using the MMNm.

(8) The monitoring of the age-appropriate development of the infant and child´s sensory-memory duration as an index of brain plasticity.

(9) The prediction of reading problems (dyslexia) emerging at the school age from MMN recordings conducted in small infants and children and the objective testing of the effectiveness of different forms of rehabilitation.

(10) The objective assessment of the functioning of the cochlear implant; MMN amplitude is highly correlated with speech perception in these patients.

(11) The use of the MMN for the pre-clinical evaluation of novel therapeutic agents.

References

Aaltonen, O., Tuomainen, J., Laine, M., & Niemi, P. (1993). Cortical differences in tonal versus vowel processing as revealed by an ERP component called mismatch negativity (MMN). *Brain and Language, 44*(2), 139–52. doi:10.1006/brln.1993.1009

Ahmed, M., Mallo, T., Leppänen, P. H. T., Hämäläinen, J., Äyräväinen, L., Ruusuvirta, T., & Astikainen, P. (2011). Mismatch brain response to speech sound changes in rats. *Frontiers in Psychology, 2*, 283.

Ahnaou, A., Huysmans, H., Biermans, R., Manyakov, N., & Drinkenburg, W. (2017). Ketamine: differential neurophysiological dynamics in functional networks in the rat brain. *Translational Psychiatry, 7*(9), e1237.

Ahveninen, J., Escera, C., Polo, M. D., Grau, C., & Jaaskelainen, I. P. (2000a). Acute and chronic effects of alcohol on preattentive auditory processing as reflected by mismatch negativity. *Audiology and Neuro-Otology, 5*(6), 303–11. doi:10.1159/000013896

Ahveninen, J., Jääskeläinen, I. P., Pekkonen, E., Hallberg, A., Hietanen, M., Mäkelä, R., et al. (1999). Suppression of mismatch negativity by backward masking predicts impaired working-memory performance in alcoholics. *Alcoholism-Clinical and Experimental Research, 23*(9), 1507–14. doi:10.1097/00000374-199909000-00013

Ahveninen, J., Jääskeläinen, I. P., Pekkonen, E., Hallberg, A., Hietanen, M., Näätänen, R., et al. (2000b). Increased distractibility by task-irrelevant sound changes in abstinent alcoholics. *Alcoholism: Clinical and Experimental Research, 24*(12), 1850–4.

Akatsuka, K., Wasaka, T., Nakata, H., Inui, K., Hoshiyama, M., & Kakigi, R. (2005). Mismatch responses related to temporal discrimination of somatosensory stimulation. *Clinical Neurophysiology, 116*(8), 1930–7. doi:10.1016/j.clinph.2005.04.021

Akatsuka, K., Wasaka, T., Nakata, H., Kida, T., Hoshiyama, M., Tamura, Y., & Kakigi, R. (2007a). Objective examination for two-point stimulation using a somatosensory oddball paradigm: An MEG study. *Clinical Neurophysiology, 118*(2), 403–11. doi:10.1016/j.clinph.2006.09.030

Akatsuka, K., Wasaka, T., Nakata, H., Kida, T., & Kakigi, R. (2007b). The effect of stimulus probability on the somatosensory mismatch field. *Experimental Brain Research, 181*(4), 607–14. doi:10.1007/s00221-007-0958-4

Alain, C., McDonald, K. L., Ostroff, J. M., & Schneider, B. (2004). Aging: a switch from automatic to controlled processing of sounds? *Psychology and Aging, 19*(1), 125–33. doi:10.1037/0882-7974.19.1.125

Alain, C., & Woods, D. L. (1999). Age-related changes in processing auditory stimuli during visual attention: Evidence for deficits in inhibitory control and sensory memory. *Psychology and Aging, 14*(3), 507–19. doi:10.1037/0882-7974.14.3.507

Alain, C., Woods, D. L., & Ogawa, K. H. (1994). Brain indices of automatic pattern processing. *NeuroReport, 6*(1), 140–4. doi:10.1097/00001756-199412300-00036

Alain, C., Zendel, B. R., Hutka, S., & Bidelman, G. M. (2014). Turning down the noise: The benefit of musical training on the aging auditory brain. *Hearing Research, 308*, 162–73. doi:10.1016/j.heares.2013.06.008

Alcantara, J. I., Weisblatt, E. J. L., Moore, B. C. J., & Bolton, P. F. (2004). Speech-in-noise perception in high-functioning individuals with autism or Asperger's syndrome. *Journal of Child Psychology and Psychiatry, 45*(6), 1107–14. doi:DOI 10.1111/j.1469-7610.2004.t01-1-00303.x

Alho, K. (1995). Cerebral generators of mismatch negativity (MMN) and its magnetic counterpart (MMNm) elicited by sound changes. *Ear and Hearing, 16*(1), 38–51.

Alho, K., Connolly, J. F., Cheour, M., Lehtokoski, A., Huotilainen, M., Virtanen, J., et al. (1998). Hemispheric lateralization in preattentive processing of speech sounds. *Neuroscience Letters, 258*(1), 9–12.

Alho, K., Donauer, N., Paavilainen, P., Reinikainen, K., Sams, M., & Näätänen, R. (1987a). Stimulus selection during auditory spatial attention as expressed by event-related potentials. *Biological Psychology, 24*(2), 153–62. doi:10.1016/0301-0511(87)90022-6

Alho, K., Escera, C., Diaz, R., Yago, E., & Serra, J. M. (1997). Effects of involuntary auditory attention on visual task performance and brain activity. *NeuroReport, 8*(15), 3233–7.

Alho, K., Sainio, K., Sajaniemi, N., Reinikainen, K., & Naatanen, R. (1990). Event-related brain potential of human newborns to pitch change of an acoustic stimulus. *Electroencephalography and Clinical Neurophysiology, 77*(2), 151–5.

Alho, K., Teder, W., Lavikainen, J., & Näätänen, R. (1994a). Strongly focused attention and auditory event-related potentials. *Biological Psychology, 38*(1), 73–90.

Alho, K., Tervaniemi, M., Huotilainen, M., Lavikainen, J., Tiitinen, H., Ilmoniemi, R. J., et al. (1996). Processing of complex sounds in the human auditory cortex as revealed by magnetic brain responses. *Psychophysiology, 33*(4), 369–75. doi:10.1111/j.1469-8986.1996.tb01061.x

Alho, K., Tottola, K., Reinikainen, K., Sams, M., & Näätänen, R. (1987b). Brain mechanism of selective listening reflected by event-related potentials. *Electroencephalography and Clinical Neurophysiology, 68*(6), 458–70.

Alho, K., Woods, D. L., Algazi, A., Knight, R. T., & Näätänen, R. (1994b). Lesions of frontal cortex diminish the auditory mismatch negativity. *Electroencephalography and Clinical Neurophysiology, 91*(5), 353–62.

Alho, K., Woods, D. L., Algazi, A., & Näätänen, R. (1992). Intermodal selective attention. II. Effects of attentional load on processing of auditory and visual stimuli in central space. *Electroencephalography and Clinical Neurophysiology, 82*(5), 356–68.

Althen, H., Grimm, S., & Escera, C. (2011). Fast detection of unexpected sound intensity decrements as revealed by human evoked potentials. *PLoS ONE, 6*(12). doi:10.1371/journal.pone.0028522

Amann, L. C., Gandal, M. J., Halene, T. B., Ehrlichman, R. S., White, S. L., McCarren, H. S., & Siegel, S. J. (2010). Mouse behavioral endophenotypes for schizophrenia. *Brain Research Bulletin, 83*(3–4), 147–61. doi:10.1016/j.brainresbull.2010.04.008

Amminger, G. P., Schäfer, M. R., Papageorgiou, K., Klier, C. M., Cotton, S. M., Harrigan M, S. M., et al. (2010). Long-chain ω-3 fatty acids for indicated prevention of psychotic disorders: A randomized, placebo-controlled trial. *Archives of General Psychiatry, 67*(2), 146–54. doi:10.1001/archgenpsychiatry.2009.192

Andersson, S., Barder, H. E., Hellvin, T., Løvdahl, H., & Malt, U. F. (2008). Neuropsychological and electrophysiological indices of neurocognitive dysfunction in bipolar II disorder. *Bipolar Disorders, 10*(8), 888–99. doi:10.1111/j.1399-5618.2008.00638.x

Aoun, P., Jones, T., Shaw, G. L., & Bodner, M. (2005). Long-term enhancement of maze learning in mice via a generalized Mozart effect. *Neurological Research, 27*(8), 791–6. doi:10.1179/016164105X63647

Arnold, P. D., Siegel-Bartelt, J., Cytrynbaum, C., Teshima, I., & Schachar, R. (2001). Velo-cardio-facial syndrome: Implications of microdeletion 22q11 for schizophrenia and mood disorders. *American Journal of Medical Genetics, 105*(4), 354–62.

Asperger, H. (1944). Die „Autistischen Psychopathen" im Kindesalter. *Archiv für psychiatrie und nervenkrankheiten, 117*(1), 76–136.

American Psychiatric Association (1994). *Diagnostic and Statistical Manual of Mental Disorders: DSM-IV*. Washington, DC.

Astikainen, P., Lillstrang, E., & Ruusuvirta, T. (2008). Visual mismatch negativity for changes in orientation - A sensory memory-dependent response. *European Journal of Neuroscience, 28*(11), 2319–24. doi:10.1111/j.1460-9568.2008.06510.x

Astikainen, P., Ruusuvirta, T., & Korhonen, T. (2000). Cortical and subcortical visual event-related potentials to oddball stimuli in rabbits. *NeuroReport, 11*(7), 1515–17. doi:Doi 10.1097/00001756-200005150-00029

Astikainen, P., Ruusuvirta, T., & Korhonen, T. (2001). Somatosensory event-related potentials in the rabbit cerebral and cerebellar cortices: a correspondence with mismatch responses in humans. *Neuroscience Letters, 298*(3), 222–4. doi:Doi 10.1016/S0304-3940(00)01747-X

Astikainen, P., Ruusuvirta, T., & Korhonen, T. (2005). Longer storage of auditory than of visual information in the rabbit brain: evidence from dorsal hippocampal electrophysiology. *Experimental Brain Research, 160*(2), 189–93. doi:10.1007/s00221-004-1999-6

Astikainen, P., Ruusuvirta, T., Wikgren, J., & Penttonen, M. (2006). Memory-based detection of rare sound feature combinations in anesthetized rats. *NeuroReport, 17*(14), 1561–4. doi:DOI 10.1097/01.wnr.0000233097.13032.7d

Astikainen, P., Stefanics, G., Nokia, M., Lipponen, A., Cong, F. Y., Penttonen, M., & Ruusuvirta, T. (2011). Memory-based mismatch response to frequency changes in rats. *PLoS ONE, 6*(9). doi:ARTN e2420810.1371/journal.pone.0024208

Atienza, M., & Cantero, J. L. (2001). Complex sound processing during human REM sleep by recovering information from long-term memory as revealed by the mismatch negativity (MMN). *Brain Research, 901*(1), 151–60. doi:10.1016/S0006-8993(01)02340-X

Atienza, M., Cantero, J. L., & Dominguez-Marin, E. (2002). Mismatch negativity (MMN): an objective measure of sensory memory and long-lasting memories during sleep. *International Journal of Psychophysiology, 46*(3), 215–25.

Atienza, M., Cantero, J. L., & Escera, C. (2001). Auditory information processing during human sleep as revealed by event-related brain potentials. *Clinical Neurophysiology, 112*(11), 2031–45. doi:10.1016/S1388-2457(01)00650-2

Atienza, M., Cantero, J. L., & Gomez, C. M. (2000). Decay time of the auditory sensory memory trace during wakefulness and REM sleep. *Psychophysiology, 37*(4), 485–93.

Atienza, M., Cantero, J. L., & Gómez, C. M. (1997). The mismatch negativity component reveals the sensory memory during REM sleep in humans. *Neuroscience Letters, 237*(1), 21–4. doi:10.1016/S0304-3940(97)00798-2

Atienza, M., Cantero, J. L., Grau, C., Gomez, C., Dominguez-Marin, E., & Escera, C. (2003). Effects of temporal encoding on auditory object formation: a mismatch negativity study. *Cognitive Brain Research, 16*(3), 359–71. doi:10.1016/S0926-6410(02)00304-X

Atienza, M., Cantero, J. L., & Quiroga, Q. R. (2005). Precise timing accounts for posttraining sleep-dependent enhancements of the auditory mismatch negativity. *NeuroImage, 26*(2), 628–34. doi:10.1016/j.neuroimage.2005.02.014

Atienza, M., Cantero, J. L., & Stickgold, R. (2004). Posttraining sleep enhances automaticity in perceptual discrimination. *Journal of Cognitive Neuroscience, 16*(1), 53–64. doi:10.1162/089892904322755557

Atkinson, R. C., & Shiffrin, R. M. (1968) Human memory: A proposed system and its control processes. In K. W. Spence & J. T. Spence (Eds), *Psychology of Learning and Motivation - Advances in Research and Theory, Volume 2* (pp. 89–195). New York: Academic Press.

Atkinson, R. J., Fulham, W. R., Michie, P. T., Ward, P. B., Todd, J., Stain, H., et al. (2017). Electrophysiological, cognitive and clinical profiles of at-risk mental state: The longitudinal minds in transition (MinT) study. *PLoS ONE, 12*(2). doi:10.1371/journal.pone.0171657

Auther, L. L., Wertz, R. T., Miller, T. A., & Kirshner, H. S. (2000). Relationships among the mismatch negativity (MMN) response, auditory comprehension, and site of lesion in aphasic adults. *Aphasiology, 14*(5–6), 461–70. doi:10.1080/026870300401243

Avissar, M., & Javitt, D. (2018). Mismatch negativity: A simple and useful biomarker of N-methyl-D-aspartate receptor (NMDAR)-type glutamate dysfunction in schizophrenia. *Schizophrenia Research, 191*, 1–4. doi:10.1016/j.schres.2017.11.006

Baddeley, A., Gathercole, S., & Papagno, C. (1998). The phonological loop as a language learning device. *Psychological Review, 105*(1), 158–73. doi:10.1037/0033-295X.105.1.158

Bajbouj, M., Lisanby, S. H., Lang, U. E., Danker-Hopfe, H., Heuser, I., & Neu, P. (2006). Evidence for impaired cortical inhibition in patients with unipolar major depression. *Biological Psychiatry, 59*(5), 395–400. doi:10.1016/j.biopsych.2005.07.036

Baker, K., Baldeweg, T., Sivagnanasundaram, S., Scambler, P., & Skuse, D. (2005). COMT Val108/158 Met modifies mismatch negativity and cognitive function in 22q11 deletion syndrome. *Biological Psychiatry, 58*(1), 23–31. doi:10.1016/j.biopsych.2005.03.020

Baldeweg, T. (2007). ERP repetition effects and mismatch negativity generation: a predictive coding perspective. *Journal of Psychophysiology, 21*(3–4), 204–13. doi:10.1027/0269-8803.21.34.204

Baldeweg, T., & Hirsch, S. R. (2015). Mismatch negativity indexes illness-specific impairments of cortical plasticity in schizophrenia: A comparison with bipolar disorder and Alzheimer's disease. *International Journal of Psychophysiology, 95*(2), 145–55. doi:10.1016/j.ijpsycho.2014.03.008

Baldeweg, T., Klugman, A., Gruzelier, J., & Hirsch, S. R. (2004). Mismatch negativity potentials and cognitive impairment in schizophrenia. *Schizophrenia Research, 69*(2–3), 203–17. doi:10.1016/j.schres.2003.09.009

Baldeweg, T., Klugman, A., Gruzelier, J. H., & Hirsch, S. R. (2002). Impairment in frontal but not temporal components of mismatch negativity in schizophrenia. *International Journal of Psychophysiology, 43*(2), 111–22. doi:10.1016/S0167-8760(01)00183-0

Baldeweg, T., Williams, J. D., & Gruzelier, J. H. (1999). Differential changes in frontal and sub-temporal components of mismatch negativity. *International Journal of Psychophysiology, 33*(2), 143–8.

Baldeweg, T., Wong, D., & Stephan, K. E. (2006). Nicotinic modulation of human auditory sensory memory: Evidence from mismatch negativity potentials. *International Journal of Psychophysiology, 59*(1), 49–58. doi:10.1016/j.ijpsycho.2005.07.014

Baltaxe, C. A. M., & Guthrie, D. (1987). The use of primary sentence stress by normal, aphasic, and autistic children. *Journal of Autism and Developmental Disorders, 17*(2), 255–71. doi:10.1007/BF01495060

Banai, K., Hornickel, J., Skoe, E., Nicol, T., Zecker, S., & Kraus, N. (2009). Reading and subcortical auditory function. *Cerebral Cortex, 19*(11), 2699–707. doi:10.1093/cercor/bhp024

Baron-Cohen, S., & Staunton, R. (1994). Do children with autism acquire the phonology of their peers? An examination of group identification through the window of bilingualism. *First Language, 14*(42–43), 241–8.

Barry, J. G., Hardiman, M. J., Line, E., White, K. B., Yasin, I., & Bishop, D. V. M. (2008). Duration of auditory sensory memory in parents of children with SLI: A mismatch negativity study. *Brain and Language, 104*(1), 75–88. doi:10.1016/j.bandl.2007.02.006

Baudena, P., Halgren, E., Heit, G., & Clarke, J. M. (1995). Intracerebral potentials to rare target and distractor auditory and visual stimuli. III. Frontal cortex. *Electroencephalography and Clinical Neurophysiology, 94*(4), 251–64.

Baudouin, S. J. (2014). Heterogeneity and convergence: the synaptic pathophysiology of autism. *European Journal of Neuroscience, 39*(7), 1107–13. doi:10.1111/ejn.12498

Bazana, P. G., & Stelmack, R. M. (2002). Intelligence and information processing during an auditory discrimination task with backward masking: an event-related potential analysis. *Journal of Personality and Social Psychology, 83*(4), 998–1008. doi:10.1037/0022-3514.83.4.998

Beal, M. F., & Robert, J. F. (2004). Experimental therapeutics in transgenic mouse models of Huntington's disease. *Nature Reviews Neuroscience, 5*(5), 373. doi:10.1038/nrn1386

Beatty, W. W. (1993). Cognitive and emotional disturbances in multiple sclerosis. *Neurologic Clinics*, *11*(1), 189–204.

Bekinschtein, T., Cologan, V., Dahmen, B., & Golombek, D. (2009a) You are only coming through in waves: wakefulness variability and assessment in patients with impaired consciousness. *Progress in Brain Research*, *177*, 171–89. doi: 10.1016/S0079-6123(09)17712-9.

Bekinschtein, T. A., Dehaene, S., Rohaut, B., Tadel, F., Cohen, L., & Naccache, L. (2009b). Neural signature of the conscious processing of auditory regularities. *Proceedings of the National Academy of Sciences of the United States of America*, *106*(5), 1672–7. doi:10.1073/pnas.0809667106

Bekinschtein, T. A., Shalom, D. E., Forcato, C., Herrera, M., Coleman, M. R., Manes, F. F., & Sigman, M. (2009c). Classical conditioning in the vegetative and minimally conscious state. *Nature Neuroscience*, *12*(10), 1343–9. doi:10.1038/nn.2391

Bellis, T. J., Nicol, T., & Kraus, N. (2000). Aging affects hemispheric asymmetry in the neural representation of speech sounds. *Journal of Neuroscience*, *20*(2), 791–7.

Benasich, A. A., & Tallal, P. (1996). Auditory temporal processing thresholds, habituation, and recognition memory over the 1st year. *Infant Behavior and Development*, *19*(3), 339–57. doi:10.1016/S0163-6383(96)90033-8

Bendixen, A., Jones, S. J., Klump, G., & Winkler, I. (2010). Probability dependence and functional separation of the object-related and mismatch negativity event-related potential components. *NeuroImage*, *50*(1), 285–90. doi:10.1016/j.neuroimage.2009.12.037

Bendixen, A., Roeber, U., & Schröger, E. (2007). Regularity extraction and application in dynamic auditory stimulus sequences. *Journal of Cognitive Neuroscience*, *19*(10), 1664–77. doi:10.1162/jocn.2007.19.10.1664

Bendixen, A., SanMiguel, I., & Schröger, E. (2012). Early electrophysiological indicators for predictive processing in audition: A review. *International Journal of Psychophysiology*, *83*(2), 120–31. doi:10.1016/j.ijpsycho.2011.08.003

Bendixen, A., & Schröger, E. (2008). Memory trace formation for abstract auditory features and its consequences in different attentional contexts. *Biological Psychology*, *78*(3), 231–41. doi:10.1016/j.biopsycho.2008.03.005

Bendixen, A., Schröger, E., & Winkler, I. (2009). I heard that coming: event-related potential evidence for stimulus-driven prediction in the auditory system. *Journal of Neuroscience*, *29*(26), 8447. doi:10.1523/JNEUROSCI.1493-09.2009

Ben-Menachem, E. (2001). Vagus nerve stimulation, side effects, and long-term safety. *Journal of Clinical Neurophysiology*, *18*(5), 415–18.

Bennemann, J., Freigang, C., Schröger, E., Rübsamen, R., & Richter, N. (2013). Resolution of lateral acoustic space assessed by electroencephalography and psychoacoustics. *Frontiers in Psychology*, *4*, 338. doi:10.3389/fpsyg.2013.00338

Berglund, M., Hagstadius, S., Risberg, J., Johanson, T. M., Bliding, A., & Mubrin, Z. (1987). Normalization of regional cerebral blood flow in alcoholics during the first 7 weeks of abstinence. *Acta Psychiatrica Scandinavica*, *75*(2), 202–8.

Berninger, V., Raskind, W., Richards, T., Abbott, R., & Stock, P. (2008). A multidisciplinary approach to understanding developmental dyslexia within working-memory architecture: genotypes, phenotypes, brain, and instruction. *Developmental Neuropsychology*, *33*(6), 707–44. doi:10.1080/87565640802418662

Berti, S. (2008a). Cognitive control after distraction: Event-related brain potentials (ERPs) dissociate between different processes of attentional allocation. *Psychophysiology*, *45*(4), 608–20. doi:10.1111/j.1469-8986.2008.00660.x

Berti, S. (2008b). Object switching within working memory is reflected in the human event-related brain potential. *Neuroscience Letters*, *434*(2), 200–5. doi:10.1016/j.neulet.2008.01.055

Berti, S. (2012). Automatic processing of rare versus novel auditory stimuli reveal different mechanisms of auditory change detection. *NeuroReport*, *23*(7), 441–6. doi:10.1097/WNR.0b013e32835308b5

Berti, S. (2013). The role of auditory transient and deviance processing in distraction of task performance: a combined behavioral and event-related brain potential study. *Frontiers in Human Neuroscience*, *7*, 352. doi:10.3389/fnhum.2013.00352

Berti, S., Roeber, U., & Schröger, E. (2004). Bottom-up influences on working memory: behavioral and electrophysiological distraction varies with distractor strength. *Journal of Experimental Psychology*, *51*(4), 249–57. doi:10.1027/1618-3169.51.4.249

Berti, S., & Schröger, E. (2001). A comparison of auditory and visual distraction effects: behavioral and event-related indices. *Cognitive Brain Research*, *10*(3), 265–73. doi:10.1016/S0926-6410(00)00044-6

Berti, S., & Schröger, E. (2003). Working memory controls involuntary attention switching: evidence from an auditory distraction paradigm. *European Journal of Neuroscience*, *17*(5), 1119–22. doi:10.1046/j.1460-9568.2003.02527.x

Berti, S., & Schröger, E. (2004). Distraction effects in vision: behavioral and event-related potential indices. *NeuroReport*, *15*(4), 665–9.

Berti, S., & Schröger, E. (2006). Visual distraction: a behavioral and event-related brain potential study in humans. *NeuroReport*, *17*(2), 151–5.

Bertoli, S., Smurzynski, J., & Probst, R. (2002). Temporal resolution in young and elderly subjects as measured by mismatch negativity and a psychoacoustic gap detection task. *Clinical Neurophysiology*, *113*(3), 396–406. doi:10.1016/S1388-2457(02)00013-5

Bertoli, S., Smurzynski, J., & Probst, R. (2005). Effects of age, age-related hearing loss, and contralateral cafeteria noise on the discrimination of small frequency changes: psychoacoustic and electrophysiological measures. *Journal of the Association for Research in Otolaryngology*, *6*(3), 207–22. doi:10.1007/s10162-005-5029-6

Beste, C., Saft, C., Güntürkün, O., & Falkenstein, M. (2008). Increased cognitive functioning in symptomatic Huntington's disease as revealed by behavioral and event-related potential indices of auditory sensory memory and attention. *Journal of Neuroscience*, *28*(45), 11695–702. doi:10.1523/JNEUROSCI.2659-08.2008

Betancur, C. (2011). Etiological heterogeneity in autism spectrum disorders: More than 100 genetic and genomic disorders and still counting. *Brain Research*, *1380*, 42–77. doi:10.1016/j.brainres.2010.11.078

Betts, T. (1997). Psychiatric aspects of nonepileptic seizures. *Epilepsy: a comprehensive textbook*, 2101–16.

Bhakta, S. G., Chou, H. H., Rana, B., Talledo, J. A., Balvaneda, B., Gaddis, L., et al. (2016). Effects of acute memantine administration on MATRICS Consensus Cognitive Battery performance in psychosis: Testing an experimental medicine strategy. *Psychopharmacology*, *233*(12), 2399–410. doi:10.1007/s00213-016-4291-0

Bishop, D. V. M. (1985). Age of onset and outcome in 'acquired aphasia with convulsive disorder' (Landau-Kleffner syndrome). *Developmental Medicine & Child Neurology*, *27*(6), 705–12. doi:10.1111/j.1469-8749.1985.tb03793.x

Bishop, D. V. M. (1997). *Uncommon Understanding: Specific Language Impairment*. Hove: Psychology Press.

Bishop, D. V. M. (2006). What causes specific language impairment in children? *Current Directions in Psychological Science*, *15*(5), 217–21. doi:10.1111/j.1467-8721.2006.00439.x

Bishop, D. V. M., & Hardiman, M. J. (2010). Measurement of mismatch negativity in individuals: A study using single-trial analysis. *Psychophysiology*, *47*(4), 697–705. doi:10.1111/j.1469-8986.2009.00970.x

Bishop, D. V. M., Hardiman, M. J., & Barry, J. G. (2010). Lower-frequency event-related desynchronization: A signature of late mismatch responses to sounds, which is reduced or absent in children with specific language impairment. *Journal of Neuroscience*, *30*(46), 15578–84. doi:10.1523/JNEUROSCI.2217-10.2010

Bishop, D. V. M., Hardiman, M. J., & Barry, J. G. (2011). Is auditory discrimination mature by middle childhood? A study using time-frequency analysis of mismatch responses from 7 years to adulthood. *Developmental Science*, *14*(2), 402–16. doi:10.1111/j.1467-7687.2010.00990.x

Bishop, D. V. M., & Snowling, M. J. (2004). Developmental dyslexia and specific language impairment: Same or different? *Psychological Bulletin*, *130*(6), 858–86. doi:10.1037/0033-2909.130.6.858

Bitz, U., Gust, K., Spitzer, M., & Kiefer, M. (2007). Phonological deficit in school children is reflected in the Mismatch Negativity. *NeuroReport*, *18*(9), 911–15. doi:10.1097/WNR.0b013e32810f2e25

Blackstock, E. G. (1978). Cerebral asymmetry and the development of early infantile autism. *Journal of Autism and Childhood Schizophrenia*, *8*(3), 339–53.

Blau, V., van Atteveldt, N., Ekkebus, M., Goebel, R., & Blomert, L. (2009). Reduced neural integration of letters and speech sounds links phonological and reading deficits in adult dyslexia. *Current Biology*, *19*(6), 503–8. doi:10.1016/j.cub.2009.01.065

Boatman, D. F., Trescher, W. H., Smith, C., Ewen, J., Los, J., Wied, H. M., et al. (2008). Cortical auditory dysfunction in benign Rolandic epilepsy. *Epilepsia*, *49*(6), 1018–26. doi:10.1111/j.1528-1167.2007.01519.x

Bodatsch, M., Brockhaus-Dumke, A., Klosterkötter, J., & Ruhrmann, S. (2015). Forecasting psychosis by event-related potentials - Systematic review and specific meta-analysis. *Biological Psychiatry*, *77*(11), 951–8. doi:10.1016/j.biopsych.2014.09.025

Bodatsch, M., Ruhrmann, S., Wagner, M., Mller, R., Schultze-Lutter, F., Frommann, I., et al. (2011). Prediction of psychosis by mismatch negativity. *Biological Psychiatry*, *69*(10), 959–66. doi:10.1016/j.biopsych.2010.09.057

Boddaert, N., Belin, P., Chabane, N., Poline, J. B., Barthelemy, C., Mouren-Simeoni, M. C., et al. (2003). Perception of complex sounds: abnormal pattern of cortical activation in autism. *American Journal of Psychiatry*, *160*(11), 2057–60. doi:10.1176/appi.ajp.160.11.2057

Boddaert, N., Chabane, N., Belin, P., Bourgeois, M., Royer, V., Barthelemy, C., et al. (2004). Perception of complex sounds in autism: abnormal auditory cortical processing in children. *American Journal of Psychiatry*, *161*(11), 2117–20. doi:10.1176/appi.ajp.161.11.2117

Boly, M., Garrido, M. I., Gosseries, O., Bruno, M. A., Boveroux, P., Schnakers, C., et al. (2011). Preserved feedforward but impaired top-down processes in the vegetative state. *Science*, *332*(6031), 858–62. doi:10.1126/science.1202043

Bomba, M. D., & Pang, E. W. (2004). Cortical auditory evoked potentials in autism: a review. *International Journal of Psychophysiology*, *53*(3), 161–9. doi:10.1016/j.ijpsycho.2004.04.001

Bonnel, A., McAdams, S., Smith, B., Berthiaume, C., Bertone, A., Ciocca, V., et al. (2010). Enhanced pure-tone pitch discrimination among persons with autism but not Asperger syndrome. *Neuropsychologia*, *48*(9), 2465–75. doi:10.1016/j.neuropsychologia.2010.04.020

Bonnel, A., Mottron, L., Peretz, I., Trudel, M., Gallun, E., & Bonnel, A. M. (2003). Enhanced pitch sensitivity in individuals with autism: a signal detection analysis. *Journal of Cognitive Neuroscience*, *15*(2), 226–35. doi:10.1162/089892903321208169

Bonte, M. L., Poelmans, H., & Blomert, L. (2007). Deviant neurophysiological responses to phonological regularities in speech in dyslexic children. *Neuropsychologia*, *45*(7), 1427–37. doi:10.1016/j.neuropsychologia.2006.11.009

Borghetti, D., Pizzanelli, C., Maritato, P., Fabbrini, M., Jensen, S., Iudice, A., et al. (2007). Mismatch negativity analysis in drug-resistant epileptic patients implanted with vagus nerve stimulator. *Brain Research Bulletin*, *73*(1–3), 81–5. doi:10.1016/j.brainresbull.2007.02.004

Botting, N., & Conti-Ramsden, G. (2001). Non-word repetition and language development in children with specific language impairment (SLI). *International Journal of Language and Communication Disorders, 36*(4), 421–32. doi:10.1080/13682820110074971

Bouras, C., Hof, P. R., Giannakopoulos, P., Michel, J. P., & Morrison, J. H. (1994). Regional distribution of neurofibrillary tangles and senile plaques in the cerebral cortex of elderly patients: a quantitative evaluation of a one-year autopsy population from a geriatric hospital. *Cerebral Cortex, 4*(2), 138–150.

Bozzi, Y., Casarosa, S., & Caleo, M. (2012). Epilepsy as a neurodevelopmental disorder. *Frontiers in Psychiatry, 3*, 19. doi:10.3389/fpsyt.2012.00019

Bradley, L., & Bryant, P. E. (1978). Difficulties in auditory organisation as a possible cause of reading backwardness. *Nature, 271*(5647), 746. doi:10.1038/271746a0

Braff, D., & Light, G. (2004). Preattentional and attentional cognitive deficits as targets for treating schizophrenia. *Psychopharmacology, 174*(1), 75–85. doi:10.1007/s00213-004-1848-0

Braff, D. L., & Light, G. A. (2005). The use of neurophysiological endophenotypes to understand the genetic basis of schizophrenia. *Dialogues in Clinical Neuroscience, 7*(2), 125–35.

Bramon, E., Croft, R. J., McDonald, C., Virdi, G. K., Gruzelier, J. G., Baldeweg, T., et al. (2004). Mismatch negativity in schizophrenia: a family study. *Schizophrenia Research, 67*(1), 1–10.

Brattico, E., Winkler, I., Näätänen, R., Paavilainen, P., & Tervaniemi, M. (2002). Simultaneous storage of two complex temporal sound patterns in auditory sensory memory. *NeuroReport, 13*(14), 1747–51.

Bregman, A. S. (1990). *Auditory Scene Analysis: The Perceptual Organization of Sound.* Cambridge: MIT Press.

Bregman, A. S., Liao, C., & Levitan, R. (1990). Auditory grouping based on fundamental frequency and formant peak frequency. *Canadian Journal of Experimental Psychology, 44*(3), 400–13.

Brewer, C. M., Leek, J. P., Green, A. J., Holloway, S., Bonthron, D. T., Markham, A. F., & FitzPatrick, D. R. (1999). A locus for isolated cleft palate, located on human chromosome 2q32. *American Journal of Human Genetics, 65*(2), 387–96. doi:10.1086/302498

Broder, H. L., Richman, L. C., & Matheson, P. B. (1998). Learning disability, school achievement, and grade retention among children with cleft: A two-center study. *Cleft Palate-Craniofacial Journal, 35*(2), 127–31. doi:10.1597/1545-1569(1998)035<0127:LDSAAG>2.3.CO2

Broen, P. A., Devers, M. C., Doyle, S. S., Prouty, J. M., & Moller, K. T. (1998). Acquisition of linguistic and cognitive skills by children with cleft palate. *Journal of Speech, Language, and Hearing Research, 41*(3), 676–687.

Bruder, G., Sutton, S., Berger-Gross, P., Quitkin, F., & Davies, S. (1981). Lateralized auditory processing in depression: Dichotic click detection. *Psychiatry Research, 4*(3), 253–66. doi:10.1016/0165-1781(81)90027-5

Bruder, G. E., Sutton, S., Babkoff, H., Gurland, B. J., Yozawitz, A., & Fleiss, J. L. (1975). Auditory signal detectability and facilitation of simple reaction time in psychiatric patients and non-patients. *Psychological Medicine, 5*(3), 260–72. doi:10.1017/S0033291700056622

Bruder, J., Leppänen, P. H., Bartling, J., Csépe, V., Demonet, J. F., & Schulte-Körne, G. (2011). Children with dyslexia reveal abnormal native language representations: evidence from a study of mismatch negativity. *Psychophysiology, 48*(8), 1107–18. doi:10.1111/j.1469-8986.2011.01179.x

Brönnick, K. S., Nordby, H., Larsen, J. P., & Aarsland, D. (2010). Disturbance of automatic auditory change detection in dementia associated with Parkinson's disease: A mismatch negativity study. *Neurobiology of Aging, 31*(1), 104–13. doi:10.1016/j.neurobiolaging.2008.02.021

Bulbena, A., & Berrios, G. E. (1993). Cognitive function in the affective disorders: A prospective study. *Psychopathology, 26*(1), 6–12. doi:10.1159/000284794

Butler, R. A. (1968). Effect of changes in stimulus frequency and intensity on habituation of the human vertex potential. *Journal of the Acoustical Society of America, 44*(4), 945–50.

Bäckman, L., Ginovart, N., Dixon, R. A., Wahlin, T.-B. R., Wahlin, Å., Halldin, C., & Farde, L. (2000). Age-related cognitive deficits mediated by changes in the striatal dopamine system. *American Journal of Psychiatry, 157*(4), 635–7. doi:10.1176/appi.ajp.157.4.635

Böttcher-Gandor, C., & Ullsperger, P. (1992). Mismatch negativity in event-related potentials to auditory stimuli as a function of varying interstimulus interval. *Psychophysiology, 29*(5), 546–550. doi:10.1111/j.1469-8986.1992.tb02028.x

Cannon, T. D., Cadenhead, K., Cornblatt, B., Woods, S. W., Addington, J., Walker, E., et al. (2008). Prediction of psychosis in youth at high clinical risk: A multisite longitudinal study in North America. *Archives of General Psychiatry, 65*(1), 28–37. doi:10.1001/archgenpsychiatry.2007.3

Cansino, S. (2009). Episodic memory decay along the adult lifespan: a review of behavioral and neurophysiological evidence. *International Journal of Psychophysiology, 71*(1), 64–9. doi:10.1016/j.ijpsycho.2008.07.005

Carral, V., Corral, M.-J., & Escera, C. (2005a). Auditory event-related potentials as a function of abstract change magnitude. *NeuroReport, 16*(3), 301–5.

Carral, V., Huotilainen, M., Ruusuvirta, T., Fellman, V., Näätänen, R., & Escera, C. (2005b). A kind of auditory 'primitive intelligence' already present at birth. *European Journal of Neuroscience, 21*(11), 3201–4. doi:10.1111/j.1460-9568.2005.04144.x

Castaneda, A. E., Tuulio-Henriksson, A., Marttunen, M., Suvisaari, J., & Lönnqvist, J. (2008). A review on cognitive impairments in depressive and anxiety disorders with a focus on young adults. *Journal of Affective Disorders, 106*(1–2), 1–27. doi:10.1016/j.jad.2007.06.006

Catts, S. V., Shelley, A. M., Ward, P. B., Liebert, B., McConaghy, N., Andrews, S., & Michie, P. T. (1995). Brain potential evidence for an auditory sensory memory deficit in schizophrenia. *American Journal of Psychiatry, 152*(2), 213–19.

Celsis, P., Boulanouar, K., Doyon, B., Ranjeva, J. P., Berry, I., Nespoulous, J. L., & Chollet, F. (1999). Differential fMRI responses in the left posterior superior temporal gyrus and left supramarginal gyrus to habituation and change detection in syllables and tones. *NeuroImage, 9*(1), 135–44. doi:10.1006/nimg.1998.0389

Čeponienė, R., Haapanen, M.-L., Ranta, R., Näätänen, R., & Hukki, J. (2002). Auditory sensory impairment in children with oral clefts as indexed by auditory event-related potentials. *Journal of Craniofacial Surgery, 13*(4), 554.

Čeponienė, R., Hukki, J., Cheour, M., Haapanen, M. L., Koskinen, M., Alho, K., & Näätänen, R. (2000). Dysfunction of the auditory cortex persists in infants with certain cleft types. *Developmental Medicine & Child Neurology, 42*(4), 258–65.

Čeponienė, R., Hukki, J., Cheour, M., Haapanen, M. L., Ranta, R., & Näätänen, R. (1999a). Cortical auditory dysfunction in children with oral clefts: Relation with cleft type. *Clinical Neurophysiology, 110*(11), 1921–6. doi:10.1016/S1388-2457(99)00152-2

Čeponienė, R., Lepistö, T., Shestakova, A., Vanhala, R., Alku, P., Näätänen, R., & Yaguchi, K. (2003). Speech-sound-selective auditory impairment in children with autism: they can perceive but do not attend.(Author Abstract). *Proceedings of the National Academy of Sciences of the United States, 100*(9), 5567.

Čeponienė, R., Service, E., Kurjenluoma, S., Cheour, M., & Näätänen, R. (1999b). Children's performance on pseudoword repetition depends on auditory trace quality: evidence from event-related potentials. *Developmental psychology, 35*(3), 709–20. doi:10.1037/0012-1649.35.3.709

Chang, E. F., & Merzenich, M. M. (2003). Environmental noise retards auditory cortical development. *Science, 300*(5618), 498–502.

Chang, Y., Xu, J., Pang, X., Sun, Y., Zheng, Y., & Liu, Y. (2015). Mismatch negativity indices of enhanced preattentive automatic processing in panic disorder as measured by a multi-feature paradigm. *Biological Psychology, 105*, 77–82. doi:10.1016/j.biopsycho.2015.01.006

Cheng, C. H., Hsu, W. Y., & Lin, Y. Y. (2013). Effects of physiological aging on mismatch negativity: A meta-analysis. *International Journal of Psychophysiology. 90*(2),165–71. doi:10.1016/j.ijpsycho.2013.06.026

Cheng, C. H., & Lin, Y. Y. (2013). Aging-related decline in somatosensory inhibition of the human cerebral cortex. *Experimental Brain Research, 226*(1), 145–52. doi:10.1007/s00221-013-3420-9

Cheng, C. H., Wang, P. N., Hsu, W. Y., & Lin, Y. Y. (2012). Inadequate inhibition of redundant auditory inputs in Alzheimer's disease: an MEG study. *Biological Psychology, 89*(2), 365–73. doi:10.1016/j.biopsycho.2011.11.010

Cheng, Y.-Y., Wu, H.-C., Tzeng, Y.-L., Yang, M.-T., Zhao, L.-L., & Lee, C.-Y. (2015). Feature-specific transition from positive mismatch response to mismatch negativity in early infancy: Mismatch responses to vowels and initial consonants. *International Journal of Psychophysiology, 96*(2), 84–94. doi:https://doi.org/10.1016/j.ijpsycho.2015.03.007

Cheour, M., Ceponiene, R., Hukki, J., Haapanen, M. L., Naatanen, R., & Alho, K. (1999). Brain dysfunction in neonates with cleft palate revealed by the mismatch negativity. *Clinical Neurophysiology, 110*(2), 324–8.

Cheour, M., Čeponienė, R., Lehtokoski, A., Luuk, A., Allik, J., Alho, K., & Näätänen, R. (1998a). Development of language-specific phoneme representations in the infant brain. *Nature Neuroscience, 1*(5), 351–3.

Cheour, M., Haapanen, M. L., Hukki, J., Ceponiene, R., Kurjenluoma, S., Alho, K., et al. (1997). The first neurophysiological evidence for cognitive brain dysfunctions in children with CATCH. *NeuroReport, 8*(7), 1785–7.

Cheour, M., Haapanen, M.-L., Čeponienė, R., Hukki, J., Ranta, R., & Näätänen, R. (1998b). Mismatch negativity (MMN) as an index of auditory sensory memory deficit in cleft-palate and CATCH syndrome children. *NeuroReport, 9*(12), 2709–12.

Cheour-Luhtanen, M., Alho, K., Kujala, T., Sainio, K., Reinikainen, K., Renlund, M., et al. (1995). Mismatch negativity indicates vowel discrimination in newborns. *Hearing Research, 82*(1), 53–8.

Choi, J. W., Lee, J. K., Ko, D., Lee, G. T., Jung, K. Y., & Kim, K. H. (2013). Fronto-temporal interactions in the theta-band during auditory deviant processing. *Neuroscience Letters, 548*, 120–5. doi:10.1016/j.neulet.2013.05.079

Choi, W., Lim, M., Kim, J. S., Kim, D. J., & Chung, C. K. (2015). Impaired pre-attentive auditory processing in fibromyalgia: A mismatch negativity (MMN) study. *Clinical Neurophysiology, 126*(7), 1310–18. doi:10.1016/j.clinph.2014.10.012

Choudhury, N., & Benasich, A. A. (2011). Maturation of auditory evoked potentials from 6 to 48 months: Prediction to 3 and 4 year language and cognitive abilities. *Clinical Neurophysiology, 122*(2), 320–38. doi:10.1016/j.clinph.2010.05.035

Chugani, D. C., Muzik, O., Rothermel, R., Behen, M., Chakraborty, P., Mangner, T., et al. (1997). Altered serotonin synthesis in the dentatothalamocortical pathway in autistic boys. *Annals of Neurology, 42*(4), 666–9. doi:10.1002/ana.410420420

Chugani, H. T., & Phelps, M. E. (1991). Imaging human brain development with positron emission tomography. *Journal of Nuclear Medicine, 32*(1), 23–6.

Clark, C. R., McFarlane, A. C., Weber, D. L., & Battersby, M. (1996). Enlarged frontal P300 to stimulus change in panic disorder. *Biological Psychiatry, 39*(10), 845–56. doi:10.1016/0006-3223(95)00288-X

Clark, E. O., Glanzer, M., & Turndorf, H. (1979). The pattern of memory loss resulting from intravenously administered diazepam. *Archives of Neurology, 36*(5), 296.

Cloninger, C. R. (1994). The genetic structure of personality and learning: a phylogenetic model. *Clinical Genetics, 46*(1), 124–37. doi:10.1111/j.1399-0004.1994.tb04214.x

Cloninger, C. R., Sigvardsson, S., Reich, T., & Bohman, M. (1986). Inheritance of risk to develop alcoholism. *NIDA Research Monograph Index, 66*, 86–96.

Cloninger, C. R., & Svrakic, D. M. (1997). Integrative psychobiological approach to psychiatric assessment and treatment. *Psychiatry, 60*(2), 120–41. doi:10.1521/00332747.1997.11024793

Coffman, J. A., Bornstein, R. A., Olson, S. C., Schwarzkopf, S. B., & Nasrallah, H. A. (1990). Cognitive impairment and cerebral structure by MRI in bipolar disorder. *Biological Psychiatry, 27*(11), 1188–96. doi:10.1016/0006-3223(90)90416-Y

Conboy, B. T., & Kuhl, P. K. (2011). Impact of second-language experience in infancy: brain measures of first- and second-language speech perception. *Developmental Science, 14*(2), 242–8. doi:10.1111/j.1467-7687.2010.00973.x

Cong, F., Sipola, T., Huttunen-Scott, T., Xu, X., Ristaniemi, T., & Lyytinen, H. (2009). Hilbert-Huang versus Morlet wavelet transformation on mismatch negativity of children in uninterrupted sound paradigm. *Nonlinear Biomedical Physics, 3*(1), 1. doi:10.1186/1753-4631-3-1

Cooper, R. J., Todd, J., McGill, K., & Michie, P. T. (2006). Auditory sensory memory and the aging brain: A mismatch negativity study. *Neurobiology of Aging, 27*(5), 752–62. doi:10.1016/j.neurobiolaging.2005.03.012

Corbera, S., Corral, M. J., Escera, C., & Idiazabal, M. A. (2005). Abnormal speech sound representation in persistent developmental stuttering. *Neurology, 65*(8), 1246–52. doi:10.1212/01.wnl.0000180969.03719.81

Corbera, S., Escera, C., & Artigas, J. (2006). Impaired duration mismatch negativity in developmental dyslexia. *NeuroReport, 17*(10), 1051–5. doi:10.1097/01.wnr.0000221846.43126.a6

Cornwell, B. R., Baas, J. M., Johnson, L., Holroyd, T., Carver, F. W., Lissek, S., & Grillon, C. (2007). Neural responses to auditory stimulus deviance under threat of electric shock revealed by spatially-filtered magnetoencephalography. *NeuroImage, 37*(1), 282–9. doi:10.1016/j.neuroimage.2007.04.055

Cotman, C., Bridges, R., Taube, J., Clark, A., Geddes, J., & Monaghan, D. (1989). The role of the NMDA receptor in central nervous system plasticity and pathology. *The Journal of NIH Research, 1*(2), 65–74.

Cowan, N. (1984). On short and long auditory stores. *Psychological Bulletin, 96*(2), 341–370.

Cowan, N. (1988). Evolving conceptions of memory storage, selective attention, and their mutual constraints within the human information-processing system. *Psychological Bulletin, 104*(2), 163–91. doi:10.1037/0033-2909.104.2.163

Cowan, N., Winkler, I., Teder, W., & Näätänen, R. (1993). Memory prerequisites of mismatch negativity in the auditory event-related potential (ERP). *Journal of Experimental Psychology: Learning, Memory, and Cognition, 19*(4), 909–21.

Cramer, S. C. (2003). Editorial comment--Implementing results of stroke recovery research into clinical practice. *Stroke, 34*(7), 1752.

Csépe, V. (1995). On the origin and development of the mismatch negativity. *Ear and Hearing, 16*(1), 91–104.

Csépe, V., Karmos, G., & Molnár, M. (1987a). Effects of signal probability on sensory evoked potentials in cats. *International Journal of Neuroscience, 33*(1–2), 61–71. doi:10.3109/00207458708985929

Csépe, V., Karmos, G., & Molnár, M. (1987b). Evoked potential correlates of stimulus deviance during wakefulness and sleep in cat - animal model of mismatch negativity. *Electroencephalography and Clinical Neurophysiology, 66*(6), 571–8. doi:10.1016/0013-4694(87)90103-9

Csépe, V., Molnár, M., Karmos, G., & Winkler, I. (1989). Effect of changes in stimulus frequency on auditory evoked potentials in awake and anaesthetized cats. *Sleep, 88*, 210–11.

Csepe, V., Osman-Sagi, J., Molnar, M., & Gosy, M. (2001). Impaired speech perception in aphasic patients: event-related potential and neuropsychological assessment. *Neuropsychologia, 39*(11), 1194–208.

Csepe, V., Pantev, C., Hoke, M., Hampson, S., & Ross, B. (1992). Evoked magnetic responses of the human auditory cortex to minor pitch changes: localization of the mismatch field. *Electroencephalography and Clinical Neurophysiology, 84*(6), 538–48.

Csépe, V., Pantev, C., Hoke, M., Ross, B., & Hampson, S. (1997). Mismatch field to tone pairs: neuromagnetic evidence for temporal integration at the sensory level. *Electroencephalography and Clinical Neurophysiology, 104*(1), 1.

Czamara, D., Bruder, J., Becker, J., Bartling, J., Hoffmann, P., Ludwig, K. U., et al. (2011). Association of a rare variant with mismatch negativity in a region between KIAA0319 and DCDC2 in dyslexia. *Behavior genetics, 41*(1), 110–19.

Czigler, I., Balazs, L., & Winkler, I. (2002). Memory-based detection of task-irrelevant visual changes. *Psychophysiology, 39*(6), 869–73. doi:10.1017/S0048577202020218

Czigler, I., Csibra, G., & Csontos, A. (1992). Age and inter-stimulus interval effects on event-related potentials to frequent and infrequent auditory stimuli. *Biological Psychology, 33*(2–3), 195–206.

Czigler, I., & Pató, L. (2009). Unnoticed regularity violation elicits change-related brain activity. *Biological Psychology, 80*(3), 339–47. doi:10.1016/j.biopsycho.2008.12.001

Czigler, I., Weisz, J., & Winkler, I. (2006a). ERPs and deviance detection: Visual mismatch negativity to repeated visual stimuli. *Neuroscience Letters, 401*(1–2), 178–82. doi:10.1016/j.neulet.2006.03.018

Czigler, I., Weisz, J., & Winkler, I. (2007). Backward masking and visual mismatch negativity: electrophysiological evidence for memory-based detection of deviant stimuli. *Psychophysiology, 44*(4), 610–19. doi:10.1111/j.1469-8986.2007.00530.x

Czigler, I., Winkler, I., Pató, L., Várnagy, A., Weisz, J., & Balázs, L. (2006b). Visual temporal window of integration as revealed by the visual mismatch negativity event-related potential to stimulus omissions. *Brain Research, 1104*(1), 129–40. doi:10.1016/j.brainres.2006.05.034

Dakin, S., & Frith, U. (2005). Vagaries of visual perception in autism. *Neuron, 48*(3), 497–507. doi:10.1016/j.neuron.2005.10.018

Daltrozzo, J., Wioland, N., Mutschler, V., & Kotchoubey, B. (2007). Predicting coma and other low responsive patients outcome using event-related brain potentials: A meta-analysis. *Clinical Neurophysiology, 118*(3), 606–14. doi:10.1016/j.clinph.2006.11.019

Datta, H., Shafer, V. L., Morr, M. L., Kurtzberg, D., & Schwartz, R. G. (2010). Electrophysiological indices of discrimination of long-duration, phonetically similar vowels in children with typical and atypical language development. *Journal of Speech, Language, and Hearing Research, 53*(3), 757–77. doi:10.1044/1092-4388(2009/08-0123)

Davids, N., Segers, E., van den Brink, D., Mitterer, H., van Balkom, H., Hagoort, P., & Verhoeven, L. (2011). The nature of auditory discrimination problems in children with specific language impairment: An MMN study. *Neuropsychologia, 49*(1), 19–28. doi:10.1016/j.neuropsychologia.2010.11.001

Davids, N., van den Brink, D., van Turennout, M., Mitterer, H., & Verhoeven, L. (2009). Towards neurophysiological assessment of phonemic discrimination: context effects of the mismatch negativity. *Clinical Neurophysiology, 120*(6), 1078–86. doi:10.1016/j.clinph.2009.01.018

Davis, H., & Zerlin, S. (1966). Acoustic relations of the human vertex potential. *The Journal of the Acoustical Society of America, 39*(1), 109.

Dawson, G., Toth, K., Abbott, R., Osterling, J., Munson, J., Estes, A., & Liaw, J. (2004). Early social attention impairments in autism: social orienting, joint attention, and attention to distress. *Developmental Psychology, 40*(2), 271–83. doi:10.1037/0012-1649.40.2.271

De Fosse, L., Hodge, S. M., Makris, N., Kennedy, D. N., Caviness, V. S., Jr., McGrath, L., et al. (2004). Language-association cortex asymmetry in autism and specific language impairment. *Annals of Neurology, 56*(6), 757–66. doi:10.1002/ana.20275

De Pascalis, V., & Varriale, V. (2012). Intelligence and Information Processing. A Mismatch Negativity Analysis Using a Passive Auditory Backward-Masking Task. *Journal of Individual Differences, 33*(2), 101–8. doi:10.1027/1614-0001/a000078

De Tommaso, M., Guido, M., Libro, G., Losito, L., Difruscolo, O., Sardaro, M., & Puca, F. M. (2004). Interictal lack of habituation of mismatch negativity in migraine. *Cephalalgia*, *24*(8), 663–8. doi:10.1111/j.1468-2982.2004.00731.x

De Tommaso, M., Navarro, J., Ricci, K., Lorenzo, M., Lanzillotti, C., Colonna, F., et al. (2013). Pain in prolonged disorders of consciousness: laser evoked potentials findings in patients with vegetative and minimally conscious states. *Brain Injury*, *27*(7–8), 962–72. doi:10.3109/02699052.2013.775507

Decasper, A. J., & Fifer, W. P. (1980). Of human bonding: Newborns prefer their mothers' voices. *Science*, *208*(4448), 1174–6. doi:10.1126/science.7375928

Dehaene-Lambertz, G. (1997). Electrophysiological correlates of categorical phoneme perception in adults. *NeuroReport*, *8*(4), 919–24.

Dehaene-Lambertz, G., & Baillet, S. (1998). A phonological representation in the infant brain. *NeuroReport*, *9*(8), 1885–8.

Dehaene-Lambertz, G., & Pena, M. (2001). Electrophysiological evidence for automatic phonetic processing in neonates. *NeuroReport*, *12*(14), 3155–8.

DeLisi, L. E., Sakuma, M., Kushner, M., Finer, D. L., Hoff, A. L., & Crow, T. J. (1997). Anomalous cerebral asymmetry and language processing in schizophrenia. *Schizophrenia Bulletin*, *23*(2), 255–71. doi:10.1093/schbul/23.2.255

Deouell, L. Y., & Bentin, S. (1998). Variable cerebral responses to equally distinct deviance in four auditory dimensions: A mismatch negativity study. *Psychophysiology*, *35*, 745–54. doi:10.1111/1469-8986.3560745

Deouell, L. Y., Bentin, S., & Giard, M. H. (1998). Mismatch negativity in dichotic listening: evidence for interhemispheric differences and multiple generators. *Psychophysiology*, *35*(4), 355–65.

Deouell, L. Y., Bentin, S., & Soroker, N. (2000a). Electrophysiological evidence for an early (pre-attentive) information processing deficit in patients with right hemisphere damage and unilateral neglect. *Brain*, *123*(2), 353–65.

Deouell, L. Y., Hämäläinen, H., & Bentin, S. (2000b). Unilateral neglect after right-hemisphere damage: Contributions from event-related potentials. *Audiology and Neuro-Otology*, *5*(3–4), 225–34.

Deouell, L. Y., Parnes, A., Pickard, N., & Knight, R. T. (2006). Spatial location is accurately tracked by human auditory sensory memory: Evidence from the mismatch negativity. *European Journal of Neuroscience*, *24*(5), 1488–94. doi:10.1111/j.1460-9568.2006.05025.x

Desjardins, N. R., Trainor, J. L., Hevenor, J. S., & Polak, P. C. (1999). Using mismatch negativity to measure auditory temporal resolution thresholds. *NeuroReport*, *10*(10), 2079–82.

Dhawan, J., Benveniste, H., Nawrocky, M., Smith, S. D., & Biegon, A. (2010). Transient focal ischemia results in persistent and widespread neuroinflammation and loss of glutamate NMDA receptors. *NeuroImage*, *51*(2), 599–605. doi:10.1016/j.neuroimage.2010.02.073

Dick, B. D., Connolly, J. F., McGrath, P. J., Finley, G. A., Stroink, G., Houlihan, M. E., & Clark, A. J. (2003). The disruptive effect of chronic pain on mismatch negativity. *Clinical Neurophysiology*, *114*(8), 1497–1506.

Dickman, S. J. (1993). Impulsivity and information processing. In W. G. McCown, J. L. Johnson & M. B. Shure, (Eds), *The Impulsive Client: Theory, Research, and Treatment* (pp. 151–184). Washington, DC: American Psychological Association.

Dickman, S. J. (2000). Impulsivity, arousal and attention. *Personality and Individual Differences*, *28*(3), 563–81. doi:10.1016/S0191-8869(99)00120-8

Dittmann-Balcar, A., Juptner, M., Jentzen, W., & Schall, U. (2001). Dorsolateral prefrontal cortex activation during automatic auditory duration-mismatch processing in humans: a positron emission tomography study. *Neuroscience Letters*, *308*(2), 119–22.

Doeller, C. F., Opitz, B., Mecklinger, A., Krick, C., Reith, W., & Schroger, E. (2003). Prefrontal cortex involvement in preattentive auditory deviance detection: neuroimaging and electrophysiological evidence. *NeuroImage, 20*(2), 1270–82. doi:10.1016/S1053-8119(03)00389-6

Donchin, E. (1981). Presidential address, 1980. Surprise!...Surprise? *Psychophysiology, 18*(5), 493–513.

Donchin, E., Ritter, W., & McCallum, W. C. (1978). Cognitive psychophysiology: The endogenous components of the ERP. In E. Callaway, P. Tueting, & S. Koslow (Eds), *Event-related Brain Potentials in Man* (pp. 349–411). New York: Academic Press.

Draganova, R., Eswaran, H., Murphy, P., Huotilainen, M., Lowery, C., & Preissl, H. (2005). Sound frequency change detection in fetuses and newborns, a magnetoencephalographic study. *NeuroImage, 28*(2), 354–61. doi:10.1016/j.neuroimage.2005.06.011

Dunbar, G., Boeijinga, P. H., Demazieres, A., Cisterni, C., Kuchibhatla, R., Wesnes, K., & Luthringer, R. (2007). Effects of TC-1734 (AZD3480), a selective neuronal nicotinic receptor agonist, on cognitive performance and the EEG of young healthy male volunteers. *Psychopharmacology (Berl), 191*(4), 919–29. doi:10.1007/s00213-006-0675-x

Dunn, M. A., Gomes, H., & Gravel, J. (2008). Mismatch negativity in children with autism and typical development. *Journal of Autism and Developmental Disorders, 38*(1), 52–71. doi:10.1007/s10803-007-0359-3

Eapen, V. (2011). Genetic basis of autism: is there a way forward? *Current Opinion in Psychiatry, 24*(3), 226. doi:10.1097/YCO.0b013e328345927e

Eason, R. G., Aiken, L. R., White, C. T., & Lichtenstein, M. (1964). Activation and behavior. II. Visually evoked cortical potentials in man as indicants of activation level. *Perceptual and motor skills, 19*, 875–95.

Eccleston, C., & Crombez, G. (1999). Pain demands attention: a cognitive–affective model of the interruptive function of pain. *Psychological Bulletin, 125*(3), 356–66. doi:10.1037/0033-2909.125.3.356

Ehrlichman, R. S., Luminais, S. N., White, S. L., Rudnick, N. D., Ma, N., Dow, H. C., et al. (2009). Neuregulin 1 transgenic mice display reduced mismatch negativity, contextual fear conditioning and social interactions. *Brain Research, 1294*, 116–27. doi:10.1016/j.brainres.2009.07.065

Ehrlichman, R. S., Maxwell, C. R., Majumdar, S., & Siegel, S. J. (2008). Deviance-elicited changes in event-related potentials are attenuated by ketamine in mice. *Journal of Cognitive Neuroscience, 20*(8), 1403–14. doi:10.1162/jocn.2008.20097

England, M. J., Liverman, C. T., Schultz, A. M., & Strawbridge, L. M. (2012). Epilepsy across the spectrum: promoting health and understanding. A summary of the Institute of Medicine report. *Epilepsy & Behavior, 25*(2), 266–76. doi:10.1016/j.yebeh.2012.06.016

Erickson, M. A., Ruffle, A., & Gold, J. M. (2016). A Meta-Analysis of Mismatch Negativity in Schizophrenia: From Clinical Risk to Disease Specificity and Progression. *Biological Psychiatry, 79*(12), 980–7. doi:10.1016/j.biopsych.2015.08.025

Escera, C., Alho, K., Schröger, E., & Winkler, I. (2000a). Involuntary attention and distractibility as evaluated with event-related brain potentials. *Audiology & Neuro-Otology, 5*(3–4), 151–66. doi:10.1159/000013877

Escera, C., Alho, K., Winkler, I., & Näätänen, R. (1998). Neural mechanisms of involuntary attention to acoustic novelty and change. *Journal of Cognitive Neuroscience, 10*(5), 590–604. doi:10.1162/089892998562997

Escera, C., Corral, M. J., & Yago, E. (2002). An electrophysiological and behavioral investigation of involuntary attention towards auditory frequency, duration and intensity changes. *Cognitive Brain Research, 14*(3), 325–32. doi:10.1016/S0926-6410(02)00135-0

Escera, C., Yago, E., & Alho, K. (2001). Electrical responses reveal the temporal dynamics of brain events during involuntary attention switching. *European Journal of Neuroscience, 14*(5), 877–83.

Escera, C., Yago, E., Corral, M. J., Corbera, S., & Nuñez, M. I. (2003). Attention capture by auditory significant stimuli: Semantic analysis follows attention switching. *European Journal of Neuroscience*, *18*(8), 2408–12. doi:10.1046/j.1460-9568.2003.02937.x

Escera, C., Yago, E., Polo, M. D., & Grau, C. (2000b). The individual replicability of mismatch negativity at short and long inter-stimulus intervals. *Clinical Neurophysiology*, *111*(3), 546–51. doi:10.1016/S1388-2457(99)00274-6

Estes, R. E., & Morris, H. L. (1970). Relationships among intelligence, speech proficiency, and hearing sensitivity in children with cleft palates. *Cleft Palate Journal*, *7*, 763–73.

Farmer, M. E., & Klein, R. M. (1995). The evidence for a temporal processing deficit linked to dyslexia: A review. *Psychonomic Bulletin & Review*, *2*(4), 460–93. doi:10.3758/BF03210983

Farooq, S., Large, M., Nielssen, O., & Waheed, W. (2009). The relationship between the duration of untreated psychosis and outcome in low-and-middle income countries: A systematic review and meta analysis. *Schizophrenia Research*, *109*(1–3), 15–23. doi:10.1016/j.schres.2009.01.008

Faugeras, F., Rohaut, B., Weiss, N., Bekinschtein, T. A., Galanaud, D., Puybasset, L., et al. (2011). Probing consciousness with event-related potentials in the vegetative state. *Neurology*, *77*(3), 264–8. doi:10.1212/WNL.0b013e3182217ee8

Featherstone, R. E., Melnychenko, O., & Siegel, S. J. (2018). Mismatch negativity in preclinical models of schizophrenia. *Schizophrenia Research*, *191*, 35–42. doi:10.1016/j.schres.2017.07.039

Featherstone, R. E., Shin, R., Kogan, J. H., Liang, Y., Matsumoto, M., & Siegel, S. J. (2015). Mice with subtle reduction of NMDA NR1 receptor subunit expression have a selective decrease in mismatch negativity: Implications for schizophrenia prodromal population. *Neurobiology of Disease*, *73*, 289–95. doi:10.1016/j.nbd.2014.10.010

Fein, G., Whitlow, B., & Finn, P. (2004). Mismatch negativity: no difference between controls and abstinent alcoholics. *Alcoholism: Clinical and Experimental Research*, *28*(1), 137–42. doi:10.1097/01.ALC.0000107199.26934.46

Fischer, C., Dailler, F., & Morlet, D. (2008). Novelty P3 elicited by the subject's own name in comatose patients. *Clinical Neurophysiology*, *119*(10), 2224–30. doi:10.1016/j.clinph.2008.03.035

Fischer, C., & Luauté, J. (2005). Evoked potentials for the prediction of vegetative state in the acute stage of coma. *Neuropsychological Rehabilitation*, *15*(3–4), 372–80.

Fischer, C., Luaute, J., Adeleine, P., & Morlet, D. (2004a). Predictive value of sensory and cognitive evoked potentials for awakening from coma. *Neurology*, *63*(4), 669–73.

Fischer, C., Luauté, J., Némoz, C., Morlet, D., Kirkorian, G., & Mauguière, F. (2006a). Editorial response: evoked potentials can be used as a prognosis factor for awakening. *Critical Care Medicine*, *34*(7), 2025.

Fischer, C., Luauté, J., Némoz, C., Morlet, D., Kirkorian, G., & Mauguière, F. (2006b). Improved prediction of awakening or nonawakening from severe anoxic coma using tree-based classification analysis. *Critical Care Medicine*, *34*(5), 1520.

Fischer, C., Morlet, D., Bouchet, P., Luaute, J., Jourdan, C., & Salord, F. (1999). Mismatch negativity and late auditory evoked potentials in comatose patients. *Clinical Neurophysiology*, *110*(9), 1601–10.

Fischer, C., Morlet, D., & Luaute, J. (2004b). Sensory and cognitive evoked potentials in the prognosis of coma. *Supplements to Clinical Neurophysiology*, *57*, 656–61.

Fisher, D. J., Grant, B., Smith, D. M., Borracci, G., Labelle, A., & Knott, V. J. (2011a). Effects of auditory hallucinations on the mismatch negativity (MMN) in schizophrenia as measured by a modified 'optimal' multi-feature paradigm. *International Journal of Psychophysiology*, *81*(3), 245–51. doi:10.1016/j.ijpsycho.2011.06.018

Fisher, D. J., Grant, B., Smith, D. M., & Knott, V. J. (2011b). Effects of deviant probability on the 'optimal' multi-feature mismatch negativity (MMN) paradigm. *International Journal of Psychophysiology*, *79*(2), 311–15. doi:10.1016/j.ijpsycho.2010.11.006

Fisher, M., Holland, C., Merzenich, M. M., & Vinogradov, S. (2009). Using neuroplasticity-based auditory training to improve verbal memory in schizophrenia. *American Journal of Psychiatry*, *166*(7), 805–11. doi:10.1176/appi.ajp.2009.08050757

Flachenecker, P. (2015). Clinical implications of neuroplasticity - the role of rehabilitation in multiple sclerosis. *Frontiers in Neurology*, *6*, 36. doi:10.3389/fneur.2015.00036

Foltynie, T., Brayne, C. E., Robbins, T. W., & Barker, R. A. (2004). The cognitive ability of an incident cohort of Parkinson's patients in the UK. The CamPaIGN study. *Brain*, *127*(Pt 3), 550–60. doi:10.1093/brain/awh067

Foong, J., Rozewicz, L., Davie, C. A., Thompson, A. J., Miller, D. H., & Ron, M. A. (1999). Correlates of executive function in multiple sclerosis: The use of magnetic resonance spectroscopy as an index of focal pathology. *Journal of Neuropsychiatry and Clinical Neurosciences*, *11*(1), 45–50.

Ford, J. M., Roth, W. T., & Kopell, B. S. (1976a). Attention effects on auditory evoked potentials to infrequent events. *Biological Psychology*, *4*(1), 65–77.

Ford, J. M., Roth, W. T., & Kopell, B. S. (1976b). Auditory evoked potentials to unpredictable shifts in pitch. *Psychophysiology*, *13*(1), 32–9.

Foster, S. M., Kisley, M. A., Davis, H. P., Diede, N. T., Campbell, A. M., & Davalos, D. B. (2013). Cognitive function predicts neural activity associated with pre-attentive temporal processing. *Neuropsychologia*, *51*(2), 211–19. doi:10.1016/j.neuropsychologia.2012.09.017

Fox, E. (1994). Grapheme-phoneme correspondence in dyslexic and matched control readers. *British Journal of Psychology*, *85*(1), 41–53.

Franken, I. H., Nijs, I., & Van Strien, J. W. (2005). Impulsivity affects mismatch negativity (MMN) measures of preattentive auditory processing. *Biological Psychology*, *70*(3), 161–7. doi:10.1016/j.biopsycho.2005.01.007

Freberg, L. (2006). *Discovering Biological Psychology*. Boston: Houghton Mifflin.

Friedman, D., Cycowicz, Y. M., & Gaeta, H. (2001). The novelty P3: an event-related brain potential (ERP) sign of the brain's evaluation of novelty. *Neuroscience & Biobehavioral Reviews*, *25*(4), 355–73.

Friedman, T., Sehatpour, P., Dias, E., Perrin, M., & Javitt, D. C. (2012). Differential relationships of mismatch negativity and visual P1 deficits to premorbid characteristics and functional outcome in schizophrenia. *Biological Psychiatry*, *71*(6), 521–9. doi:10.1016/j.biopsych.2011.10.037

Friedrich, M., Weber, C., & Friederici, A. D. (2004). Electrophysiological evidence for delayed mismatch response in infants at-risk for specific language impairment. *Psychophysiology*, *41*(5), 772–82. doi:10.1111/j.1469-8986.2004.00202.x

Friel-Patti, S., & Finitzo, T. (1990). Language learning in a prospective study of otitis media with effusion in the first two years of life. *Journal of Speech Language and Hearing Research*, *33*(1), 188. doi:10.1044/jshr.3301.188

Frisina, D. R., Frisina, R. D., Snell, K. B., Burkard, R., Walton, J. P., & Ison, J. R. (2001). Auditory temporal processing during aging. In P. R. Hof & C. V. Mobbs (Eds), *Functional Neurobiology of Aging* (pp. 565–79). Academic Press: San Diego.

Friston, K. (2005). A theory of cortical responses. *Philosophical Transactions of the Royal Society of London. Series B, Biological Sciences*, *360*(1456), 815–36. doi:10.1098/rstb.2005.1622

Frodl-Bauch, T., Kathmann, N., Moller, H. J., & Hegerl, U. (1997). Dipole localization and test-retest reliability of frequency and duration mismatch negativity generator processes. *Brain Topography*, *10*(1), 3–8.

Froyen, D., Van Atteveldt, N., Bonte, M., & Blomert, L. (2008). Cross-modal enhancement of the MMN to speech-sounds indicates early and automatic integration of letters and speech-sounds. *Neuroscience Letters*, *430*(1), 23–8. doi:10.1016/j.neulet.2007.10.014

Froyen, D., Willems, G., & Blomert, L. (2011). Evidence for a specific cross-modal association deficit in dyslexia: an electrophysiological study of letter-speech sound processing. *Developmental Science*, *14*(4), 635–48. doi:10.1111/j.1467-7687.2010.01007.x

Fruhstorfer, H., & Bergström, R. M. (1969). Human vigilance and auditory evoked responses. *Electroencephalography and Clinical Neurophysiology*, *27*(4), 346–55. doi:10.1016/0013-4694(69)91443-6

Fusar-Poli, P., & Borgwardt, S. (2012). Predictive power of attenuated psychosis syndrome: Is it really low? The case of mild cognitive impairment. *Schizophrenia Research*, *135*(1–3), 192–3. doi:10.1016/j.schres.2011.11.023

Gaeta, H., Friedman, D., Ritter, W., & Cheng, J. (1998). An event-related potential study of age-related changes in sensitivity to stimulus deviance. *Neurobiology of Aging, 19*(5), 447–59.

Gaeta, H., Friedman, D., Ritter, W., & Cheng, J. (1999). Changes in sensitivity to stimulus deviance in Alzheimer's disease: an ERP perspective. *NeuroReport, 10*(2), 281–7.

Gaeta, H., Friedman, D., Ritter, W., & Hunt, G. (2002). Age-related changes in neural trace generation of rule-based auditory features. *Neurobiology of Aging, 23*(3), 443–55.

Gallon, N., Harris, J., & van der Lely, H. (2007). Non-word repetition: An investigation of phonological complexity in children with grammatical SLI. *Clinical Linguistics and Phonetics, 21*(6), 435–55. doi:10.1080/02699200701299982

Gandour, J., Tong, Y., Wong, D., Talavage, T., Dzemidzic, M., Xu, Y., et al. (2004). Hemispheric roles in the perception of speech prosody. *NeuroImage, 23*(1), 344–57. doi:10.1016/j.neuroimage.2004.06.004

Garrido, M. I., Kilner, J. M., Kiebel, S. J., & Friston, K. J. (2007). Evoked brain responses are generated by feedback loops. *Proceedings of the National Academy of Sciences of the United States, 104*(52), 20961–6.

Garrido, M. I., Kilner, J. M., Kiebel, S. J., & Friston, K. J. (2009). Dynamic causal modeling of the response to frequency deviants. *Journal of Neurophysiology, 101*(5), 2620–31. doi:10.1152/jn.90291.2008

Ge, Y., Wu, J., Sun, X., & Zhang, K. (2011). Enhanced mismatch negativity in adolescents with posttraumatic stress disorder (PTSD). *International Journal of Psychophysiology, 79*(2), 231–5. doi:10.1016/j.ijpsycho.2010.10.012

Gendry Meresse, I., Zilbovicius, M., Boddaert, N., Robel, L., Philippe, A., Sfaello, I., et al. (2005). Autism severity and temporal lobe functional abnormalities. *Annals of Neurology, 58*(3), 466–9. doi:10.1002/ana.20597

Gene-Cos, N., Pottinger, R., Barrett, G., Trimble, M. R., & Ring, H. A. (2005). A comparative study of mismatch negativity (MMN) in epilepsy and non-epileptic seizures. *Epileptic Disorders, 7*(4), 363–72.

George, M. S., Costa, D. C., Kouris, K., Ring, H. A., & Ell, P. J. (1992). Cerebral blood flow abnormalities in adults with infantile autism. *Journal of Nervous and Mental Disease, 180*(7), 413–17.

Gervais, H., Belin, P., Boddaert, N., Leboyer, M., Coez, A., Sfaello, I., et al. (2004). Abnormal cortical voice processing in autism. *Nature Neuroscience, 7*(8), 801–2. doi:10.1038/nn1291

Giard, M. H., Lavikahen, J., Reinikainen, K., Perrin, F., Bertrand, O., Pernier, J., & Näätänen, R. (1995). Separate representation of stimulus frequency, intensity, and duration in auditory sensory memory: an event-related potential and dipole-model analysis. *Journal of Cognitive Neuroscience, 7*(2), 133–43. doi:10.1162/jocn.1995.7.2.133

Giard, M. H., Perrin, F., Pernier, J., & Bouchet, P. (1990). Brain generators implicated in the processing of auditory stimulus deviance: a topographic event-related potential study. *Psychophysiology, 27*(6), 627–40.

Gil, R., Zai, L., Neau, J. P., Jonveaux, T., Agbo, C., Rosolacci, T., et al. (1993). Event-related auditory evoked potentials and multiple sclerosis. *Electroencephalography and Clinical Neurophysiology*, *88*(3), 182–7.

Gil-Da-Costa, R., Stoner, G. R., Fung, R., & Albright, T. D. (2013). Nonhuman primate model of schizophrenia using a noninvasive EEG method. *Proceedings of the National Academy of Sciences of the United States of America*, *110*(38), 15425–30. doi:10.1073/pnas.1312264110

Gillberg, C., & Coleman, M. (2000). *The Biology of the Autistic Syndromes* (3rd ed.). London: Mac Keith Press.

Glass, E., Sachse, S., & von Suchodoletz, W. (2008a). Auditory sensory memory in 2-year-old children: an event-related potential study. *NeuroReport*, *19*(5), 569–73. doi:10.1097/WNR.0b013e3282f97867

Glass, E., Sachse, S., & von Suchodoletz, W. (2008b). Development of auditory sensory memory from 2 to 6 years: an MMN study. *Journal of Neural Transmission*, *115*(8), 1221–9. doi:10.1007/s00702-008-0088-6

Goff, D. C., & Coyle, J. T. (2001). The emerging role of glutamate in the pathophysiology and treatment of schizophrenia. *American Journal of Psychiatry*, *158*(9), 1367–77. doi:10.1176/appi.ajp.158.9.1367

Goldberg, R., Motzkin, B., Marion, R., Scambler, P. J., & Shprintzen, R. J. (1993). Velo-cardio-facial syndrome: a review of 120 patients. *American Journal of Medical Genetics Part A*, *45*(3), 313–19. doi:10.1002/ajmg.1320450307

Golding-Kushner, K. J., Weller, G., & Shprintzen, R. J. (1985). Velo-cardio-facial syndrome: Language and psychological profiles. *Journal of Craniofacial Genetics and Developmental Biology*, *5*(3), 259–66.

Gomes, H., Bernstein, R., Ritter, W., Vaughan, H. G., Jr., & Miller, J. (1997). Storage of feature conjunctions in transient auditory memory. *Psychophysiology*, *34*(6), 712–16.

Gomes, H., Ritter, W., & Vaughan, H. G., Jr. (1995). The nature of preattentive storage in the auditory system. *Journal of Cognitive Neuroscience*, *7*(1), 81–94. doi:10.1162/jocn.1995.7.1.81

Gomot, M., Blanc, R., Clery, H., Roux, S., Barthelemy, C., & Bruneau, N. (2011). Candidate electrophysiological endophenotypes of hyper-reactivity to change in autism. *Journal of Autism and Developmental Disorders*, *41*(6), 705–14. doi:10.1007/s10803-010-1091-y

Gomot, M., Giard, M. H., Adrien, J. L., Barthelemy, C., & Bruneau, N. (2002). Hypersensitivity to acoustic change in children with autism: electrophysiological evidence of left frontal cortex dysfunctioning. *Psychophysiology*, *39*(5), 577–84. doi:10.1017.S0048577202394058

Gomot, M., Giard, M. H., Roux, S., Barthelemy, C., & Bruneau, N. (2000). Maturation of frontal and temporal components of mismatch negativity (MMN) in children. *NeuroReport*, *11*(14), 3109–12.

Gould, H. J. (1990). Hearing loss and cleft palate: the perspective of time. *The Cleft Palate-Craniofacial Journal*, *27*(1), 36–9.

Granholm, E., McQuaid, J. R., McClure, F. S., Auslander, L. A., Perivoliotis, D., Pedrelli, P., et al. (2005). A randomized, controlled trial of cognitive behaviors social skills training for middle-aged and older outpatients with chronic schizophrenia. *American Journal of Psychiatry*, *162*(3), 520–9. doi:10.1176/appi.ajp.162.3.520

Grant, A. C., Zangaladze, A., Thiagarajah, M. C., & Sathian, K. (1999). Tactile perception in developmental dyslexia: a psychophysical study using gratings. *Neuropsychologia*, *37*(10), 1201–11. doi:10.1016/S0028-3932(99)00013-5

Granö, N., Virtanen, M., Vahtera, J., Elovainio, M., & Kivimäki, M. (2004). Impulsivity as a predictor of smoking and alcohol consumption. *Personality and Individual Differences*, *37*(8), 1693–700. doi:10.1016/j.paid.2004.03.004

Grau, C., Escera, C., Yago, E., & Polo, M. D. (1998). Mismatch negativity and auditory sensory memory evaluation: a new faster paradigm. *NeuroReport*, *9*(11), 2451–6.

Grau, C., Polo, M. D., Yago, E., Gual, A., & Escera, C. (2001). Auditory sensory memory as indicated by mismatch negativity in chronic alcoholism. *Clinical Neurophysiology, 112*(5), 728–31. doi:10.1016/S1388-2457(01)00490-4

Gray, J. A. (1976). The behavioural inhibition system: A possible substrate for anxiety. In M. P. B. Feldman, A. (Ed.), *Theoretical and Experimental Bases of the Behaviour Therapies* (pp. 3–41). London: Wiley.

Green, M. (1996). What are the functional consequences of neurocognitive deficits in schizophrenia? *American Journal of Psychiatry, 153*(3), 321–30.

Green, M. F., Kern, R. S., Braff, D. L., & Mintz, J. (2000). Neurocognitive deficits and functional outcome in schizophrenia: are we measuring the "right stuff"? *Schizophrenia Bulletin, 26*(1), 119–36.

Greenwood, L.-M., Leung, S., Michie, P. T., Green, A., Nathan, P. J., Fitzgerald, P., et al. (2018). The effects of glycine on auditory mismatch negativity in schizophrenia. *Schizophrenia Research, 191*, 61–9.

Grillon, C., Sinha, R., & O'Malley, S. S. (1995). Effects of ethanol on the processing of low probability stimuli: an ERP study. *Psychopharmacology (Berl), 119*(4), 455–65.

Grimm, S., Bendixen, A., Deouell, L. Y., & Schröger, E. (2009). Distraction in a visual multi-deviant paradigm: behavioral and event-related potential effects. *International Journal of Psychophysiology, 72*(3), 260–6.

Grimm, S., & Escera, C. (2012). Auditory deviance detection revisited: evidence for a hierarchical novelty system. *International Journal of Psychophysiology, 85*(1), 88–92. doi:10.1016/j.ijpsycho.2011.05.012

Grimm, S., Recasens, M., Althen, H., & Escera, C. (2012). Ultrafast tracking of sound location changes as revealed by human auditory evoked potentials. *Biological Psychology, 89*(1), 232–9. doi:10.1016/j.biopsycho.2011.10.014

Grimm, S., Schroger, E., Bendixen, A., Bass, P., Roye, A., & Deouell, L. Y. (2008). Optimizing the auditory distraction paradigm: behavioral and event-related potential effects in a lateralized multi-deviant approach. *Clinical Neurophysiology, 119*(4), 934–47. doi:10.1016/j.clinph.2007.12.011

Grimm, S., & Schröger, E. (2007). The processing of frequency deviations within sounds: evidence for the predictive nature of the Mismatch Negativity (MMN) system. *Restorative Neurology and Neuroscience, 25*(3–4), 241.

Grimm, S., Widmann, A., & Schröger, E. (2004). Differential processing of duration changes within short and long sounds in humans. *Neuroscience Letters, 356*(2), 83–6. doi:10.1016/j.neulet.2003.11.035

Groenen, P., Snik, A., & van den Broek, P. (1996). On the clinical relevance of mismatch negativity: results from subjects with normal hearing and cochlear implant users. *Audiology & Neurotology, 1*(2), 112–24.

Grossheinrich, N., Kademann, S., Bruder, J., Bartling, J., & Von Suchodoletz, W. (2010). Auditory sensory memory and language abilities in former late talkers: A mismatch negativity study. *Psychophysiology, 47*(5), 822–30. doi:10.1111/j.1469-8986.2010.00996.x

Guimarães, J., & Sá, M. J. (2012). Cognitive Dysfunction in Multiple Sclerosis. *Frontiers in Neurology, 3*, 74. doi:10.3389/fneur.2012.00074

Gumenyuk, V., Korzyukov, O., Alho, K., Escera, C., Schröger, E., Ilmoniemi, R. J., & Näätänen, R. (2001). Brain activity index of distractibility in normal school-age children. *Neuroscience Letters, 314*(3), 147–50. doi:10.1016/S0304-3940(01)02308-4

Gumenyuk, V., Korzyukov, O., Alho, K., Winkler, I., Paavilainen, P., & Näätänen, R. (2003). Electric brain responses indicate preattentive processing of abstract acoustic regularities in children. *NeuroReport, 14*(11), 1411–15. doi:10.1097/00001756-200308060-00001

Gumenyuk, V., Korzyukov, O., Escera, C., Hamalainen, M., Huotilainen, M., Hayrinen, T., et al. (2005). Electrophysiological evidence of enhanced distractibility in ADHD children. *Neuroscience Letters*, *374*(3), 212–17. doi:10.1016/j.neulet.2004.10.081

Gustafsson, L. (1997). Inadequate cortical feature maps: a neural circuit theory of autism. *Biological Psychiatry*, *42*(12), 1138–47.

Haenschel, C., Vernon, D. J., Dwivedi, P., Gruzelier, J. H., & Baldeweg, T. (2005). Event-related brain potential correlates of human auditory sensory memory-trace formation. *Journal of Neuroscience*, *25*(45), 10494–501. doi:10.1523/JNEUROSCI.1227-05.2005

Hagberg, C., Larson, O., & Milerad, J. (1998). Incidence of cleft lip and palate and risks of additional malformations. *Cleft Palate-Craniofacial Journal*, *35*(1), 40.

Haigh, S. M., Coffman, B. A., & Salisbury, D. F. (2017). Mismatch negativity in first-episode schizophrenia. *Clinical EEG and Neuroscience*, *48*(1), 3–10. doi:10.1177/1550059416645980

Halgren, E., Baudena, P., Clarke, J. M., Heit, G., Liégeois, C., Chauvel, P., & Musolino, A. (1995). Intracerebral potentials to rare target and distractor auditory and visual stimuli. I. Superior temporal plane and parietal lobe. *Electroencephalography and Clinical Neurophysiology*, *94*(3), 191–220. doi:10.1016/0013-4694(94)00259-N

Halgren, E., Marinkovic, K., & Chauvel, P. (1998). Generators of the late cognitive potentials in auditory and visual oddball tasks. *Electroencephalography and Clinical Neurophysiology*, *106*(2), 156–64.

Hall, M. H., Rijsdijk, F., Kalidindi, S., Schulze, K., Kravariti, E., Kane, F., et al. (2007). Genetic overlap between bipolar illness and event-related potentials. *Psychological Medicine*, *37*(5), 667–78. doi:10.1017/S003329170600972X

Hall, M. H., Schulze, K., Rijsdijk, F., Kalidindi, S., McDonald, C., Bramon, E., et al. (2009). Are auditory P300 and duration MMN heritable and putative endophenotypes of psychotic bipolar disorder? A Maudsley Bipolar Twin and Family Study. *Psychological Medicine*, *39*(8), 1277–87. doi:10.1017/S0033291709005261

Hall, M. H., Schulze, K., Rijsdijk, F., Picchioni, M., Ettinger, U., Bramon, E., et al. (2006). Heritability and reliability of P300, P50 and duration mismatch negativity. *Behavior Genetics*, *36*(6), 845–57. doi:10.1007/s10519-006-9091-6

Hamilton, H. K., D'Souza, D. C., Ford, J. M., Roach, B. J., Kort, N. S., Ahn, K. H et al. (2018). Interactive effects of an N-methyl-D-aspartate receptor antagonist and a nicotinic acetylcholine receptor agonist on mismatch negativity: Implications for schizophrenia. *Schizophrenia Research*, *191*, 87–94. doi:10.1016/j.schres.2017.06.040

Hämäläinen, M., Hari, R., Ilmoniemi, R. J., Knuutila, J., & Lounasmaa, O. V. (1993). Magnetoencephalography theory, instrumentation, and applications to noninvasive studies of the working human brain. *Reviews of Modern Physics*, *65*(2), 413–97. doi:10.1103/RevModPhys.65.413

Hammar, Å., & Årdal, G. (2009). Cognitive functioning in major depression - A summary. *Frontiers in Human Neuroscience*, *3*:26. doi:10.3389/neuro.09.026.2009

Hanagasi, H. A., Gurvit, I. H., Ermutlu, N., Kaptanoglu, G., Karamursel, S., Idrisoglu, H. A., et al. (2002). Cognitive impairment in amyotrophic lateral sclerosis: evidence from neuropsychological investigation and event-related potentials. *Brain Research. Cognitive Brain Research*, *14*(2), 234–44.

Hansen, J. C., & Hillyard, S. A. (1980). Endogenous brain potentials associated with selective auditory attention. *Electroencephalography and Clinical Neurophysiology*, *49*(3–4), 277.

Hansen, J. C., & Hillyard, S. A. (1983). Selective attention to multidimensional auditory stimuli. *Journal of Experimental Psychology: Human Perception and Performance*, *9*(1), 1–19. doi:10.1037/0096-1523.9.1.1

Hansen, J. C., & Hillyard, S. A. (1984). Effects of stimulation rate and attribute cuing on event-related potentials during selective auditory attention. *Psychophysiology*, *21*(4), 394–405. doi:10.1111/j.1469-8986.1984.tb00216.x

Hansenne, M. (1999). P300 and personality: an investigation with the Cloninger's model. *Biological Psychology, 50*(2), 143–55.

Hansenne, M., Pinto, E., Scantamburlo, G., Couvreur, A., Reggers, J., Fuchs, S., et al. (2003). Mismatch negativity is not correlated with neuroendocrine indicators of catecholaminergic activity in healthy subjects. *Human Psychopharmacology, 18*(3), 201–5. doi:10.1002/hup.468

Happé, F., & Frith, U. (1996). The neuropsychology of autism. *Brain, 119*(4), 1377–1400.

Happe, F., & Frith, U. (2006). The weak coherence account: detail-focused cognitive style in autism spectrum disorders. *Journal of Autism and Developmental Disorders, 36*(1), 5–25. doi:10.1007/s10803-005-0039-0

Hara, K., Ohta, K., Miyajima, M., Hara, M., Iino, H., Matsuda, A., et al. (2012). Mismatch negativity for speech sounds in temporal lobe epilepsy. *Epilepsy Behaviour, 23*(3), 335–41. doi:10.1016/j.yebeh.2012.01.019

Hari, R., Hamalainen, M., Ilmoniemi, R., Kaukoranta, E., Reinikainen, K., Salminen, J., et al. (1984). Responses of the primary auditory cortex to pitch changes in a sequence of tone pips: Neuromagnetic recordings in man. *Neuroscience Letters, 50*(1–3), 127–32.

Hari, R., Rif, J., Tiihonen, J., & Sams, M. (1992). Neuromagnetic mismatch fields to single and paired tones. *Electroencephalography and Clinical Neurophysiology, 82*(2), 152–4.

Harkrider, A. W., & Hedrick, M. S. (2005). Acute effect of nicotine on auditory gating in smokers and non-smokers. *Hearing Research, 202*(1–2), 114–28. doi:10.1016/j.heares.2004.11.009

Harms, L. (2016). Mismatch responses and deviance detection in N-methyl-D-aspartate (NMDA) receptor hypofunction and developmental models of schizophrenia. *Biological Psychology, 116*, 75–81. doi:10.1016/j.biopsycho.2015.06.015

Hawkins, H. L., & Presson, J. C. (1977). Masking and preperceptual selectivity in auditory recognition. In S. Dornic (Ed.), *Attention and Performance* (Vol. 6, pp. 195–211). Hillsdale, New Jersey: Lawrence Erlbaum Associates.

Hay, R. A., Roach, B. J., Srihari, V. H., Woods, S. W., Ford, J. M., & Mathalon, D. H. (2015). Equivalent mismatch negativity deficits across deviant types in early illness schizophrenia-spectrum patients. *Biological Psychology, 105*, 130–7. doi:10.1016/j.biopsycho.2015.01.004

He, W., Chai, H., Zheng, L., Yu, W., Chen, W., Li, J., et al. (2010). Mismatch negativity in treatment-resistant depression and borderline personality disorder. *Progress in Neuro-Psychopharmacology & Biological Psychiatry, 34*(2), 366–71. doi:10.1016/j.pnpbp.2009.12.021

He, C., Hotson, L., & Trainor, L. J. (2009). Maturation of cortical mismatch responses to occasional pitch change in early infancy: Effects of presentation rate and magnitude of change. *Neuropsychologia, 47*(1), 218–229. doi:10.1016/j.neuropsychologia.2008.07.019

Heaton, P. (2003). Pitch memory, labelling and disembedding in autism. *Journal of Child Psychology and Psychiatry, 44*(4), 543–51.

Heaton, P. (2005). Interval and contour processing in autism. *Journal of Autism and Developmental Disorders, 35*(6), 787–93. doi:10.1007/s10803-005-0024-7

Heaton, P., Pring, L., & Hermelin, B. (1999). A pseudo-savant: A case of exceptional musical splinter skills. *Neurocase, 5*(6), 503–9. doi:10.1080/13554799908402745

Heaton, P., Pring, L., & Hermelin, B. (2001). Musical processing in high functioning children with autism. *Annals of the New York Academy of Sciences, 930*, 443–4.

Heaton, P., Williams, K., Cummins, O., & Happe, F. (2008). Autism and pitch processing splinter skills: A group and subgroup analysis. *Autism, 12*(2), 203–19. doi:10.1177/1362361307085270

Heinke, W., Kenntner, R., Gunter, T. C., Sammler, D., Olthoff, D., & Koelsch, S. (2004). Sequential effects of increasing propofol sedation on frontal and temporal cortices as indexed by auditory event-related potentials. *Anesthesiology, 100*(3), 617–25. doi:10.1097/00000542-200403000-00023

Heinke, W., & Koelsch, S. (2005). The effects of anesthetics on brain activity and cognitive function. *Current Opinion in Anaesthesiology, 18*(6), 625.

Herbert, M. R., Harris, G. J., Adrien, K. T., Ziegler, D. A., Makris, N., Kennedy, D. N., et al. (2002). Abnormal asymmetry in language association cortex in autism. *Annals of Neurology, 52*(5), 588–96. doi:10.1002/ana.10349

Hermanutz, M., Cohen, R., & Sommer, W. (1981). The effects of serial order in long sequences of auditory stimuli on event-related potentials. *Psychophysiology, 18*(4), 415–23.

Hermens, D. F., Ward, P. B., Hodge, M. A., Kaur, M., Naismith, S. L., & Hickie, I. B. (2010). Impaired MMN/P3a complex in first-episode psychosis: Cognitive and psychosocial associations. *Progress in Neuro-Psychopharmacology & Biological Psychiatry, 34*(6), 822–9. doi:10.1016/j.pnpbp.2010.03.019

Hillyard, S. A., Hink, R. F., Schwent, V. L., & Picton, T. W. (1973). Electrical signs of selective attention in the human brain. *Science, 182*(4108), 177–80.

Hirose, Y., Hara, K., Miyajima, M., Matsuda, A., Maehara, T., Hara, M., et al. (2014). Changes in the duration and frequency of deviant stimuli engender different mismatch negativity patterns in temporal lobe epilepsy. *Epilepsy Behavior, 31*, 136–42. doi:10.1016/j.yebeh.2013.11.026

Hirvonen, J., Jääskelainen, I. P., Näätänen, R., & Sillanaukee, P. (2000). Adenosine A1/A2a receptors mediate suppression of mismatch negativity by ethanol in humans. *Neuroscience Letters, 278*(1–2), 57–60.

Ho, B. C., Alicata, D., Ward, J., Moser, D. J., O'Leary, D. S., Arndt, S., & Andreasen, N. C. (2003a). Untreated initial psychosis: Relation to cognitive deficits and brain morphology in first-episode schizophrenia. *American Journal of Psychiatry, 160*(1), 142–8. doi:10.1176/appi.ajp.160.1.142

Ho, B. C., Andreasen, N. C., Nopoulos, P., Arndt, S., Magnotta, V., & Flaum, M. (2003b). Progressive structural brain abnormalities and their relationship to clinical outcome: A longitudinal magnetic resonance imaging study early in schizophrenia. *Archives of General Psychiatry, 60*(6), 585–94. doi:10.1001/archpsyc.60.6.585

Holeckova, I., Fischer, C., Morlet, D., Delpuech, C., Costes, N., & Mauguière, F. (2008). Subject's own name as a novel in a MMN design: A combined ERP and PET study. *Brain Research, 1189*(1), 152–65. doi:10.1016/j.brainres.2007.10.091

Holopainen, I. E., Korpilahti, P., Juottonen, K., Lang, H., & Sillanpää, M. (1998). Abnormal frequency mismatch negativity in mentally retarded children and in children with developmental dysphasia. *Journal of Child Neurology, 13*(4), 178–83. doi:10.1177/088307389801300406

Hommet, C., Vidal, J., Roux, S., Blanc, R., Barthez, M. A., De Becque, B., et al. (2009). Topography of syllable change-detection electrophysiological indices in children and adults with reading disabilities. *Neuropsychologia, 47*(3), 761–70. doi:10.1016/j.neuropsychologia.2008.12.010

Honbolygo, F., Csepe, V., Fekeshazy, A., Emri, M., Marian, T., Sarkozy, G., & Kalmanchey, R. (2006). Converging evidences on language impairment in Landau-Kleffner Syndrome revealed by behavioral and brain activity measures: A case study. *Clin Neurophysiol, 117*(2), 295–305. doi:10.1016/j.clinph.2005.10.016

Hong, L. E., Moran, L. V., Du, X., O'Donnell, P., & Summerfelt, A. (2012). Mismatch negativity and low frequency oscillations in schizophrenia families. *Clinical Neurophysiology, 123*(10), 1980–8. doi:10.1016/j.clinph.2012.03.011

Horton, J., Millar, A., Labelle, A., & Knott, V. J. (2011). MMN responsivity to manipulations of frequency and duration deviants in chronic, clozapine-treated schizophrenia patients. *Schizophrenia Research, 126*(1–3), 202–11. doi:10.1016/j.schres.2010.11.028

Horváth, J., Czigler, I., Winkler, I., & Teder-Sälejärvi, W. A. (2007). The temporal window of integration in elderly and young adults. *Neurobiology of Aging, 28*(6), 964–75. doi:10.1016/j.neurobiolaging.2006.05.002

Houlihan, M., & Stelmack, R. M. (2012). Mental ability and mismatch negativity: pre-attentive discrimination of abstract feature conjunctions in auditory sequences. *Intelligence, 40*(3), 239–44. doi:10.1016/j.intell.2012.02.003

Howell, T. J., **Conduit, R.**, Toukhsati, S., & **Bennett, P.** (2012). Auditory stimulus discrimination recorded in dogs, as indicated by mismatch negativity (MMN). *Behavioural Processes, 89*(1), 8–13. doi:10.1016/j.beproc.2011.09.009

Hsiao, F. J., Cheng, C. H., Liao, K. K., & **Lin, Y. Y.** (2010). Cortico-cortical phase synchrony in auditory mismatch processing. *Biological Psychology, 84*(2), 336–45. doi:10.1016/j.biopsycho.2010.03.019

Hughes, L. E., Ghosh, B. C., & **Rowe, J. B.** (2013). Reorganisation of brain networks in frontotemporal dementia and progressive supranuclear palsy. *Neuroimage Clinical, 2*, 459–68. doi:10.1016/j.nicl.2013.03.009

Hughes, L. E., & **Rowe, J. B.** (2013). The impact of neurodegeneration on network connectivity: A study of change detection in frontotemporal dementia. *Journal of Cognitive Neuroscience, 25*(5), 802.

Huotilainen, M., **Ilmoniemi, R.**, Lavikainen, J., Tiitinen, H., Alho, K., Sinkkonen, J., et al. (1993). Interaction between representations of different features of auditory sensory memory. *NeuroReport, 4*(11), 1279–81.

Huotilainen, M., **Kujala, A.**, Hotakainen, M., Parkkonen, L., Taulu, S., Simola, J., et al. (2005). Short-term memory functions of the human fetus recorded with magnetoencephalography. *NeuroReport, 16*(1), 81–4.

Huotilainen, M., **Winkler, I.**, Alho, K., Escera, C., Virtanen, J., Ilmoniemi, R. J., et al. (1998). Combined mapping of human auditory EEG and MEG responses. *Electroencephalography and Clinical Neurophysiology, 108*(4), 370–9.

Huttenlocher, P. R., & **Dabholkar, A. S.** (1997). Regional differences in synaptogenesis in human cerebral cortex. *Journal of Comparative Neurology, 387*(2), 167–78.

Huttunen-Scott, T., **Kaartinen, J.**, Tolvanen, A., & **Lyytinen, H.** (2008). Mismatch negativity (MMN) elicited by duration deviations in children with reading disorder, attention deficit or both. *International Journal of Psychophysiology, 69*(1), 69–77. doi:10.1016/j.ijpsycho.2008.03.002

Ilvonen, T. M., **Kujala, T.**, Kiesiläinen, A., Salonen, O., Kozou, H., Pekkonen, E., et al. (2003). Auditory discrimination after left-hemisphere stroke: A mismatch negativity follow-up study. *Stroke, 34*(7), 1746–51. doi:10.1161/01.STR.0000078836.26328.3B

Imada, T., **Hari, R.**, Loveless, N., McEvoy, L., & **Sams, M.** (1993). Determinants of the auditory mismatch response. *Electroencephalography and Clinical Neurophysiology, 87*(3), 144–53.

Inami, R., **Kirino, E.**, Inoue, R., & **Arai, H.** (2005). Transdermal nicotine administration enhances automatic auditory processing reflected by mismatch negativity. *Pharmacology Biochemistry and Behavior, 80*(3), 453–61. doi:10.1016/j.pbb.2005.01.001

Jääskeläinen, I. P., **Hirvonen, J.**, Kujala, T., Alho, K., Eriksson, C. J., Lehtokoski, A., et al. (1998). Effects of naltrexone and ethanol on auditory event-related brain potentials. *Alcohol, 15*(2), 105–11.

Jääskelainen, I. P., **Schröger, E.**, & **Näätänen, R.** (1999). Electrophysiological indices of acute effects of ethanol on involuntary attention shifting. *Psychopharmacology, 141*(1), 16–21.

Jablensky, A. (1997). The 100-year epidemiology of schizophrenia. *Schizophrenia Research, 28*(2–3), 111–25.

Jacobs, B., & **Schneider, S.** (2003). Analysis of lexical-semantic processing and extensive neurological, electrophysiological, speech perception, and language evaluation following a unilateral left hemisphere lesion: Pure word deafness? *Aphasiology, 17*(2), 123–41. doi:10.1080/729255217

Jacobsen, T., & **Schröger, E.** (2003). Measuring duration mismatch negativity. *Clinical Neurophysiology, 114*(6), 1133–43. doi:10.1016/S1388-2457(03)00043-9

Jacobsen, T., **Schröger, E.**, & **Alter, K.** (2004). Pre-attentive perception of vowel phonemes from variable speech stimuli. *Psychophysiology, 41*(4), 654–9. doi:10.1111/1469-8986.2004.00175.x

Jacobsen, T., **Schröger, E.**, Horenkamp, T., & **Winkler, I.** (2003). Mismatch negativity to pitch change: varied stimulus proportions in controlling effects of neural refractoriness on human auditory event-related brain potentials. *Neuroscience Letters, 344*(2), 79–82.

Jacobsen, T., Schröger, E., Winkler, I., & Horváth, J. (2005). Familiarity affects the processing of task-irrelevant auditory deviance. *Journal of Cognitive Neuroscience, 17*(11), 1704–13. doi:10.1162/089892905774589262

Jahshan, C., Cadenhead, K. S., Rissling, A. J., Kirihara, K., Braff, D. L., & Light, G. A. (2012). Automatic sensory information processing abnormalities across the illness course of schizophrenia. *Psychological Medicine, 42*(1), 85–97. doi:10.1017/S0033291711001061

Jahshan, C., Wynn, J. K., & Green, M. F. (2013). Relationship between auditory processing and affective prosody in schizophrenia. *Schizophrenia Research, 143*(2–3), 348–53. doi:10.1016/j.schres.2012.11.025

James, W. (1890). *The Principles of Psychology.* New York: Holt and company.

Jankowiak, S., & Berti, S. (2007). Behavioral and event-related potential distraction effects with regularly occurring auditory deviants. *Psychophysiology, 44*(1), 79–85. doi:10.1111/j.1469-8986.2006.00479.x

Jansson-Verkasalo, E., Eggers, K., Järvenpää, A., Suominen, K., Van Den Bergh, B., De Nil, L., & Kujala, T. (2014). Atypical central auditory speech-sound discrimination in children who stutter as indexed by the mismatch negativity. *Journal of Fluency Disorders, 41*, 1–11. doi:10.1016/j.jfludis.2014.07.001

Jansson-Verkasalo, E., Kujala, T., Jussila, K., Mattila, M. L., Moilanen, I., Näätänen, R., et al. (2005). Similarities in the phenotype of the auditory neural substrate in children with Asperger syndrome and their parents. *European Journal of Neuroscience, 22*(4), 986–90. doi:10.1111/j.1460-9568.2005.04216.x

Javitt, D. C. (2015). Neurophysiological models for new treatment development in schizophrenia: Early sensory approaches. *Annals of the New York Academy of Sciences, 1344*(1), 92–104. doi:10.1111/nyas.12689

Javitt, D. C., Doneshka, P., Grochowski, S., & Ritter, W. (1995). Impaired mismatch negativity generation reflects widespread dysfunction of working memory in schizophrenia. *Archives of General Psychiatry, 52*(7), 550–8. doi:10.1001/archpsyc.1995.03950190032005

Javitt, D. C., Grochowski, S., Shelley, A.-M., & Ritter, W. (1998). Impaired mismatch negativity (MMN) generation in schizophrenia as a function of stimulus deviance, probability, and interstimulus/interdeviant interval. *Electroencephalography and Clinical Neurophysiology/ Evoked Potentials Section, 108*(2), 143–53. doi:10.1016/S0168-5597(97)00073-7

Javitt, D. C., Schroeder, C. E., Steinschneider, M., Arezzo, J. C., & Vaughan, H. G., Jr. (1992). Demonstration of mismatch negativity in the monkey. *Electroencephalography and Clinical Neurophysiology, 83*(1), 87–90.

Javitt, D. C., Spencer, K. M., Thaker, G. K., Winterer, G., & Hajos, M. (2008). Neurophysiological biomarkers for drug development in schizophrenia. *Nature Reviews Drug Discovery, 7*(1), 68–83. doi:10.1038/nrd2463

Javitt, D. C., Steinschneider, M., Schroeder, C. E., & Arezzo, J. C. (1996). Role of cortical N-methyl-D-aspartate receptors in auditory sensory memory and mismatch negativity generation: implications for schizophrenia. *Proceedings of the National Academy of Sciences, 93*(21), 11962–7.

Javitt, D. C., & Zukin, S. R. (1991). Recent advances in the phencyclidine model of schizophrenia. *American Journal of Psychiatry, 148*(10), 1301–8.

Javitt, D. C., Zukin, S. R., Heresco-Levy, U., & Umbricht, D. (2012). Has an angel shown the way? Etiological and therapeutic implications of the PCP/NMDA model of schizophrenia. *Schizophrenia Bulletin, 38*(5), 958–66. doi:10.1093/schbul/sbs069

Javitt, D. C., Zylberman, I., Zukin, S. R., Heresco-Levy, U., & Lindenmayer, J. P. (1994). Amelioration of negative symptoms in schizophrenia by glycine. *American Journal of Psychiatry, 151*(8), 1234–6. doi:10.1176/ajp.151.8.1234

Jemel, B., Achenbach, C., Muller, B. W., Ropcke, B., & Oades, R. D. (2002). Mismatch negativity results from bilateral asymmetric dipole sources in the frontal and temporal lobes. *Brain Topography*, *15*(1), 13–27.

Jessen, F., Fries, T., Kucharski, C., Nishimura, T., Hoenig, K., Maier, W., et al. (2001). Amplitude reduction of the mismatch negativity in first-degree relatives of patients with schizophrenia. *Neuroscience Letters*, *309*(3), 185–8.

Jing, H., & Benasich, A. A. (2006). Brain responses to tonal changes in the first two years of life. *Brain & Development*, *28*(4), 247–56. doi:10.1016/j.braindev.2005.09.002

Johnson, J. M. (2009). Late auditory event-related potentials in children with cochlear implants: A review. *Developmental Neuropsychology*, *34*(6), 701–20. doi:10.1080/87565640903265152

Johnston, M. C., Bronsky, P. T., & Millicovsky, G. (1990). Embryogenesis of cleft lip and palate. *Plastic Surgery. Cleft Lip and Palate and Craniofacial Anomalies*, *4*, 2515–22.

Jones, C. R. G., Happe, F., Baird, G., Simonoff, E., Marsden, A. J. S., Tregay, J., et al. (2009). Auditory discrimination and auditory sensory behaviours in autism spectrum disorders. *Neuropsychologia*, *47*(13), 2850–8. doi:10.1016/j.neuropsychologia.2009.06.015

Joshi, Y. B., Breitenstein, B., Tarasenko, M., Thomas, M. L., Chang, W. L., Sprock, J., et al. (2018). Mismatch negativity impairment is associated with deficits in identifying real-world environmental sounds in schizophrenia. *Schizophrenia Research*, *191*, 5–9. doi:10.1016/j.schres.2017.05.020

Jung, J., Morlet, D., Mercier, B., Confavreux, C., & Fischer, C. (2006). Mismatch negativity (MMN) in multiple sclerosis: An event-related potentials study in 46 patients. *Clinical Neurophysiology*, *117*(1), 85–93. doi:10.1016/j.clinph.2005.09.013

Jusczyk, P. W. (1997). Finding and remembering words: Some beginnings by English-learning infants. *Current Directions in Psychological Science*, *6*(6), 170–4. doi:10.1111/1467-8721.ep10772947

Jusczyk, P. W., & Bertoncini, J. (1988). Viewing the development of speech perception as an innately guided learning process. *Language and Speech*, *31*(3), 217–38.

Jääskeläinen, I. P., Alho, K., Escera, C., Winkler, I., Sillanaukee, P., & Näätänen, R. (1996a). Effects of ethanol and auditory distraction on forced choice reaction time. *Alcohol*, *13*(2), 153–6.

Jääskeläinen, I. P., Lehtokoski, A., Alho, K., Kujala, T., Pekkonen, E., Sinclair, J. D., et al. (1995b). Low dose of ethanol suppresses mismatch negativity of auditory event-related potentials. *Alcoholism: Clinical and Experimental Research*, *19*(3), 607–10.

Jääskeläinen, I. P., Näätänen, R., & Sillanaukee, P. (1996b). Effect of acute ethanol on auditory and visual event-related potentials: A review and reinterpretation. *Biological Psychiatry*, *40*(4), 284–91.

Jääskeläinen, I. P., Pekkonen, E., Alho, K., Sinclair, J. D., Sillanaukee, P., & Näätänen, R. (1995). Dose-related effect of alcohol on mismatch negativity and reaction time performance. *Alcohol*, *12*(6), 491–5.

Jääskeläinen, I. P., Pekkonen, E., Hirvonen, J., Sillanaukee, P., & Näätänen, R. (1996c). Mismatch negativity subcomponents and ethyl alcohol. *Biological Psychology*, *43*(1), 13–25.

Kaaden, S., & Helmstaedter, C. (2009). Age at onset of epilepsy as a determinant of intellectual impairment in temporal lobe epilepsy. *Epilepsy and Behavior*, *15*(2), 213–17. doi:10.1016/j.yebeh.2009.03.027

Kähkönen, S., Yamashita, H., Rytsälä, H., Suominen, K., Ahveninen, J., & Isometsä, E. (2007). Dysfunction in early auditory processing in major depressive disorder revealed by combined MEG and EEG. *Journal of Psychiatry & Neuroscience: JPN*, *32*(5), 316.

Kaipio, M. L., Alho, K., Winkler, I., Escera, C., Surma-Aho, O., & Näätänen, R. (1999). Event-related brain potentials reveal covert distractibility in closed head injuries. *NeuroReport*, *10*(10), 2125–9.

Kaipio, M.-L., Cheour, M., Ceponiene, R., Öhman, J., Alku, P., & Näätänen, R. (2000). Increased distractibility in closed head injury as revealed by event-related potentials. *NeuroReport*, *11*(7), 1463–8.

Kaipio, M.-L., Novitski, N., Tervaniemi, M., Alho, K., Öhman, J., Salonen, O., & Näätänen, R. (2001). Fast vigilance decrement in closed head injury patients as reflected by the mismatch negativity (MMN). *NeuroReport, 12*(7), 1517–22.

Kalyakin, I., González, N., Ivannikov, A., & Lyytinen, H. (2009). Extraction of the mismatch negativity elicited by sound duration decrements: A comparison of three procedures. *Data & Knowledge Engineering, 68*(12), 1411–26. doi:10.1016/j.datak.2009.07.004

Kalyakin, I., González, N., Joutsensalo, J., Huttunen, T., Kaartinen, J., & Lyytinen, H. (2007). Optimal digital filtering versus difference waves on the mismatch negativity in an uninterrupted sound paradigm. *Developmental Neuropsychology, 31*(3), 429–52. doi:10.1080/87565640701229607

Kalyakin, I., González, N., Kärkkäinen, T., & Lyytinen, H. (2008). Independent component analysis on the mismatch negativity in an uninterrupted sound paradigm. *Journal of Neuroscience Methods, 174*(2), 301–12. doi:10.1016/j.jneumeth.2008.07.012

Kane, N., Curry, S., Rowlands, C., Manara, A., Lewis, T., Moss, T., et al. (1996). Event-related potentials —neurophysiological tools for predicting emergence and early outcome from traumatic coma. *Intensive Care Medicine, 22*(1), 39–46. doi:10.1007/BF01728329

Kane, N. M., Butler, S. R., & Simpson, T. (2000). Coma Outcome Prediction Using Event-Related Potentials: P3 and Mismatch Negativity. *Audiology & Neurotology, 5*(3–4), 186–91. doi:10.1159/000013879

Kane, N. M., Curry, S. H., Butler, S. R., & Cummins, B. H. (1993). Electrophysiological indicator of awakening from coma. *Lancet, 341*(8846), 688.

Kanner, L. (1943). Autistic disturbances of affective contact. *Nervous child, 2*(3), 217–50.

Kantrowitz, J. T., & Javitt, D. C. (2010). Thinking glutamatergically: Changing concepts of schizophrenia based upon changing neurochemical models. *Clinical Schizophrenia and Related Psychoses, 4*(3), 189–200. doi:10.3371/CSRP.4.3.6

Kantrowitz, J., & Javitt, D. C. (2012). Glutamatergic transmission in schizophrenia: From basic research to clinical practice. *Current Opinion in Psychiatry, 25*(2), 96–102. doi:10.1097/YCO.0b013e32835035b2

Karl, A., Malta, L. S., & Maercker, A. (2006). Meta-analytic review of event-related potential studies in post-traumatic stress disorder. *Biological Psychology, 71*(2), 123–47. doi:10.1016/j.biopsycho.2005.03.004

Kasai, K., Hashimoto, O., Kawakubo, Y., Yumoto, M., Kamio, S., Itoh, K., et al. (2005). Delayed automatic detection of change in speech sounds in adults with autism: A magnetoencephalographic study. *Clinical Neurophysiology, 116*(7), 1655–64. doi:10.1016/j.clinph.2005.03.007

Kasai, K., Nakagome, K., Itoh, K., Koshida, I., Hata, A., Iwanami, A., et al. (2002a). Impaired cortical network for preattentive detection of change in speech sounds in schizophrenia: A high-resolution event-related potential study. *American Journal of Psychiatry, 159*(4), 546–53. doi:10.1176/appi.ajp.159.4.546

Kasai, K., Okazawa, K., Nakagome, K., Hiramatsu, K.-I., Hata, A., Fukuda, M., et al. (1999). Mismatch negativity and N2b attenuation as an indicator for dysfunction of the preattentive and controlled processing for deviance detection in schizophrenia: a topographic event-related potential study. *Schizophrenia Research, 35*(2), 141–56. doi:10.1016/S0920-9964(98)00116-9

Kasai, K., Yamada, H., Kamio, S., Nakagome, K., Iwanami, A., Fukuda, M., et al. (2002b). Do high or low doses of anxiolytics and hypnotics affect mismatch negativity in schizophrenic subjects? An EEG and MEG study. *Clinical Neurophysiology, 113*(1), 141–50. doi:10.1016/S1388-2457(01)00710-6

Kathmann, N., Frodl-Bauch, T., & Hegerl, U. (1999). Stability of the mismatch negativity under different stimulus and attention conditions. *Clinical Neurophysiology, 110*(2), 317–23. doi:10.1016/S1388-2457(98)00011-X

Kathmann, N., Wagner, M., Rendtorff, N., & Engel, R. R. (1995). Delayed peak latency of the mismatch negativity in schizophrenics and alcoholics. *Biological Psychiatry, 37*(10), 754–7. doi:10.1016/0006-3223(94)00309-Q

Kaukoranta, E., Sams, M., Hari, R., Hämäläinen, M., & Näätänen, R. (1989). Reactions of human auditory cortex to a change in tone duration. *Hearing Research*, *41*(1), 15–21. doi:10.1016/0378-5955(89)90174-3

Kaur, M., Battisti, R. A., Lagopoulos, J., Ward, P. B., Hickie, I. B., & Hermens, D. F. (2012). Neurophysiological biomarkers support bipolar-spectrum disorders within psychosis cluster. *Journal of Psychiatry and Neuroscience*, *37*(5), 313–21. doi:10.1503/jpn.110081

Kawakubo, A. Y., Kasai, A. K., Kudo, A. N., Rogers, A. M., Nakagome, A. K., Itoh, A. K., & Kato, A. N. (2006). Phonetic mismatch negativity predicts verbal memory deficits in schizophrenia. *NeuroReport*, *17*(10), 1043–6. doi:10.1097/01.wnr.0000221828.10846.ba

Kawakubo, Y., Kamio, S., Nose, T., Iwanami, A., Nakagome, K., Fukuda, M., et al. (2007). Phonetic mismatch negativity predicts social skills acquisition in schizophrenia. *Psychiatry Research*, *152*(2–3), 261–5. doi:10.1016/j.psychres.2006.02.010

Kawakubo, Y., & Kasai, K. (2006). Support for an association between mismatch negativity and social functioning in schizophrenia. *Progress in Neuro-Psychopharmacology and Biological Psychiatry*, *30*(7), 1367–8.

Kazmerski, V. A., Friedman, D., & Ritter, W. (1997). Mismatch negativity during attend and ignore conditions in Alzheimer's disease. *Biological Psychiatry*, *42*(5), 382–402. doi:10.1016/S0006-3223(96)00344-7

Kekoni, J., Hämäläinen, H., Saarinen, M., Gröhn, J., Reinikainen, K., Lehtokoski, A., & Näätänen, R. (1997). Rate effect and mismatch responses in the somatosensory system: ERP-recordings in humans. *Biological Psychology*, *46*(2), 125–42. doi:10.1016/S0301-0511(97)05249-6

Kelly, A. S., Purdy, S. C., & Thorne, P. R. (2005). Electrophysiological and speech perception measures of auditory processing in experienced adult cochlear implant users. *Clinical Neurophysiology*, *116*(6), 1235–46. doi:10.1016/j.clinph.2005.02.011

Kenemans, J. L., Hebly, W., van den Heuvel, E., & Grent-'T-Jong, T. (2010). Moderate alcohol disrupts a mechanism for detection of rare events in human visual cortex. *Journal of Psychopharmacology*, *24*(6), 839–45.

Kenemans, L. J., Jong, G.-T. T., & Verbaten, N. M. (2003). Detection of visual change: mismatch or rareness? *NeuroReport*, *14*(9), 1239–42.

Kennedy, N., Foy, K., Sherazi, R., McDonough, M., & McKeon, P. (2007). Long-term social functioning after depression treated by psychiatrists: A review. *Bipolar Disorders*, *9*(1–2), 25–37. doi:10.1111/j.1399-5618.2007.00326.x

Kere, J. (2011). Molecular genetics and molecular biology of dyslexia. *Wiley Interdisciplinary Reviews: Cognitive Science*, *2*(4), 441–8. doi:10.1002/wcs.138

Kessler, R. C., Aguilar-Gaxiola, S., Alonso, J., Chatterji, S., Lee, S., Ormel, J., et al. (2009). The global burden of mental disorders: An update from the WHO World Mental Health (WMH) surveys. *Epidemiology and Psychiatric Sciences*, *18*(1), 23–33. doi:10.1017/S1121189X00001421

Khalfa, S., Bruneau, N., Rogé, B., Georgieff, N., Veuillet, E., Adrien, J.-L., et al. (2004). Increased perception of loudness in autism. *Hearing Research*, *198*(1), 87–92. doi:10.1016/j.heares.2004.07.006

Kiang, M., Braff, D. L., Sprock, J., & Light, G. A. (2009). The relationship between preattentive sensory processing deficits and age in schizophrenia patients. *Clinical Neurophysiology*, *120*(11), 1949–57. doi:10.1016/j.clinph.2009.08.019

Kiang, M., Light, G. A., Prugh, J., Coulson, S., Braff, D. L., & Kutas, M. (2007). Cognitive, neurophysiological, and functional correlates of proverb interpretation abnormalities in schizophrenia. *Journal of the International Neuropsychological Society*, *13*(4), 653–63. doi:10.1017/S1355617707070816

Kileny, P. R., Boerst, A., & Zwolan, T. (1997). Cognitive evoked potentials to speech and tonal stimuli in children with implants. *Otolaryngology - Head and Neck Surgery*, *117*(3), 161–9. doi:10.1016/S0194-5998(97)70169-4

Kilpeläinen, R., Partanen, J., & Karhu, J. (1999). Reduced mismatch negativity (MMN) suggests deficits in pre-attentive auditory processing in distractible children. *NeuroReport, 10*(16), 3341–5. doi:10.1097/00001756-199911080-00016

Kim, M., Kim, S. N., Lee, S., Byun, M. S., Shin, K. S., Park, H. Y., et al. (2014). Impaired mismatch negativity is associated with current functional status rather than genetic vulnerability to schizophrenia. *Psychiatry Research: Neuroimaging, 222*(1–2), 100–6. doi:10.1016/j.pscychresns.2014.02.012

Kim, H., Lee, M. H., Chang, H. K., Lee, T. H., Lee, H. H., Shin, M. C., et al. (2006). Influence of prenatal noise and music on the spatial memory and neurogenesis in the hippocampus of developing rats. *Brain and Development, 28*(2), 109–14. doi:10.1016/j.braindev.2005.05.008

Kimura, M., Katayama, J., & Murohashi, H. (2006a). An ERP study of visual change detection: Effects of feature and spatial attention on the changerelated posterior positivity. *Psychophysiology, 43*, S52.

Kimura, M., Katayama, J., & Murohashi, H. (2008a). Involvement of memory-comparison-based change detection in visual distraction. *Psychophysiology, 45*(3), 445–57. doi:10.1111/j.1469-8986.2007.00640.x

Kimura, M., Katayama, J., & Murohashi, H. (2008b). Attention switching function of memory-comparison-based change detection system in the visual modality. *International Journal of Psychophysiology, 67*(2), 101–13. doi:10.1016/j.ijpsycho.2007.10.009

Kimura, M., Katayama, J. I., & Murohashi, H. (2006b). Probability-independent and -dependent ERPs reflecting visual change detection. *Psychophysiology, 43*(2), 180–9. doi:10.1111/j.1469-8986.2006.00388.x

Kimura, M., Katayama, J. I., Ohira, H., & Schröger, E. (2009). Visual mismatch negativity: New evidence from the equiprobable paradigm. *Psychophysiology, 46*(2), 402–9. doi:10.1111/j.1469-8986.2008.00767.x

Kimura, M., Ohira, H., & Schröger, E. (2010a). Localizing sensory and cognitive systems for pre-attentive visual deviance detection: An sLORETA analysis of the data of Kimura et al. (2009). *Neuroscience Letters, 485*(3), 198–203. doi:10.1016/j.neulet.2010.09.011

Kimura, M., Schröger, E., & Czigler, I. (2011). Visual mismatch negativity and its importance in visual cognitive sciences. *NeuroReport, 22*(14), 669–73. doi:10.1097/WNR.0b013e32834973ba

Kimura, M., Schröger, E., Czigler, I., & Ohira, H. (2010b). Human visual system automatically encodes sequential regularities of discrete events. *Journal of Cognitive Neuroscience, 22*(6), 1124–39. doi:10.1162/jocn.2009.21299

Kimura, M., Widmann, A., & Schröger, E. (2010c). Human visual system automatically represents large-scale sequential regularities. *Brain Research, 1317*, 165–79. doi:10.1016/j.brainres.2009.12.076

King, C., McGee, T., Rubel, E. W., Nicol, T., & Kraus, N. (1995). Acoustic features and acoustic change are represented by different central pathways. *Hearing Research, 85*(1), 45–52. doi:10.1016/0378-5955(95)00028-3

King, J. R., Faugeras, F., Gramfort, A., Schurger, A., El Karoui, I., Sitt, J. D., et al. (2013a). Single-trial decoding of auditory novelty responses facilitates the detection of residual consciousness. *NeuroImage, 83*, 726–38. doi:10.1016/j.neuroimage.2013.07.013

King, J.-R., Sitt, Jacobo d., Faugeras, F., Rohaut, B., El karoui, I., Cohen, L., et al. (2013b). Information sharing in the brain indexes consciousness in noncommunicative patients. *Current Biology, 23*(19), 1914–19. doi:10.1016/j.cub.2013.07.075

Kisley, M. A., Davalos, D. B., Engleman, L. L., Guinther, P. M., & Davis, H. P. (2005). Age-related change in neural processing of time-dependent stimulus features. *Cognitive Brain Research, 25*(3), 913–25. doi:10.1016/j.cogbrainres.2005.09.014

Klin, A. (1991). Young autistic children's listening preferences in regard to speech: A possible characterization of the symptom of social withdrawal. *Journal of Autism and Developmental Disorders, 21*(1), 29–42. doi:10.1007/BF02206995

Knight, R. T. (1991). Capacity in human frontal lobe lesions. In H. S. Levin, H. M. Eisenberg, & A. L. Benton (Eds), *Frontal Lobe Function And Dysfunction* (pp. 139–156). New York: Oxford University Press.

Knight, R. T., Scabini, D., & Woods, D. L. (1989). Prefrontal cortex gating of auditory transmission in humans. *Brain Research, 504*(2), 338–42. doi:10.1016/0006-8993(89)91381-4

Koelsch, S., Heinke, W., Sammler, D., & Olthoff, D. (2006). Auditory processing during deep propofol sedation and recovery from unconsciousness. *Clinical Neurophysiology, 117*(8), 1746–59. doi:10.1016/j.clinph.2006.05.009

Koelsch, S., Schröger, E., & Tervaniemi, M. (1999). Superior pre-attentive auditory processing in musicians. *NeuroReport, 10*(6), 1309–13.

Koelsch, S., Wittfoth, M., Wolf, A., Müller, J., & Hahne, A. (2004). Music perception in cochlear implant users: An event-related potential study. *Clinical Neurophysiology, 115*(4), 966–72. doi:10.1016/j.clinph.2003.11.032

Kohlmetz, C., Altenmüller, E., Schuppert, M., Wieringa, B. M., & Münte, T. F. (2001). Deficit in automatic sound-change detection may underlie some music perception deficits after acute hemispheric stroke. *Neuropsychologia, 39*(11), 1121–4. doi:10.1016/S0028-3932(01)00079-3

Kok, L. L., & Solman, R. T. (1995). Velocardiofacial syndrome: Learning difficulties and intervention. *Journal of Medical Genetics, 32*(8), 612–8. doi:10.1136/jmg.32.8.612

Korkman, M., Granström, M.-L., Appelqvist, K., & Liukkonen, E. (1998). Neuropsychological characteristics of five children with the Landau-Kleffner syndrome: Dissociation of auditory and phonological discrimination. *Journal of the International Neuropsychological Society, 4*(6), 566–75.

Korostenskaja, M., Dapsys, K., Siurkute, A., Maciulis, V., Ruksenas, O., & Kähkönen, S. (2005). Effects of olanzapine on auditory P300 and mismatch negativity (MMN) in schizophrenia spectrum disorders. *Progress in Neuro-Psychopharmacology and Biological Psychiatry, 29*(4), 543–8. doi:10.1016/j.pnpbp.2005.01.019

Korostenskaja, M., Pardos, M., Fujiwara, H., Kujala, T., Horn, P., Rose, D., et al. (2010). Neuromagnetic evidence of impaired cortical auditory processing in pediatric intractable epilepsy. *Epilepsy Research, 92*(1), 63–73. doi:10.1016/j.eplepsyres.2010.08.008

Korpilahti, P., Jansson-Verkasalo, E., Mattila, M.-L., Kuusikko, S., Suominen, K., Rytky, S., et al. (2007). Processing of affective speech prosody is impaired in Asperger syndrome. *Journal of Autism and Developmental Disorders, 37*(8), 1539–49. doi:10.1007/s10803-006-0271-2

Korpilahti, P., Krause, C. M., Holopainen, I., & Lang, A. H. (2001). Early and late mismatch negativity elicited by words and speech-like stimuli in children. *Brain and Language, 76*(3), 332–9. doi:10.1006/brln.2000.2426

Korpilahti, P., & Lang, H. A. (1994). Auditory ERP components and mismatch negativity in dysphasic children. *Electroencephalography and Clinical Neurophysiology, 91*(4), 256–64. doi:10.1016/0013-4694(94)90189-9

Korzyukov, O., Alho, K., Kujala, A., Gumenyuk, V., Ilmoniemi, R. J., Virtanen, J., et al. (1999). Electromagnetic responses of the human auditory cortex generated by sensory-memory based processing of tone-frequency changes. *Neuroscience Letters, 276*(3), 169–72. doi:10.1016/S0304-3940(99)00807-1

Koshiyama, D., Kirihara, K., Tada, M., Nagai, T., Fujioka, M., Koike, S., et al. (2017a). Association between mismatch negativity and global functioning is specific to duration deviance in early stages of psychosis. *Schizophrenia Research, 195*, 373–84. doi:10.1016/j.schres.2017.09.045

Koshiyama, D., Kirihara, K., Tada, M., Nagai, T., Koike, S., Suga, M., et al. (2017b). Duration and frequency mismatch negativity shows no progressive reduction in early stages of psychosis. *Schizophrenia Research, 190*, 32–38. doi:10.1016/j.schres.2017.03.015

Kotchoubey, B., Lang, S., Herb, E., Maurer, P., Schmalohr, D., Bostanov, V., & Birbaumer, N. (2003). Stimulus complexity enhances auditory discrimination in patients with extremely severe brain injuries. *Neuroscience Letters, 352*(2), 129–32. doi:10.1016/j.neulet.2003.08.045

Krauel, K., Schott, P., Sojka, B., Pause, B. M., & Ferstl, R. (1999). Is there a mismatch negativity analogue in the olfactory event-related potential? *Journal of Psychophysiology, 13*(1), 49–55. doi:10.1027//0269-8803.13.1.49

Kraus, N., & Cheour, M. (2000). Speech sound representation in the brain. *Audiology and Neurotology, 5*(3–4), 140–50.

Kraus, N., McGee, T., Carrell, T., King, C., Littman, T., & Nicol, T. (1994a). Discrimination of speech-like contrasts in the auditory thalamus and cortex. *The Journal of the Acoustical Society of America, 96*(5), 2758–68.

Kraus, N., McGee, T., Carrell, T. D., King, C., Tremblay, K., & Nicol, T. (1995a). Central auditory system plasticity associated with speech discrimination training. *Journal of Cognitive Neuroscience, 7*(1), 25–32. doi:10.1162/jocn.1995.7.1.25

Kraus, N., McGee, T., Carrell, T. D., & Sharma, A. (1995b). Neurophysiologic bases of speech discrimination. *Ear and Hearing, 16*(1), 19–37. doi:10.1097/00003446-199502000-00003

Kraus, N., McGee, T., Littman, T., Nicol, T., & King, C. (1994b). Nonprimary auditory thalamic representation of acoustic change. *Journal of Neurophysiology, 72*(3), 1270–7.

Kraus, N., Micco, A. G., Koch, D. B., McGee, T., Carrell, T., Sharma, A., et al. (1993). The mismatch negativity cortical evoked potential elicited by speech in cochlear-implant users. *Hearing Research, 65*(1), 118–24. doi:10.1016/0378-5955(93)90206-G

Kreitschmann-Andermahr, I., Rosburg, T., Demme, U., Gaser, E., Nowak, H., & Sauer, H. (2001). Effect of ketamine on the neuromagnetic mismatch field in healthy humans. *Cognitive Brain Research, 12*(1), 109–16. doi:10.1016/S0926-6410(01)00043-X

Kropotov, J. D., Alho, K., Näätänen, R., Ponomarev, V. A., Kropotova, O. V., Anichkov, A. D., & Nechaev, V. B. (2000). Human auditory-cortex mechanisms of preattentive sound discrimination. *Neuroscience Letters, 280*(2), 87–90. doi:10.1016/S0304-3940(00)00765-5

Kropotov, J. D., Näätänen, R., Sevostianov, A. V., Alho, K., Reinikainen, K., & Kropotova, O. V. (1995). Mismatch negativity to auditory stimulus change recorded directly from the human temporal cortex. *Psychophysiology, 32*(4), 418–22. doi:10.1111/j.1469-8986.1995.tb01226.x

Krystal, J. H., Karper, L. P., Seibyl, J. P., Freeman, G. K., Delaney, R., Bremner, J. D., et al. (1994). Subanesthetic effects of the noncompetitive NMDA antagonist, ketamine, in humans: Psychotomimetic, perceptual, cognitive, and neuroendocrine responses. *Archives of General Psychiatry, 51*(3), 199–214. doi:10.1001/archpsyc.1994.03950030035004

Kuhl, P. K. (2004). Early language acquisition: cracking the speech code. *Nature Reviews Neuroscience, 5*(11), 831. doi:10.1038/nrn1533

Kuhl, P. K., Coffey-Corina, S., Padden, D., & Dawson, G. (2005). Links between social and linguistic processing of speech in preschool children with autism: Behavioral and electrophysiological measures. *Developmental Science, 8*(1), F1–F12. doi:10.1111/j.1467-7687.2004.00384.x

Kujala, T., Aho, E., Lepistö, T., Jansson-Verkasalo, E., Nieminen-Von Wendt, T., Von Wendt, L., & Näätänen, R. (2007a). Atypical pattern of discriminating sound features in adults with Asperger syndrome as reflected by the mismatch negativity. *Biological Psychology, 75*(1), 109–14. doi:10.1016/j.biopsycho.2006.12.007

Kujala, T., Belitz, S., Tervaniemi, M., & Näätänen, R. (2003). Auditory sensory memory disorder in dyslexic adults as indexed by the mismatch negativity. *European Journal of Neuroscience, 17*(6), 1323–7. doi:10.1046/j.1460-9568.2003.02559.x

Kujala, T., & Brattico, E. (2009). Detrimental noise effects on brain's speech functions. *Biological Psychology, 81*(3), 135–43. doi:10.1016/j.biopsycho.2009.03.010

Kujala, T., Halmetoja, J., Näätänen, R., Alku, P., Lyytinen, H., & Sussman, E. (2006a). Speech- and sound-segmentation in dyslexia: evidence for a multiple-level cortical impairment. *European Journal of Neuroscience, 24*(8), 2420–7. doi:10.1111/j.1460-9568.2006.05100.x

Kujala, A., Huotilainen, M., Hotakainen, M., Lennes, M., Parkkonen, L., Fellman, V., & Näätänen, R. (2004). Speech-sound discrimination in neonates as measured with MEG. *NeuroReport*, *15*(13), 2089–92.

Kujala, T., Karma, K., Ceponiene, R., Belitz, S., Turkkila, P., Tervaniemi, M., & Näätänen, R. (2001). Plastic neural changes and reading improvement caused by audiovisual training in reading-impaired children. *Proceedings of the National Academy of Sciences of the United States of America*, *98*(18), 10509–14.

Kujala, T., Kuuluvainen, S., Saalasti, S., Jansson-Verkasalo, E., Wendt, L. V., & Lepistö, T. (2010). Speech-feature discrimination in children with Asperger syndrome as determined with the multi-feature mismatch negativity paradigm. *Clinical Neurophysiology*, *121*(9), 1410–19. doi:10.1016/j.clinph.2010.03.017

Kujala, T., Lepistö, T., Nieminen-Von Wendt, T., Näätänen, P., & Näätänen, R. (2005). Neurophysiological evidence for cortical discrimination impairment of prosody in Asperger syndrome. *Neuroscience Letters*, *383*(3), 260–65. doi:10.1016/j.neulet.2005.04.048

Kujala, T., Lovio, R., Lepistö, T., Laasonen, M., & Näätänen, R. (2006b). Evaluation of multi-attribute auditory discrimination in dyslexia with the mismatch negativity. *Clinical Neurophysiology*, *117*(4), 885–93. doi:10.1016/j.clinph.2006.01.002

Kujala, T., Myllyviita, K., Tervaniemi, M., Alho, K., Kallio, J., & Näätänen, R. (2000). Basic auditory dysfunction in dyslexia as demonstrated by brain activity measurements. *Psychophysiology*, *37*(2), 262–6.

Kujala, T., Shtyrov, Y., Winkler, I., Saher, M., Tervaniemi, M., Sallinen, M., et al. (2004). Long-term exposure to noise impairs cortical sound processing and attention control. *Psychophysiology*, *41*(6), 875–81.

Kujala, T., Tervaniemi, M., & Schröger, E. (2007b). The mismatch negativity in cognitive and clinical neuroscience: Theoretical and methodological considerations. *Biological Psychology*, *74*(1), 1–19. doi:10.1016/j.biopsycho.2006.06.001

Kuuluvainen, S., Alku, P., Makkonen, T., Lipsanen, J., & Kujala, T. (2016). Cortical speech and non-speech discrimination in relation to cognitive measures in preschool children. *European Journal of Neuroscience*, *43*(6), 738–50. doi:10.1111/ejn.13141

Kuuluvainen, S., Nevalainen, P., Sorokin, A., Mittag, M., Partanen, E., Putkinen, V., et al. (2014). The neural basis of sublexical speech and corresponding nonspeech processing: A combined EEG–MEG study. *Brain and Language*, *130*, 19–32. doi:10.1016/j.bandl.2014.01.008

Kwon, J. S., Youn, T., Park, H.-J., Kong, S. W., & Kim, M. S. (2002). Temporal association of MMN multiple generators: High density recording (128 channels). *International Congress Series*, *1232*, 335–8. doi:10.1016/S0531-5131(01)00727-0

Kähkönen, S., Marttinen Rossi, E., & Yamashita, H. (2005). Alcohol impairs auditory processing of frequency changes and novel sounds: A combined MEG and EEG study. *Psychopharmacology*, *177*(4), 366–72. doi:10.1007/s00213-004-1960-1

Lachmann, T., Berti, S., Kujala, T., & Schröger, E. (2005). Diagnostic subgroups of developmental dyslexia have different deficits in neural processing of tones and phonemes. *International Journal of Psychophysiology*, *56*(2), 105–20. doi:10.1016/j.ijpsycho.2004.11.005

Landau, W. M., & Kleffner, F. R. (1957). Syndrome of acquired aphasia with convulsive disorder in children. *Neurology*, *7*(8), 523–30.

Lang, A. H., Eerola, O., Korpilahti, P., Holopainen, I., Salo, S., & Aaltonen, O. (1995). Practical issues in the clinical application of mismatch negativity. *Ear and Hearing*, *16*(1), 118–30.

Lang, A. H., Nyrke, T., Ek, M., Aaltonen, O., Raimo, I., & Näätänen, R. (1990). Pitch discrimination performance and auditive event related potentials. In C. Brunia, A. W. K. Gaillard, & A. Kok (Eds), *Psychophysiological Brain Research: Vol. 2* (pp. 294–8). Tilburg: Tilburg University Press.

Lauritsen, M. B. (2013). Autism spectrum disorders. *European Child & Adolescent Psychiatry*, *22*(1), S37–42.

Lavikainen, J., Huotilainen, M., Ilmoniemi, R. J., Simola, J. T., & Näätänen, R. (1995). Pitch change of a continuous tone activates two distinct processes in human auditory cortex: a study with whole-head magnetometer. *Electroencephalography and Clinical Neurophysiology*, *96*(1), 93–96.

Lavikainen, J. J., Huotilainen, J. M., Pekkonen, J. E., Ilmoniemi, J. R., & Näätänen, J. R. (1994). Auditory stimuli activate parietal brain regions: A whole-head MEG study. *NeuroReport*, *6*(1), 182–4.

Lavoie, S., Murray, M., Deppen, P., Knyazeva, M. G., Berk, M., Boulat, O., et al. (2007). Glutathione precursor, n-acetyl-cysteine, improves mismatch negativity in schizophrenia patients. *Neuropsychopharmacology*, *33*(9), 2187–99. doi:10.1038/sj.npp.1301624

Lavoie, S., Murray, M. M., Deppen, P., Knyazeva, M. G., Berk, M., Boulat, O., et al. (2008). Glutathione precursor, N-acetyl-cysteine, improves mismatch negativity in schizophrenia patients. *Neuropsychopharmacology*, *33*(9), 2187–99. doi:10.1038/sj.npp.1301624

Lee, C. Y., Yen, H. L., Yeh, P. W., Lin, W. H., Cheng, Y. Y., Tzeng, Y. L., & Wu, H. C. (2012). Mismatch responses to lexical tone, initial consonant, and vowel in Mandarin-speaking preschoolers. *Neuropsychologia*, *50*(14), 3228–39. doi:10.1016/j.neuropsychologia.2012.08.025

Lee, M., Balla, A., Sershen, H., Sehatpour, P., Lakatos, P., & Javitt, D. C. (2018). Rodent mismatch negativity/theta neuro-oscillatory response as a translational neurophysiological biomarker for N-methyl-d-aspartate receptor-based new treatment development in schizophrenia. *Neuropsychopharmacology*, *43*(3), 571–82.

Lee, S. H., Sung, K., Lee, K. S., Moon, E., & Kim, C. G. (2014). Mismatch negativity is a stronger indicator of functional outcomes than neurocognition or theory of mind in patients with schizophrenia. *Progress in Neuro-Psychopharmacology and Biological Psychiatry*, *48*, 213–19. doi:10.1016/j.pnpbp.2013.10.010

Leekam, S., Nieto, C., Libby, S., Wing, L., & Gould, J. (2007). Describing the sensory abnormalities of children and adults with autism. *Journal of Autism and Developmental Disorders*, *37*(5), 894–910. doi:10.1007/s10803-006-0218-7

Leitman, D. I., Sehatpour, P., Higgins, B. A., Foxe, J. J., Silipo, G., & Javitt, D. C. (2010). Sensory deficits and distributed hierarchical dysfunction in schizophrenia. *American Journal of Psychiatry*, *167*(7), 818–27. doi:10.1176/appi.ajp.2010.09030338

Leminen, A., Lehtonen, M., Leminen, M., Nevalainen, P., Mäkelä, J., & Kujala, T. (2013). The role of attention in processing morphologically complex spoken words: an EEG/MEG study. *Frontiers in Human Neuroscience*, *6*,353. doi:10.3389/fnhum.2012.00353

Leonard, L. (1998). *Children with Specific Language Impairment*. Cambridge, MA: MIT Press.

Lepistö, T., Kajander, M., Vanhala, R., Alku, P., Huotilainen, M., Näätänen, R., & Kujala, T. (2008). The perception of invariant speech features in children with autism. *Biological Psychology*, *77*(1), 25–31. doi:10.1016/j.biopsycho.2007.08.010

Lepistö, T., Kujala, T., Vanhala, R., Alku, P., Huotilainen, M., & Näätänen, R. (2005). The discrimination of and orienting to speech and non-speech sounds in children with autism. *Brain Research*, *1066*(1), 147–57. doi:10.1016/j.brainres.2005.10.052

Lepistö, T., Nieminen-Von Wendt, T., Von Wendt, L., Näätänen, R., & Kujala, T. (2007). Auditory cortical change detection in adults with Asperger syndrome. *Neuroscience Letters*, *414*(2), 136–40. doi:10.1016/j.neulet.2006.12.009

Lepistö, T., Silokallio, S., Nieminen-Von Wendt, T., Alku, P., Näätänen, R., & Kujala, T. (2006). Auditory perception and attention as reflected by the brain event-related potentials in children with Asperger syndrome. *Clinical Neurophysiology*, *117*(10), 2161–71. doi:10.1016/j.clinph.2006.06.709

Lepistö, T., Soininen, M., Čeponiene, R., Almqvist, F., Näätänen, R., & Aronen, E. T. (2004). Auditory event-related potential indices of increased distractibility in children with major depression. *Clinical Neurophysiology, 115*(3), 620–7. doi:10.1016/j.clinph.2003.10.020

Leppänen, P. T., Eklund, K., & Lyytinen, H. (1997). Event-related brain potentials to change in rapidly presented acoustic stimuli in newborns. *Developmental Neuropsychology, 13*(2), 175–204. doi:10.1080/87565649709540677

Leppänen, P. H. T., Guttorm, T. K., Pihko, E., Takkinen, S., Eklund, K. M., & Lyytinen, H. (2004). Maturational effects on newborn ERPs measured in the mismatch negativity paradigm. *Experimental Neurology, 190*, 91–101. doi:https://doi.org/10.1016/j.expneurol.2004.06.002

Leppänen, P. H. T., Pihko, E., Eklund, K. M., & Lyytinen, H. (1999). Cortical responses of infants with and without a genetic risk for dyslexia: II. Group effects. *NeuroReport, 10*(5), 969–73. doi:10.1097/00001756-199904060-00014

Leppänen, P. H. T., Richardson, U., Pihko, E., Eklund, K. M., Guttorm, T. K., Aro, M., & Lyytinen, H. (2002). Brain responses to changes in speech sound durations differ between infants with and without familial risk for dyslexia. *Developmental Neuropsychology, 22*(1), 407–22. doi:10.1207/S15326942dn2201_4

Leung, S., Croft, R. J., Baldeweg, T., & Nathan, P. J. (2007). Acute dopamine D1 and D2 receptor stimulation does not modulate mismatch negativity (MMN) in healthy human subjects. *Psychopharmacology, 194*(4), 443–51. doi:10.1007/s00213-007-0865-1

Leung, S., Croft, R. J., Guille, V., Scholes, K., O'Neill, B. V., Phan, K. L., & Nathan, P. J. (2010). Acute dopamine and/or serotonin depletion does not modulate mismatch negativity (MMN) in healthy human participants. *Psychopharmacology, 208*(2), 233–44. doi:10.1007/s00213-009-1723-0

Levänen, S., Ahonen, A., Hari, R., McEvoy, L., & Sams, M. (1996). Deviant auditory stimuli activate human left and right auditory cortex differently. *Cerebral Cortex, 6*(2), 288–96. doi:10.1093/cercor/6.2.288

Levänen, S., Hari, R., McEvoy, L., & Sams, M. (1993). Responses of the human auditory cortex to changes in one versus two stimulus features. *Experimental Brain Research, 97*(1), 177–83. doi:10.1007/BF00228828

Li, X., Lu, Y., Sun, G., Gao, L., & Zhao, L. (2012). Visual mismatch negativity elicited by facial expressions: New evidence from the equiprobable paradigm. *Behavioral and Brain Functions, 8*, 7. doi:10.1186/1744-9081-8-7

Liang, M., Zhang, X., Chen, T., Zheng, Y., Zhao, F., Yang, H., et al. (2014). Evaluation of auditory cortical development in the early stages of post cochlear implantation using mismatch negativity measurement. *Otology and Neurotology, 35*(1), e7–e14. doi:10.1097/MAO.0000000000000181

Liasis, A., Bamiou, D. E., Boyd, S., & Towell, A. (2006). Evidence for a neurophysiologic auditory deficit in children with benign epilepsy with centro-temporal spikes. *Journal of Neural Transmission, 113*(7), 939–49. doi:10.1007/s00702-005-0357-6

Liasis, A., Towell, A., Alho, K., & Boyd, S. (2001). Intracranial identification of an electric frontal-cortex response to auditory stimulus change: a case study. *Cognitive Brain Research, 11*(2), 227–33. doi:10.1016/S0926-6410(00)00077-X

Liasis, A., Towell, A., & Boyd, S. (1999). Intracranial auditory detection and discrimination potentials as substrates of echoic memory in children. *Cognitive Brain Research, 7*(4), 503–6. doi:10.1016/S0926-6410(98)00049-4

Liasis, A., Towell, A., & Boyd, S. (2000). Intracranial evidence for differential encoding of frequency and duration discrimination responses. *Ear and Hearing, 21*(3), 252–6.

Liberman, I. Y. (1973). 1. Segmentation of the spoken word and reading acquisition. *Bulletin of the Orton Society, 23*(1), 64–77. doi:10.1007/BF02653842

Lichtenstein, P., Carlstrom, E., Rastam, M., Gillberg, C., & Anckarsater, H. (2010). The genetics of autism spectrum disorders and related neuropsychiatric disorders in childhood. *American Journal of Psychiatry, 167*(11), 1357–63.

Lieberman, J., Chakos, M., Wu, H., Alvir, J., Hoffman, E., Robinson, D., & Bilder, R. (2001). Longitudinal study of brain morphology in first episode schizophrenia. *Biological Psychiatry, 49*(6), 487–99. doi:10.1016/S0006-3223(01)01067-8

Light, G., & Braff, D. L. (2005a). Mismatch negativity deficits are associated with poor functioning in schizophrenia patients. *Biological Psychiatry, 55*, 74S–75S.

Light, G. A., & Braff, D. L. (2005b). Stability of mismatch negativity deficits and their relationship to functional impairments in chronic schizophrenia. *American Journal of Psychiatry, 162*(9), 1741–3.

Light, G., Greenwood, T. A., Swerdlow, N. R., Calkins, M. E., Freedman, R., Green, M. F., et al. (2014). Comparison of the heritability of schizophrenia and endophenotypes in the COGS-1 family study. *Schizophrenia Bulletin, 40*(6), 1404–11. doi:10.1093/schbul/sbu064

Light, G. A., & Makeig, S. (2015). Electroencephalographic biomarkers of psychosis: present and future. *Biological Psychiatry, 77*(2), 87–9. doi:10.1016/j.biopsych.2014.11.002

Light, G. A., & Näätänen, R. (2013). Mismatch negativity is a breakthrough biomarker for understanding and treating psychotic disorders. *Proceedings of the National Academy of Sciences of the United States of America, 110*(38), 15175–6. doi:10.1073/pnas.1313287110

Light, G. A., & Swerdlow, N. R. (2015). Future clinical uses of neurophysiological biomarkers to predict and monitor treatment response for schizophrenia. *Annals of the New York Academy of Sciences, 1344*(1), 105–19. doi:10.1111/nyas.12730

Light, G. A., Swerdlow, N. R., & Braff, D. L. (2007). Preattentive sensory processing as indexed by the MMN and P3a brain responses is associated with cognitive and psychosocial functioning in healthy adults. *Journal of Cognitive Neuroscience, 19*(10), 1624–32. doi:10.1162/jocn.2007.19.10.1624

Light, G. A., Swerdlow, N. R., Rissling, A. J., Radant, A., Sugar, C. A., Sprock, J., et al. (2012). Characterization of neurophysiologic and neurocognitive biomarkers for use in genomic and clinical outcome studies of schizophrenia. *PLoS ONE, 7*(7). doi:10.1371/journal.pone.0039434

Light, G. A., Swerdlow, N. R., Thomas, M. L., Calkins, M. E., Green, M. F., Greenwood, T. A., et al. (2015). Validation of mismatch negativity and P3a for use in multi-site studies of schizophrenia: Characterization of demographic, clinical, cognitive, and functional correlates in COGS-2. *Schizophrenia Research, 163*(1–3), 63–72. doi:10.1016/j.schres.2014.09.042

Lin, Y.-Y., Hsiao, F.-J., Shih, Y.-H., Yiu, C.-H., Yen, D.-J., Kwan, S.-Y., et al. (2007). Plastic phase-locking and magnetic mismatch response to auditory deviants in temporal lobe epilepsy. *Cerebral Cortex, 17*(11), 2516–25. doi:10.1093/cercor/bhl157

Lindenberger, U., & Baltes, P. B. (1994). Sensory functioning and intelligence in old age: A strong connection. *Psychology and Aging, 9*(3), 339–55. doi:10.1037/0882-7974.9.3.339

Lindín, M., Correa, K., Zurrón, M., & Díaz, F. (2013). Mismatch negativity (MMN) amplitude as a biomarker of sensory memory deficit in amnestic mild cognitive impairment. *Frontiers in Aging Neuroscience, 5*, 79. doi:10.3389/fnagi.2013.00079

Liu, H. M., Chen, Y., & Tsao, F. M. (2014). Developmental changes in mismatch responses to Mandarin consonants and lexical tones from early to middle childhood. *PLoS ONE, 9*(4). doi:10.1371/journal.pone.0095587

Liu, T., Shi, J., Zhang, Q., Zhao, D., & Yang, J. (2007). Neural mechanisms of auditory sensory processing in children with high intelligence. *NeuroReport, 18*(15), 1571–5. doi:10.1097/WNR.0b013e3282ef7640

Liu, T., Xiao, T., & Shi, J. (2016). Automatic change detection to facial expressions in adolescents: Evidence from visual mismatch negativity responses. *Frontiers in Psychology, 7*, 462. doi:10.3389/fpsyg.2016.00462

Lonka, E., Kujala, T., Lehtokoski, A., Johansson, R., Rimmanen, S., Alho, K., & Näätänen, R. (2004). Mismatch negativity brain response as an index of speech perception recovery in cochlear-implant recipients. *Audiology & Neurotology*, *9*(3), 160–2. doi:10.1159/000077265

Lord, C., & Paul, R. (1977). Language and communication in autism. In D. J. Cohen & F. R. Volkmar (Eds), *Handbook of Autism and Pervasive Developmental Disorders* (2nd ed., pp. 195–225). New York: John Wiley & Sons.

Lorenzo-López, L., Amenedo, E., Pazo-Alvarez, P., & Cadaveira, F. (2004). Pre-attentive detection of motion direction changes in normal aging. *NeuroReport*, *15*(17), 2633–6.

Louis, E. D. (2009). Essential tremors: A family of neurodegenerative disorders? *Archives of Neurology*, *66*(10), 1202–8. doi:10.1001/archneurol.2009.217

Loveless, N. (1983). The orienting response and evoked potentials in man. In D. Siddle (Ed.), *Orienting and Habituation: Perspectives in Human Research* (pp. 71–108). New York: John Wiley & Sons.

Loveless, N., Levänen, S., Jousmäki, V., Sams, M., & Hari, R. (1996). Temporal integration in auditory sensory memory: Neuromagnetic evidence. *Electroencephalography and Clinical Neurophysiology/ Evoked Potentials Section*, *100*(3), 220–8. doi:10.1016/0168-5597(95)00271-5

Lovio, R., Halttunen, A., Lyytinen, H., Näätänen, R., & Kujala, T. (2012). Reading skill and neural processing accuracy improvement after a 3-hour intervention in preschoolers with difficulties in reading-related skills. *Brain Research*, *1448*, 42–55. doi:10.1016/j.brainres.2012.01.071

Lovio, R., Näätänen, R., & Kujala, T. (2010). Abnormal pattern of cortical speech feature discrimination in 6-year-old children at risk for dyslexia. *Brain Research*, *1335*, 53–62. doi:10.1016/ j.brainres.2010.03.097

Lovio, R., Pakarinen, S., Huotilainen, M., Alku, P., Silvennoinen, S., Näätänen, R., & Kujala, T. (2009). Auditory discrimination profiles of speech sound changes in 6-year-old children as determined with the multi-feature MMN paradigm. *Clinical Neurophysiology*, *120*(5), 916–21. doi:10.1016/ j.clinph.2009.03.010

Luauté, J., Fischer, C., Adeleine, P., Morlet, D., Tell, L., & Boisson, D. (2005). Late auditory and event-related potentials can be useful to predict good functional outcome after coma. *Archives of physical medicine and rehabilitation*, *86*(5), 917–23.

Lütkenhöner, B., & Steinsträter, O. (1998). High-precision neuromagnetic study of the functional organization of the human auditory cortex. *Audiology & Neurotology*, *3*(2–3), 191–213. doi:10.1159/ 000013790

Lyytinen, H., Blomberg, A. P., & Näätänen, R. (1992). Event-related potentials and autonomic responses to a change in unattended auditory stimuli. *Psychophysiology*, *29*(5), 523–34. doi:10.1111/ j.1469-8986.1992.tb02025.x

Lyytinen, H., Erskine, J., Kujala, J., Ojanen, E., & Richardson, U. (2009). In search of a science-based application: A learning tool for reading acquisition. *Scandinavian Journal of Psychology*, *50*(6), 668–75. doi:10.1111/j.1467-9450.2009.00791.x

Lyytinen, H., & Näätänen, R. (1987). Autonomic and ERP responses to deviant stimuli: Analysis of covariation. *Electroencephalography and Clinical Neurophysiology. Supplement*, *40*, 108–117.

Lyytinen, H., Ronimus, M., Alanko, A., Poikkeus, A.-M., & Taanila, M. (2007). Early identification of dyslexia and the use of computer game-based practice to support reading acquisition. *Nordic Psychology*, *59*(2), 109–26. doi:10.1027/1901-2276.59.2.109

Lövdén, M., Schaefer, S., Noack, H., Bodammer, N. C., Kühn, S., Heinze, H.-J., et al. (2012). Spatial navigation training protects the hippocampus against age-related changes during early and late adulthood. *Neurobiology of Aging*, *33*(3), 620.e9–620.e22. doi:https://doi.org/10.1016/ j.neurobiolaging.2011.02.013

Macmillan, N. A. (1973). Detection and recognition of intensity changes in tone and noise: The detection-recognition disparity. *Perception & Psychophysics*, *13*(1), 65–75. doi:10.3758/BF03207236

Maekawa, T., Tobimatsu, S., Ogata, K., Onitsuka, T., & Kanba, S. (2009). Preattentive visual change detection as reflected by the mismatch negativity (MMN)—Evidence for a memory-based process. *Neuroscience Research, 65*(1), 107–12. doi:10.1016/j.neures.2009.06.005

Maestro, S., Muratori, F., Cavallaro, M. C., Pei, F., Stern, D., Golse, B., & Palacio-Espasa, F. (2002). Attentional skills during the first 6 months of age in autism spectrum disorder. *Journal of the American Academy of Child & Adolescent Psychiatry, 41*(10), 1239–45. doi:10.1097/00004583-200210000-00014

Magnusson, K. R. (1998). The aging of the NMDA receptor complex. *Frontiers in Bioscience: a Journal and Virtual Library, 3,* e70–e80. doi:10.2741/A368

Magnusson, K. R., Brim, B. L., & Das, S. R. (2010). Selective vulnerabilities of N-methyl-D-aspartate (NMDA) receptors during brain aging. *Frontiers in Aging Neuroscience, 19,* 2:11. doi:10.3389/fnagi.2010.00011

Mahmoudian, S., Farhadi, M., Najafi-Koopaie, M., Darestani-Farahani, E., Mohebbi, M., Dengler, R., et al. (2013). Central auditory processing during chronic tinnitus as indexed by topographical maps of the mismatch negativity obtained with the multi-feature paradigm. *Brain Research, 1527,* 161–73. doi:10.1016/j.brainres.2013.06.019

Mäkelä, J. P., Salmelin, R., Hokkanen, L., Launes, J., & Hari, R. (1998a). Neuromagnetic sequelae of herpes simplex encephalitis. *Electroencephalography and Clinical Neurophysiology, 106*(3), 251–8. doi:10.1016/S0013-4694(97)00132-6

Mäkelä, J. P., Salmelin, R., Kotila, M., Salonen, O., Laaksonen, R., Hokkanen, L., & Hari, R. (1998b). Modification of neuromagnetic cortical signals by thalamic infarctions. *Electroencephalography and Clinical Neurophysiology, 106*(5), 433–43. doi:10.1016/S0013-4694(98)00005-4

Marco-Pallarés, J., Ruffini, G., Polo, M. D., Gual, A., Escera, C., & Grau, C. (2007). Mismatch negativity impairment associated with alcohol consumption in chronic alcoholics: A scalp current density study. *International Journal of Psychophysiology, 65*(1), 51–7. doi:10.1016/j.ijpsycho.2007.03.001

Marler, J. A., Champlin, C. A., & Gillam, R. B. (2002). Auditory memory for backward masking signals in children with language impairment. *Psychophysiology, 39*(6), 767–80.

Marshall, M., Lewis, S., Lockwood, A., Drake, R., Jones, P., & Croudace, T. (2005). Association between duration of untreated psychosis and outcome in cohorts of first-episode patients: A systematic review. *Archives of General Psychiatry, 62*(9), 975–83. doi:10.1001/archpsyc.62.9.975

Martin, L. F., Davalos, D. B., & Kisley, M. A. (2009). Nicotine enhances automatic temporal processing as measured by the mismatch negativity waveform. *Nicotine & Tobacco Research, 11*(6), 698–706. doi:10.1093/ntr/ntp052

Massaro, D. W. (1970). Preperceptual auditory images. *Journal of Experimental Psychology, 85*(3), 411–17. doi:10.1037/h0029712

Massaro, D. W. (1975). Backward recognition masking. *Journal of the Acoustical Society of America, 58*(5), 1059–65. doi:10.1121/1.380765

Mathalon, D. H., Ahn, K. H., Perry, E. B., Cho, H. S., Roach, B. J., Blais, R. K., et al. (2014). Effects of nicotine on the neurophysiological and behavioral effects of ketamine in humans. *Frontiers in Psychiatry, 5,* 3. doi:10.3389/fpsyt.2014.00003

Matsubayashi, J., Kawakubo, Y., Suga, M., Takei, Y., Kumano, S., Fukuda, M., et al. (2008). The influence of gender and personality traits on individual difference in auditory mismatch: A magnetoencephalographic (MMNm) study. *Brain Research, 1236,* 159–65. doi:10.1016/j.brainres.2008.07.120

Mattson, M. P. (2008) Glutamate and neurotrophic factors in neuronal plasticity and disease. *Annals of the New York Academy of Sciences, 1144,* 97–112.

Matuoka, T., Yabe, H., Ren, A., Hara, E., & Kaneko, S. (2008). Memory trace dependence on number of stimuli in magnetic mismatch negativity. *NeuroReport, 19*(10), 1003–7. doi:10.1097/WNR.0b013e328303ba66

Maurer, U., Bucher, K., Brem, S., Benz, R., Kranz, F., Schulz, E., et al. (2009). Neurophysiology in preschool improves behavioral prediction of reading ability throughout primary school. *Biological Psychiatry*, 66(4), 341–8. doi:10.1016/j.biopsych.2009.02.031

Maurer, U., Bucher, K., Brem, S., & Brandeis, D. (2003). Development of the automatic mismatch response: From frontal positivity in kindergarten children to the mismatch negativity. *Clinical Neurophysiology*, 114(5), 808–17. doi:10.1016/S1388-2457(03)00032-4

May, P. J. C., & Tiitinen, H. (2010). Mismatch negativity (MMN), the deviance-elicited auditory deflection, explained. *Psychophysiology*, 47(1), 66–122. doi:10.1111/j.1469-8986.2009.00856.x

McAdams, S., & Bertoncini, J. (1997). Organization and discrimination of repeating sound sequences by newborn infants. *Journal of the Acoustical Society of America*, 102(5 I), 2945–53. doi:10.1121/1.420349

McCann, J., & Peppé, S. (2003). Prosody in autism spectrum disorders: A critical review. *International Journal of Language & Communication Disorders*, 38(4), 325–50.

McGee, T., Kraus, N., & Nicol, T. (1997). Is it really a mismatch negativity? An assessment of methods for determining response validity in individual subjects. *Electroencephalography and Clinical Neurophysiology - Evoked Potentials*, 104(4), 359–68. doi:10.1016/S0168-5597(97)00024-5

McGorry, P. D., Nelson, B., Phillips, L. J., Yuen, H. P., Francey, S. M., Thampi, A., et al. (2013). Randomized controlled trial of interventions for young people at ultra-high risk of psychosis: Twelve-month outcome. *Journal of Clinical Psychiatry*, 74(4), 349–56. doi:10.4088/JCP.12m07785

McGorry, P. D., Yung, A. R., Phillips, L. J., Yuen, H. P., Francey, S., Cosgrave, E. M., et al. (2002). Randomized controlled trial of interventions designed to reduce the risk of progression to first-episode psychosis in a clinical sample with subthreshold symptoms. *Archives of General Psychiatry*, 59(10), 921–8.

McGurk, S. R., Twamley, E. W., Sitzer, D. I., McHugo, G. J., & Mueser, K. T. (2007). A meta-analysis of cognitive remediation in schizophrenia. *American Journal of Psychiatry*, 164(12), 1791–1802.

Menning, E. H., Roberts, E. L., & Pantev, E. C. (2000). Plastic changes in the auditory cortex induced by intensive frequency discrimination training. *NeuroReport*, 11(4), 817–22.

Metz-Lutz, M. N., & Filippini, M. (2006). Neuropsychological findings in Rolandic epilepsy and Landau-Kleffner syndrome. *Epilepsia*, 47(s2), 71–5.

Michie, P. T., Budd, T. W., Todd, J., Rock, D., Wichmann, H., Box, J., & Jablensky, A. V. (2000). Duration and frequency mismatch negativity in schizophrenia. *Clinical Neurophysiology*, 111(6), 1054–65. doi:10.1016/S1388-2457(00)00275-3

Michie, P. T., Innes-Brown, H., Todd, J., & Jablensky, A. V. (2002). Duration mismatch negativity in biological relatives of patients with schizophrenia spectrum disorders. *Biological Psychiatry*, 52(7), 749–58. doi:10.1016/S0006-3223(02)01379-3

Miller, T. J., McGlashan, T. H., Rosen, J. L., Somjee, L., Markovich, P. J., Stein, K., & Woods, S. W. (2002). Prospective diagnosis of the initial prodrome for schizophrenia based on the structured interview for prodromal syndromes: Preliminary evidence of interrater reliability and predictive validity. *American Journal of Psychiatry*, 159(5), 863–5. doi:10.1176/appi.ajp.159.5.863

Minks, E., Jurák, P., Chládek, J., Chrastina, J., Halámek, J., Shaw, D., & Bareš, M. (2014). Mismatch negativity-like potential (MMN-like) in the subthalamic nuclei in Parkinson's disease patients. *Journal of Neural Transmission*, 121(12), 1507–22. doi:10.1007/s00702-014-1221-3

Mitsumoto, H. (2000). GDNF is trophic for mouse motoneurons that express a mutant superoxide dismutase (SOD1) gene. *Amyotrophic Lateral Sclerosis and Other Motor Neuron Disorders*, 1(2), 69–70.

Mittag, M., Takegata, R., & Kujala, T. (2011). The effects of visual material and temporal synchrony on the processing of letters and speech sounds. *Experimental Brain Research*, 211(2), 287–98. doi:10.1007/s00221-011-2686-z

Mittag, M., Thesleff, P., Laasonen, M., & Kujala, T. (2013). The neurophysiological basis of the integration of written and heard syllables in dyslexic adults. *Clinical Neurophysiology, 124*(2), 315–26. doi:10.1016/j.clinph.2012.08.003

Miyajima, M., Ohta, K., Hara, K., Iino, H., Maehara, T., Hara, M., et al. (2011). Abnormal mismatch negativity for pure-tone sounds in temporal lobe epilepsy. *Epilepsy Research, 94*(3), 149–57. doi:10.1016/j.eplepsyres.2011.01.009

Moberget, T., Karns, C. M., Deouell, L. Y., Lindgren, M., Knight, R. T., & Ivry, R. B. (2008). Detecting violations of sensory expectancies following cerebellar degeneration: A mismatch negativity study. *Neuropsychologia, 46*(10), 2569–79. doi:10.1016/j.neuropsychologia.2008.03.016

Moeller, F. G., Barratt, E. S., Dougherty, D. M., Schmitz, J. M., & Swann, A. C. (2001). Psychiatric aspects of impulsivity. *American journal of psychiatry, 158*(11), 1783–93.

Molfese, D. L. (2000). Predicting dyslexia at 8 years of age using neonatal brain responses. *Brain and Language, 72*(3), 238–45. doi:10.1006/brln.2000.2287

Molholm, S., Martinez, A., Ritter, W., Javitt, D. C., & Foxe, J. J. (2005). The neural circuitry of pre-attentive auditory change-detection: An fMRI study of pitch and duration mismatch negativity generators. *Cerebral Cortex, 15*(5), 545–51.

Moore, B. C. J. (1989). *An Introduction to the Psychology of Hearing.* New York: Academic Press.

Moore, J. K. (2002). Maturation of human auditory cortex: Implications for speech perception. *Annals of Otology, Rhinology & Laryngology, 111*(5), 7–10.

Moore, J. K., & Guan, Y.-L. (2001). Cytoarchitectural and axonal maturation in human auditory cortex. *Journal of the Association for Research in Otolaryngology, 2*(4), 297–311. doi:10.1007/s101620010052

Morgan, C. A., & Grillon, C. (1999). Abnormal mismatch negativity in women with sexual assault-related posttraumatic stress disorder. *Biological Psychiatry, 45*(7), 827–32. doi:10.1016/S0006-3223(98)00194-2

Morlet, D., Demarquay, G., Brudon, F., Fischer, C., & Caclin, A. (2014a). Attention orienting dysfunction with preserved automatic auditory change detection in migraine. *Clinical Neurophysiology, 125*(3), 500–11. doi:10.1016/j.clinph.2013.05.032

Morlet, D., & Fischer, C. (2014b). MMN and novelty P3 in coma and other altered states of consciousness: A review. *Brain Topography, 27*(4), 467–79. doi:10.1007/s10548-013-0335-5

Morr, M. L., Shafer, V. L., Kreuzer, J. A., & Kurtzberg, D. (2002). Maturation of mismatch negativity in typically developing infants and preschool children. *Ear and Hearing, 23*(2), 118–36.

Morrison, A. P., French, P., Parker, S., Roberts, M., Stevens, H., Bentall, R. P., & Lewis, S. W. (2007). Three-year follow-up of a randomized controlled trial of cognitive therapy for the prevention of psychosis in people at ultrahigh risk. *Schizophrenia Bulletin, 33*(3), 682–7. doi:10.1093/schbul/sbl042

Morrison, A. P., French, P., Stewart S.L., Birchwood M., Fowler D., Gumley A.I., et al. (2012). Early detection and intervention evaluation for people at risk of psychosis: multisite randomised controlled trial. *BMJ 344*:e2233.

Mottron, L., Dawson, M., Soulieres, I., Hubert, B., & Burack, J. (2006). Enhanced perceptual functioning in autism: An update, and eight principles of autistic perception. *Journal of Autism and Developmental Disorders, 36*(1), 27–43. doi:10.1007/s10803-005-0040-7

Mottron, L., Peretz, I., Belleville, S., & Rouleau, N. (1999). Absolute pitch in autism: A case study. *Neurocase, 5*(6), 485–501. doi:10.1080/13554799908402744

Mottron, L., Peretz, I., & Mnard, E. (2000). Local and global processing of music in high-functioning persons with autism: beyond central coherence? *Journal of Child Psychology and Psychiatry, 41*(8), 1057–65.

Mowszowski, L., Diamond, K., Norrie, L., Lewis, S. J. G., Naismith, S. L., Hermens, D. F., & Hickie, I. B. (2012). Reduced mismatch negativity in mild cognitive impairment: Associations with neuropsychological performance. *Journal of Alzheimer's Disease, 30*(1), 209–19. doi:10.3233/JAD-2012-111868

Mundy, P., & Neal, A.R. (2000). Neural plasticity, joint attention, and a transactional social-orienting model of autism. In: *Vol. 23. International Review of Research in Mental Retardation* (pp. 139–68).

Mundy, P., & Neal, R. (2001). Neural plasticity, joint attention and autistic developmental pathology. *International Review of Research in Mental Retardation, 23*, 139–68.

Müller, B. W., Jüptner, M., Jentzen, W., & Müller, S. P. (2002). Cortical activation to auditory mismatch elicited by frequency deviant and complex novel sounds: a PET study. *NeuroImage, 17*(1), 231–9. doi:10.1006/nimg.2002.1176

Müller, D., Widmann, A., & Schröger, E. (2005b). Deviance-repetition effects as a function of stimulus feature, feature value variation, and timing: A mismatch negativity study. *Biological Psychology, 68*(1), 1–14. doi:10.1016/j.biopsycho.2004.03.018

Müller, R. A., Behen, M., Rothermel, R., Chugani, D., Muzik, O., Mangner, T., & Chugani, H. (1999). Brain mapping of language and auditory perception in high-functioning autistic adults: A PET study. *Journal of Autism and Developmental Disorders, 29*(1), 19–31. doi:10.1023/A:1025914515203

Murphy, K., Jones, L., & Owen, M. (1999). High rates of schizophrenia in adults with velo-cardio-facial syndrome. *Archives of General Psychiatry 56*, 940–5.

Näätänen, R. (1975). Selective attention and evoked potentials in humans—A critical review. *Biological Psychology, 2*(4), 237–307. doi:10.1016/0301-0511(75)90038-1

Näätänen, R. (1982). Processing negativity: an evoked-potential reflection of selective attention. *Psychological Bulletin, 92*(3), 605–640.

Näätänen, R. (1984). In search of a short-duration memory trace of a stimulus in the human brain. In L. Pulkkinen & H. Lyytinen (Eds), *Human Action and Personality. Essays in Honour of Martti Takala.* Jyväskylä: University of Jyväskylä.

Näätänen, R. (1985). Selective attention and stimulus processing: Reflections in event-related potentials, magnetoencephalogram, and regional cerebral blood flow. In M. I. Posner & O. S. M. Marin (Eds), *Attention and Performance XI* (pp. 355–73). Hillsdale, New Jersey: Lawrence Erlbaum Associates.

Näätänen, R. (1988). Implications of ERP data for psychological theories of attention. *Biological Psychology, 26*(1–3), 117–63. doi:10.1016/0301-0511(88)90017-8

Näätänen, R. (1990). The role of attention in auditory information processing as revealed by event-related potentials and other brain measures of cognitive function. *Behavioral and Brain Sciences, 13*(2), 201–33. doi:10.1017/S0140525X00078407

Näätänen, R. (1992). *Attention and Brain Function.* Hillsdale, New Jersey: Lawrence Erlbaum Associates.

Näätänen, R. (1995). The mismatch negativity: A powerful tool for cognitive neuroscience. *Ear and hearing, 16*(1), 6–18.

Näätänen, R. (1999). Phoneme representations of the human brain as reflected by event-related potentials. *Electroencephalography and clinical neurophysiology. Supplement, 49*, 170–3.

Näätänen, R. (2001). The perception of speech sounds by the human brain as reflected by the mismatch negativity (MMN) and its magnetic equivalent (MMNm). *Psychophysiology, 38*(1), 1–21.

Näätänen, R. (2008). Mismatch negativity (MMN) as an index of central auditory system plasticity. *International Journal of Audiology, 47*(2), S16–S20. doi:10.1080/14992020802340116

Näätänen, R., Astikainen, P., Ruusuvirta, T., & Huotilainen, M. (2010). Automatic auditory intelligence: An expression of the sensory–cognitive core of cognitive processes. *Brain Research Reviews, 64*(1), 123–36. doi:10.1016/j.brainresrev.2010.03.001

Näätänen, R., & Gaillard, A. W. K. (1983). 5 The orienting reflex and the N2 deflection of the event-related potential (ERP). *Advances in Psychology, 10*, 119–41. 10.1016/S0166-4115(08)62036-1.

Näätänen, R., Gaillard, A. W. K., & Mäntysalo, S. (1978). Early selective-attention effect on evoked potential reinterpreted. *Acta Psychologica, 42*(4), 313–29.

Näätänen, R., Ilmoniemi, R. J., & Alho, K. (1994). Magnetoencephalography in studies of human cognitive brain function. *Trends in Neurosciences, 17*(9), 389–95. doi:10.1016/0166-2236(94)90048-5

Näätänen, R., & Kreegipuu, K. (2010). The mismatch negativity as an index of different forms of memory in audition. In L. Bäckman & L. Nyberg (Eds), *Memory, Aging and the Brain: A Festschrift in Honour of Lars-Göran Nilsson* (pp. 287–99). London: Psychology Press.

Näätänen, R., & Kreegipuu, K. (2011). The mismatch negativity (MMN). In S. J. Luck, E. S. Kappenman, (Eds), *Oxford Handbook of Event-Related Potential Components* (pp.143–58). New York: Oxford University Press.

Näätänen, R., Kujala, T., Escera, C., Baldeweg, T., Kreegipuu, K., Carlson, S., & Ponton, C. (2012). The mismatch negativity (MMN) - A unique window to disturbed central auditory processing in ageing and different clinical conditions. *Clinical Neurophysiology, 123*(3), 424–58.

Näätänen, R., Kujala, T., Kreegipuu, K., Carlson, S., Escera, C., Baldeweg, T., & Ponton, C. (2011). The mismatch negativity: An index of cognitive decline in neuropsychiatric and neurological diseases and in ageing. *Brain, 134*(12), 3432–50. doi:10.1093/brain/awr064

Näätänen, R., Kujala, T., & Winkler, I. (2011). Auditory processing that leads to conscious perception: A unique window to central auditory processing opened by the mismatch negativity and related responses. *Psychophysiology, 48*(1), 4–22. doi:10.1111/j.1469-8986.2010.01114.x

Näätänen, R., Lehtokoski, A., Lennes, M., Cheour, M., Huotilainen, M., Iivonen, A., et al. (1997). Language-specific phoneme representations revealed by electric and magnetic brain responses. *Nature, 385*(6615), 432. doi:10.1038/385432a0

Näätänen, R., & Michie, P. T. (1979). Early selective-attention effects on the evoked potential: A critical review and reinterpretation. *Biological Psychology, 8*(2), 81–136. doi:10.1016/0301-0511(79)90053-X

Näätänen, R., Paavilainen, P., Alho, K., Reinikainen, K., & Sams, M. (1987). The mismatch negativity to intensity changes in an auditory stimulus sequence. *Electroencephalography and Clinical Neurophysiology. Supplement, 40*, 125–31.

Näätänen, R., Paavilainen, P., Alho, K., Reinikainen, K., & Sams, M. (1989). Do event-related potentials reveal the mechanism of the auditory sensory memory in the human brain? *Neuroscience Letters, 98*(2), 217–21. doi:10.1016/0304-3940(89)90513-2

Näätänen, R., Paavilainen, P., & Reinikainen, K. (1989). Do event-related potentials to infrequent decrements in duration of auditory stimuli demonstrate a memory trace in man? *Neuroscience Letters, 107*(1), 347–52. doi:10.1016/0304-3940(89)90844-6

Näätänen, R., Paavilainen, P., Rinne, T., & Alho, K. (2007). The mismatch negativity (MMN) in basic research of central auditory processing: A review. *Clinical Neurophysiology, 118*(12), 2544–90. doi:10.1016/j.clinph.2007.04.026

Näätänen, R., Pakarinen, S., Rinne, T., & Takegata, R. (2004). The mismatch negativity (MMN): towards the optimal paradigm. *Clinical Neurophysiology, 115*(1), 140–4. doi:10.1016/j.clinph.2003.04.001

Näätänen, R., Petersen, B., Torppa, R., Lonka, E., & Vuust, P. (2017). The MMN as a viable and objective marker of auditory development in CI users. *Hearing Research, 353*, 57–75. doi:https://doi.org/10.1016/j.heares.2017.07.007

Näätänen, R., & Picton, R. (1987). The N1 wave of the human electric and magnetic response to sound: A review and an analysis of the component structure. *Psychophysiology, 24*(4), 375–425. doi:doi:10.1111/j.1469-8986.1987.tb00311.x

Näätänen, R., & Rinne, T. (2002). Electric brain response to sound repetition in humans: an index of long-term-memory – trace formation? *Neuroscience Letters, 318*(1), 49–51. doi:10.1016/S0304-3940(01)02438-7

Näätänen, R., Schröger, E., Karakas, S., Tervaniemi, M., & Paavilainen, P. (1993). Development of a memory trace for a complex sound in the human brain. *NeuroReport, 4*(5), 503–6.

Näätänen, R., Simpson, M., & Loveless, N. E. (1982). Stimulus deviance and evoked potentials. *Biological Psychology, 14*(1), 53–98. doi:10.1016/0301-0511(82)90017-5

Näätänen, R., & Summala, H. (1976). *Road-user Behavior and Traffic Accidents.* Amsterdam: North-Holland Publishing Co.

Näätänen, R., Sussman, E., Salisbury, D., & Shafer, V. (2014). Mismatch negativity (MMN) as an index of cognitive dysfunction. *Brain Topography, 27*(4), 451–66. doi:10.1007/s10548-014-0374-6

Näätänen, R., Tervaniemi, M., Sussman, E., Paavilainen, P., & Winkler, I. (2001). 'Primitive intelligence' in the auditory cortex. *Trends in Neurosciences, 24*(5), 283–88. doi:10.1016/S0166-2236(00)01790-2

Näätänen, R., & Winkler, I. (1999). The concept of auditory stimulus representation in cognitive neuroscience. *Psychological Bulletin, 125*(6), 826–59. doi:10.1037/0033-2909.125.6.826

Naccache, L., Puybasset, L., Gaillard, R., Serve, E., & Willer, J. C. (2005). Auditory mismatch negativity is a good predictor of awakening in comatose patients: a fast and reliable procedure. *Clinical neurophysiology, 116*(4), 988–9.

Nagai, T., Kirihara, K., Tada, M., Koshiyama, D., Koike, S., Suga, M., et al. (2017). Reduced mismatch negativity is associated with increased plasma level of glutamate in first-episode psychosis. *Scientific Reports, 7*(1), 2258. doi:10.1038/s41598-017-02267-1

Nagai, T., Tada, M., Kirihara, K., Araki, T., Jinde, S., & Kasai, K. (2013a). Mismatch negativity as a 'translatable' brain marker toward early intervention for psychosis: A review. *Frontiers in Psychiatry, 4*, 115. doi:10.3389/fpsyt.2013.00115

Nagai, T., Tada, M., Kirihara, K., Yahata, N., Hashimoto, R., Araki, T., & Kasai, K. (2013b). Auditory mismatch negativity and P3a in response to duration and frequency changes in the early stages of psychosis. *Schizophrenia Research, 150*(2–3), 547–54. doi:10.1016/j.schres.2013.08.005

Nager, F. W., Teder-Sälejärvi, F. W., Kunze, F. S., & Münte, F. T. (2003). Preattentive evaluation of multiple perceptual streams in human audition. *NeuroReport, 14*(6), 871–4.

Nager, W., Kohlmetz, C., Joppich, G., Möbes, J., & Münte, T. F. (2003). Tracking of multiple sound sources defined by interaural time differences: brain potential evidence in humans. *Neuroscience Letters, 344*(3), 181–4. doi:10.1016/S0304-3940(03)00439-7

Nager, W., Münte, T. F., Bohrer, I., Lenarz, T., Dengler, R., Möbes, J., et al. (2007). Automatic and attentive processing of sounds in cochlear implant patients - electrophysiological evidence. *Restorative Neurology and Neuroscience, 25*(3–4), 391–6.

Naismith, S. L., Mowszowski, L., Ward, P. B., Diamond, K., Paradise, M., Kaur, M., et al. (2012). Reduced temporal mismatch negativity in late-life depression: An event-related potential index of cognitive deficit and functional disability? *Journal of Affective Disorders, 138*(1–2), 71–8. doi:10.1016/j.jad.2011.12.028

Nashida, T., Yabe, H., Sato, Y., Hiruma, T., Sutoh, T., Shinozaki, N., & Kaneko, S. (2000). Automatic auditory information processing in sleep. *Sleep, 23*(6), 821–8.

Nearing, K., Madhavan, D., & Devinsky, O. (2007). Temporal lobe epilepsy: a progressive disorder? *Rev Neurol Dis, 4*(3), 122–7.

Neumann, N., & Kotchoubey, B. (2004). Assessment of cognitive functions in severely paralysed and severely brain-damaged patients: Neuropsychological and electrophysiological methods. *Brain Research Protocols, 14*(1), 25–36. doi:10.1016/j.brainresprot.2004.09.001

Niemitalo-Haapola, E., Lapinlampi, S., Kujala, T., Alku, P., Kujala, T., Suominen, K., & Jansson-Verkasalo, E. (2013). Linguistic multi-feature paradigm as an eligible measure of central auditory processing and novelty detection in 2-year-old children. *Cognitive Neuroscience, 4*(2), 99–106. doi:10.1080/17588928.2013.781146

Nordby, H., Roth, W. T., & Pfefferbaum, A. (1988). Event-related potentials to time-deviant and pitch-deviant tones. *Psychophysiology, 25*(3), 249–61.

Normann, C., Schmitz, D., Fürmaier, A., Döing, C., & Bach, M. (2007). Long-term plasticity of visually evoked potentials in humans is altered in major depression. *Biological Psychiatry, 62*(5), 373–80. doi:10.1016/j.biopsych.2006.10.006

Norton, E. S., & Wolf, M. (2012). Rapid automatized naming (RAN) and reading fluency: Implications for understanding and treatment of reading disabilities. *Annual Review of Psychology, 63*, 427–52.

Nousak, J. M. K., Deacon, D., Ritter, W., & Vaughan, H. G. (1996). Storage of information in transient auditory memory. *Cognitive Brain Research, 4*(4), 305–17. doi:10.1016/S0926-6410(96)00068-7

Nudel, R., Simpson, N. H., Baird, G., O'Hare, A., Conti-Ramsden, G., Bolton, P. F., et al. (2014). Genome-wide association analyses of child genotype effects and parent-of-origin effects in specific language impairment. *Genes, Brain and Behavior, 13*(4), 418–29. doi:10.1111/gbb.12127

Nyman, G., Alho, K., Laurinen, P., Paavilainen, P., Radil, T., Reinikainen, K., et al. (1990). Mismatch negativity (MMN) for sequences of auditory and visual stimuli: Evidence for a mechanism specific to the auditory modality. *Electroencephalography and Clinical Neurophysiology, 77*(6), 436–44.

Oceák, A., Winkler, I., Sussman, E., & Alho, K. (2006). Loudness summation and the mismatch negativity event-related brain potential in humans. *Psychophysiology, 43*(1), 13–20. doi:10.1111/j.1469-8986.2006.00372.x

Ogura, C., Nageishi, Y., Fukao, K., Shimoji, Y., Hirano, K., Hokama, H., et al. (1991). Deviate N200 component of event-related potentials in shuchaku-seikaku, a premorbid personality of depression. *Psychiatry and Clinical Neurosciences, 45*(3), 641–51. doi:10.1111/j.1440-1819.1991.tb01185.x

Ogura, C., Nageishi, Y., Omura, F., Fukao, K., Ohta, H., Kishimoto, A., & Matsubayashi, M. (1993). N200 component of event-related potentials in depression. *Biological Psychiatry, 33*(10), 720–6. doi:10.1016/0006-3223(93)90122-T

Ohnishi, T., Matsuda, H., Hashimoto, T., Kunihiro, T., Nishikawa, M., Uema, T., & Sasaki, M. (2000). Abnormal regional cerebral blood flow in childhood autism. *Brain, 123*(9), 1838–44.

Okazaki, S., Kanoh, S., Takaura, K., Tsukada, M., & Oka, K. (2006). Change detection and difference detection of tone duration discrimination. *NeuroReport, 17*(4), 395–9. doi:10.1097/01.wnr.0000204979.91253.7a

Okazaki, S., Kanoh, S. i., Tsukada, M., & Oka, K. (2010). Neural substrate of sound duration discrimination during an auditory sequence in the guinea pig primary auditory cortex. *Hearing Research, 259*(1), 107–16. doi:10.1016/j.heares.2009.10.011

Okita, T., Konishi, K., & Inamori, R. (1983). Attention-related negative brain potential for speech words and pure tones. *Biological Psychology, 16*(1), 29–47. doi:10.1016/0301-0511(83)90053-4

Olof Dahlgren, S., & Gillberg, C. (1989). Symptoms in the first two years of life - A preliminary population study of infantile autism. *European Archives of Psychiatry and Neurological Sciences, 238*(3), 169–74. doi:10.1007/BF00451006

O'Neill, M., & Jones, R. (1997). Sensory-perceptual abnormalities in autism: A case for more research? *Journal of Autism and Developmental Disorders, 27*(3), 283–93. doi:10.1023/A:1025850431170

Opitz, B., Rinne, T., Mecklinger, A., Von Cramon, D. Y., & Schröger, E. (2002). Differential contribution of frontal and temporal cortices to auditory change detection: fMRI and ERP results. *NeuroImage, 15*(1), 167–74. doi:10.1006/nimg.2001.0970

Opitz, B., Schröger, E., & Von Cramon, D. Y. (2005). Sensory and cognitive mechanisms for preattentive change detection in auditory cortex. *European Journal of Neuroscience, 21*(2), 531–5. doi:10.1111/j.1460-9568.2005.03839.x

Oram Cardy, E. J., Flagg, J. E., Roberts, P. L. W., & Roberts, P. L. T. (2005). Delayed mismatch field for speech and non-speech sounds in children with autism. *NeuroReport, 16*(5), 521–5.

Oranje, B., Aggernaes, B., Rasmussen, H., Ebdrup, B. H., & Glenthoj, B. Y. (2017). Selective attention and mismatch negativity in antipsychotic-naïve, first-episode schizophrenia patients before and after 6 months of antipsychotic monotherapy. *Psychological Medicine, 47*(12), 2155–65. doi:10.1017/S0033291717000599

O'Riordan, M., & Passetti, F. (2006). Discrimination in autism within different sensory modalities. *Journal of Autism and Developmental Disorders, 36*(5), 665–75. doi:10.1007/s10803-006-0106-1

Ortmann, M., Dobel, C., Knief, A., Deuster, D., Brinkheetker, S., Zehnhoff-Dinnesen, A., & Zwitserlood, P. (2013). Neural correlates of speech processing in prelingually deafened children and adolescents with cochlear implants. *PLoS ONE, 8*(7), e67696. doi:10.1371/journal.pone.0067696

Paavilainen, P. (2013). The mismatch-negativity (MMN) component of the auditory event-related potential to violations of abstract regularities: A review. *International Journal of Psychophysiology, 88*(2), 109–23.

Paavilainen, P., Alho, K., Reinikainen, K., Sams, M., & Näätänen, R. (1991). Right hemisphere dominance of different mismatch negativities. *Electroencephalography and Clinical Neurophysiology, 78*(6), 466–79. doi:10.1016/0013-4694(91)90064-B

Paavilainen, P., Arajärvi, P., & Takegata, R. (2007). Preattentive detection of nonsalient contingencies between auditory features. *NeuroReport, 18*(2), 159–63. doi:10.1097/WNR.0b013e328010e2ac

Paavilainen, P., Jaramillo, M., Näätänen, R., & Winkler, I. (1999). Neuronal populations in the human brain extracting invariant relationships from acoustic variance. *Neuroscience Letters, 265*(3), 179–82. doi:10.1016/S0304-3940(99)00237-2

Paavilainen, P., Jiang, D., Lavikainen, J., & Näätänen, R. (1993). Stimulus duration and the sensory memory trace: An event-related potential study. *Biological Psychology, 35*(2), 139–52. doi:10.1016/0301-0511(93)90010-6

Paavilainen, P., Karlsson, M.-L., Reinikainen, K., & Näätänen, R. (1989). Mismatch negativity to change in spatial location of an auditory stimulus. *Electroencephalography and Clinical Neurophysiology, 73*(2), 129–41. doi:10.1016/0013-4694(89)90192-2

Paavilainen, P., Saarinen, J., Tervaniemi, M., & Näätänen, R. (1995). Mismatch negativity to changes in abstract sound features during dichotic listening. *Journal of Psychophysiology, 9*(3), 243–9.

Pakarinen, S., Lovio, R., Huotilainen, M., Alku, P., Näätänen, R., & Kujala, T. (2009). Fast multi-feature paradigm for recording several mismatch negativities (MMNs) to phonetic and acoustic changes in speech sounds. *Biological Psychology, 82*(3), 219–26. doi:10.1016/j.biopsycho.2009.07.008

Pakarinen, S., Takegata, R., Rinne, T., Huotilainen, M., & Näätänen, R. (2007). Measurement of extensive auditory discrimination profiles using the mismatch negativity (MMN) of the auditory event-related potential (ERP). *Clinical Neurophysiology, 118*(1), 177–85. doi:10.1016/j.clinph.2006.09.001

Palmer, B., Dawes, S., & Heaton, R. (2009). What do we know about neuropsychological aspects of schizophrenia? *Neuropsychology Review, 19*(3), 365–84. doi:10.1007/s11065-009-9109-y

Pang, E. W., & Fowler, B. (1999). Dissociation of the mismatch negativity and processing negativity attentional waveforms with nitrous oxide. Psychophysiology, 36(5), 552–8.

Partanen, E., Kujala, T., Näätänen, R., Liitola, A., Sambeth, A., & Huotilainen, M. (2013a). Learning-induced neural plasticity of speech processing before birth. *Proceedings of the National Academy of Sciences of the United States of America, 110*(37), 15145–50. doi:10.1073/pnas.1302159110

Partanen, E., Kujala, T., Tervaniemi, M., & Huotilainen, M. (2013b). Prenatal music exposure induces long-term neural effects. *PLoS ONE, 8*(10), e78946. doi:10.1371/journal.pone.0078946

Partanen, E., Pakarinen, S., Kujala, T., & Huotilainen, M. (2013c). Infants' brain responses for speech sound changes in fast multifeature MMN paradigm. *Clinical Neurophysiology, 124*(8), 1578–85. doi:10.1016/j.clinph.2013.02.014

Partanen, E., Torppa, R., Pykäläinen, J., Kujala, T., & Huotilainen, M. (2013d). Children's brain responses to sound changes in pseudo words in a multifeature paradigm. *Clinical Neurophysiology*, *124*(6), 1132–8. doi:10.1016/j.clinph.2012.12.005

Paul, R., Augustyn, A., Klin, A., & Volkmar, F. R. (2005). Perception and production of prosody by speakers with autism spectrum disorders. *Journal of Autism and Developmental Disorders*, *35*(2), 205–20. doi:10.1007/s10803-004-1999-1

Pauletti, C., Mannarelli, D., Locuratolo, N., Vanacore, N., De Lucia, M. C., & Fattapposta, F. (2014). Mismatch negativity in essential tremor: Role of age at onset in pre-attentive auditory discrimination. *Clinical Neurophysiology*, *125*(4), 708–14. doi:10.1016/j.clinph.2013.09.008

Pause, B. M., & Krauel, K. (2000). Chemosensory event-related potentials (CSERP) as a key to the psychology of odors. *International Journal of Psychophysiology*, *36*(2), 105–22. doi:10.1016/S0167-8760(99)00105-1

Pazo-Álvarez, P., Amenedo, E., & Cadaveira, F. (2004a). Automatic detection of motion direction changes in the human brain. *European Journal of Neuroscience*, *19*(7), 1978–86. doi:10.1111/j.1460-9568.2004.03273.x

Pazo-Álvarez, P., Amenedo, E., Lorenzo-López, L., & Cadaveira, F. (2004b). Effects of stimulus location on automatic detection of changes in motion direction in the human brain. *Neuroscience Letters*, *371*(2), 111–16. doi:10.1016/j.neulet.2004.08.073

Peach, R. K., & Newhoff, M. (1994). A topographic event-related potential analysis of the attention deficit for auditory processing in aphasia. *Clinical Aphasiology*, *22*, 81–96.

Peach, R. K., Newhoff, M., & Rubin, S. S. (1992). Attention in aphasia as revealed by event-related potentials: a preliminary investigation. *Clinical Aphasiology*, *21*, 323–33.

Pekkonen, E., Ahveninen, J., Jääskeläinen, I. P., Seppä, K., Näätänen, R., & Sillanaukee, P. (1998a). Selective acceleration of auditory processing in chronic alcoholics during abstinence. *Alcoholism: Clinical and Experimental Research*, *22*(3), 605–9. doi:10.1111/j.1530-0277.1998.tb04299.x

Pekkonen, E., Huotilainen, M., Virtanen, J., Näätänen, R., Ilmoniemi, R. J., & Erkinjuntti, T. (1996a). Alzheimer's disease affects parallel processing between the auditory cortices. *NeuroReport*, *7*(8), 1365–8.

Pekkonen, E., Jousmäki, V., Könönen, M., Reinikainen, K., & Partanen, J. (1994). Auditory sensory memory impairment in Alzheimer's disease: an event-related potential study. *NeuroReport*, *5*(18), 2537–40.

Pekkonen, E., Jousmäki, V., Partanen, J., & Karhu, J. (1993). Mismatch negativity area and age-related auditory memory. *Electroencephalography and Clinical Neurophysiology*, *87*(5), 321–5. doi:10.1016/0013-4694(93)90185-X

Pekkonen, E., Jousmäki, V., Reinikainen, K., & Partanen, J. (1995a). Automatic auditory discrimination is impaired in Parkinson's disease. *Electroencephalography and Clinical Neurophysiology*, *95*(1), 47–52. doi:10.1016/0013-4694(94)00304-4

Pekkonen, E., Osipova, D., & Laaksovirta, H. (2004). Magnetoencephalographic evidence of abnormal auditory processing in amyotrophic lateral sclerosis with bulbar signs. *Clinical Neurophysiology*, *115*(2), 309–15. doi:10.1016/S1388-2457(03)00360-2

Pekkonen, E., Rinne, T., & Näätänen, R. (1995b). Variability and replicability of the mismatch negativity. *Electroencephalography and Clinical Neurophysiology*, *96*(6), 546–54.

Pekkonen, E., Rinne, T., Reinikainen, K., Kujala, T., Alho, K., & Näätänen, R. (1996b). Aging effects on auditory processing: an event-related potential study. *Experimental Aging Research*, *22*(2), 171–84. doi:10.1080/03610739608254005

Pekkonen, E., Teräväinen, H., Jyrki Ahveninen, J., Virtanen, E., Pekkonen, J., & Virtanen, J. (1998b). Parkinson's disease selectively impairs preattentive auditory processing: An MEG study. *NeuroReport*, *9*(13), 2949–52.

Perez, V. B., Swerdlow, N. R., Braff, D. L., Näätänen, R., & Light, G. A. (2014a). Using biomarkers to inform diagnosis, guide treatments and track response to interventions in psychotic illnesses. *Biomarkers in Medicine*, *8*(1), 9–14. doi:10.2217/bmm.13.133

Perez, V. B., Tarasenko, M., Miyakoshi, M., Pianka, S. T., Makeig, S. D., Braff, D. L., et al. (2017). Mismatch negativity is a sensitive and predictive biomarker of perceptual learning during auditory cognitive training in schizophrenia. *Neuropsychopharmacology*, *42*(11), 2206–13. doi:10.1038/npp.2017.25

Perez, V. B., Woods, S. W., Roach, B. J., Ford, J. M., McGlashan, T. H., Srihari, V. H., & Mathalon, D. H. (2014b). Automatic auditory processing deficits in schizophrenia and clinical high-risk patients: Forecasting psychosis risk with mismatch negativity. *Biological Psychiatry*, *75*(6), 459–69. doi:10.1016/j.biopsych.2013.07.038

Perkell, J., Lane, H., Svirsky, M., & Webster, J. (1992). Speech of cochlear implant patients: a longitudinal study of vowel production. *Journal of the Acoustical Society of America*, *91*(5), 2961–78. doi:10.1121/1.402932

Perkins, D. O., Gu, H., Boteva, K., & Lieberman, J. A. (2005). Relationship between duration of untreated psychosis and outcome in first-episode schizophrenia: A critical review and meta-analysis. *American Journal of Psychiatry*, *162*(10), 1785–1804. doi:10.1176/appi.ajp.162.10.1785

Petermann, M., Kummer, P., Burger, M., Lohscheller, J., Eysholdt, U., & Döllinger, M. (2009). Statistical detection and analysis of mismatch negativity derived by a multi-deviant design from normal hearing children. *Hearing Research*, *247*(2), 128–36. doi:10.1016/j.heares.2008.11.001

Petersen, B., Weed, E., Hansen, M., Vuust, P., Sørensen, S. D., Sandmann, P., & Brattico, E. (2015). Brain responses to musical feature changes in adolescent cochlear implant users. *Frontiers in Human Neuroscience*, *9*, 7. doi:10.3389/fnhum.2015.00007

Peterson, L., & Peterson, M. J. (1959). Short-term retention of individual verbal items. *Journal of Experimental Psychology*, *58*(3), 193–8.

Pettigrew, C., Murdoch, B., Kei, J., Ponton, C., Alku, P., & Chenery, H. (2005). The mismatch negativity (MMN) response to complex tones and spoken words in individuals with aphasia. *Aphasiology*, *19*(2), 131–63. doi:10.1080/02687030444000642

Pfefferbaum, A., Sullivan, E. V., Mathalon, D. H., & Lim, K. O. (1997). Frontal lobe volume loss observed with magnetic resonance imaging in older chronic alcoholics. *Alcoholism: Clinical and Experimental Research*, *21*(3), 521–9. doi:10.1111/j.1530-0277.1997.tb03798.x

Pfefferbaum, A., Sullivan, E. V., Rosenbloom, M. J., Mathalon, D. H., & Lim, K. O. (1998). A controlled study of cortical gray matter and ventricular changes in alcoholic men over a 5-year interval. *Archives of General Psychiatry*, *55*(10), 905–12.

Pichora-Fuller, M. K. (2003). Cognitive aging and auditory information processing. *International Journal of Audiology*, *42*(sup2), 26–32.

Pihko, E., Leppäsaari, T., & Lyytinen, H. (1995). Brain reacts to occasional changes in duration of elements in a continuous sound. *NeuroReport*, *6*(8), 1215–8.

Pihko, E., Mickos, A., Kujala, T., Pihlgren, A., Westman, M., Alku, P., et al. (2007). Group intervention changes brain activity in bilingual language-impaired children. *Cerebral Cortex*, *17*(4), 849–58. doi:10.1093/cercor/bhk037

Pincze, Z., Lakatos, P., Rajkai, C., Ulbert, I., & Karmos, G. (2001). Separation of mismatch negativity and the N1 wave in the auditory cortex of the cat: a topographic study. *Clinical Neurophysiology*, *112*(5), 778–84. doi:10.1016/S1388-2457(01)00509-0

Pincze, Z., Lakatos, P., Rajkai, C., Ulbert, I., & Karmos, G. (2002). Effect of deviant probability and interstimulus/interdeviant interval on the auditory N1 and mismatch negativity in the cat auditory cortex. *Cognitive Brain Research*, *13*(2), 249–53. doi:10.1016/S0926-6410(01)00105-7

Pitkänen, A., & Sutula, T. P. (2002). Is epilepsy a progressive disorder? Prospects for new therapeutic approaches in temporal-lobe epilepsy. *Lancet Neurology*, *1*(3), 173–81. doi:10.1016/S1474-4422(02)00073-X

Polo, M. D., Escera, C., Gual, A., & Grau, C. (1999). Mismatch negativity and auditory sensory memory in chronic alcoholics. *Alcoholism: Clinical and Experimental Research, 23*(11), 1744–50. doi:10.1111/j.1530-0277.1999.tb04069.x

Polo, M. D., Escera, C., Yago, E., Alho, K., Gual, A., & Grau, C. (2003). Electrophysiological evidence of abnormal activation of the cerebral network of involuntary attention in alcoholism. *Clinical Neurophysiology, 114*(1), 134–46. doi:10.1016/S1388-2457(02)00336-X

Polo, M. D., Newton, P., Rogers, D., Escera, C., & Butler, S. (2002). ERPs and behavioural indices of long-term preattentive and attentive deficits after closed head injury. *Neuropsychologia, 40*(13), 2350–9. doi:10.1016/S0028-3932(02)00127-6

Ponton, C., Bernstein, L., & Auer, E. (2009). Mismatch negativity with visual-only and audiovisual speech. *Brain Topography, 21*(3), 207–15. doi:10.1007/s10548-009-0094-5

Ponton, C., Eggermont, J. J., Khosla, D., Kwong, B., & Don, M. (2002). Maturation of human central auditory system activity: separating auditory evoked potentials by dipole source modeling. *Clinical Neurophysiology, 113*(3), 407–20. doi:10.1016/S1388-2457(01)00733-7

Ponton, C. W., & Don, M. (1995). The mismatch negativity in cochlear implant users. *Ear and Hearing, 16*(1), 131–46.

Ponton, C. W., & Don, M. (2003). Cortically-evoked activity recorded from cochlear implant users: Methods and applications. In: *Cochlear Implants Objective Measures*, 187–230. In: H. Cullington (Ed.) Whurr Publishers Ltd, London

Ponton, C. W., Don, M., Eggermont, J. J., & Kwong, B. (1997). Integrated mismatch negativity (MMN(i)): A noise-free representation of evoked responses allowing single-point distribution-free statistical tests. *Electroencephalography and Clinical Neurophysiology - Evoked Potentials, 104*(2), 143–50. doi:10.1016/S0168-5597(97)96104-9

Ponton, C. W., Eggermont, J. J., Don, M., Waring, M. D., Kwong, B., Cunningham, J., & Trautwein, P. (2000). Maturation of the mismatch negativity: Effects of profound deafness and cochlear implant use. *Audiology & Neuro-Otology, 5*(3–4), 167–85. doi:10.1159/000013878

Preskorn, S. H., Gawryl, M., Dgetluck, N., Palfreyman, M., Bauer, L. O., & Hilt, D. C. (2014). Normalizing effects of EVP-6124, an alpha-7 nicotinic partial agonist, on event-related potentials and cognition: a proof of concept, randomized trial in patients with schizophrenia. *Journal of Psychiatric Practice, 20*(1), 12–24.

Price, G. W., Michie, P. T., Johnston, J., Innes-Brown, H., Kent, A., Clissa, P., & Jablensky, A. V. (2006). A multivariate electrophysiological endophenotype, from a unitary cohort, shows greater research utility than any single feature in the Western Australian family study of schizophrenia. *Biological Psychiatry, 60*(1), 1–10.

Pulvermüller, F., & Assadollahi, R. (2007). Grammar or serial order? Discrete combinatorial brain mechanisms reflected by the syntactic mismatch negativity. *Journal of Cognitive Neuroscience, 19*(6), 971–80. doi:10.1162/jocn.2007.19.6.971

Pulvermüller, F., Kujala, T., Shtyrov, Y., Simola, J., Tiitinen, H., Alku, P., et al. (2001). Memory traces for words as revealed by the mismatch negativity. *NeuroImage, 14*(3), 607–16. doi:10.1006/nimg.2001.0864

Pulvermüller, F., & Shtyrov, Y. (2006). Language outside the focus of attention: The mismatch negativity as a tool for studying higher cognitive processes. *Progress in Neurobiology, 79*(1), 49–71. doi:10.1016/j.pneurobio.2006.04.004

Pulvermüller, F., Shtyrov, Y., Hasting, A. S., & Carlyon, R. P. (2008). Syntax as a reflex: neurophysiological evidence for early automaticity of grammatical processing. *Brain and Language, 104*(3), 244–53. doi:10.1016/j.bandl.2007.05.002

Putkinen, V., Niinikuru, R., Lipsanen, J., Tervaniemi, M., & Huotilainen, M. (2012). Fast measurement of auditory event-related potential profiles in 2–3-year-olds. *Developmental Neuropsychology, 37*(1), 51–75. doi:10.1080/87565641.2011.615873

Qin, P., Di, H., Yan, X., Yu, S., Yu, D., Laureys, S., & Weng, X. (2008). Mismatch negativity to the patient's own name in chronic disorders of consciousness. *Neuroscience Letters, 448*(1), 24–8. doi:10.1016/j.neulet.2008.10.029

Raglio, A., Filippi, S., Bellandi, D., & Stramba-Badiale, M. (2014). Global music approach to persons with dementia: evidence and practice. *Clinical Interventions in Aging, 9*, 1669–76.

Ramus, F. (2004). Neurobiology of dyslexia: a reinterpretation of the data. *Trends in Neurosciences, 27*(12), 720–6. doi:10.1016/j.tins.2004.10.004

Ramus, F., Marshall, C. R., Rosen, S., & Van Der Lely, H. K. J. (2013). Phonological deficits in specific language impairment and developmental dyslexia: Towards a multidimensional model. *Brain, 136*(2), 630–45. doi:10.1093/brain/aws356

Ramus, F., Rosen, S., Dakin, S. C., Day, B. L., Castellote, J. M., White, S., & Frith, U. (2003). Theories of developmental dyslexia: insights from a multiple case study of dyslexic adults. *Brain, 126*(4), 841–65.

Rapin, I. (2002). The autistic-spectrum disorders. *New England Journal of Medicine, 347*(5), 302–3. doi:10.1056/NEJMp020062

Rapin, I., & Dunn, M. (2003). Update on the language disorders of individuals on the autistic spectrum. *Brain and Development, 25*(3), 166–72. doi:10.1016/S0387-7604(02)00191-2

Rapin, I., Schimmel, H., Tourk, L. M., Krasnegor, N. A., & Pollak, C. (1966). Evoked responses to clicks and tones of varying intensity in waking adults. *Electroencephalography and Clinical Neurophysiology, 21*(4), 335–44.

Rascovsky, K., Salmon, D. P., Hansen, L. A., Thal, L. J., & Galasko, D. (2007). Disparate letter and semantic category fluency deficits in autopsy-confirmed frontotemporal dementia and Alzheimer's disease. *Neuropsychology, 21*(1), 20–30. doi:10.1037/0894-4105.21.1.20

Rasser, P. E., Schall, U., Todd, J., Michie, P. T., Ward, P. B., Johnston, P., et al. (2011). Gray matter deficits, mismatch negativity, and outcomes in schizophrenia. *Schizophrenia Bulletin, 37*(1), 131–40. doi:10.1093/schbul/sbp060

Realmuto, G., Begleiter, H., Odencrantz, J., & Porjesz, B. (1993). Event-related potential evidence of dysfunction in automatic processing in abstinent alcoholics. *Biological Psychiatry, 33*(8), 594–601. doi:10.1016/0006-3223(93)90097-W

Reite, M., Teale, P., Rojas, D. C., Reite, E., Asherin, R., & Hernandez, O. (2009). MEG auditory evoked fields suggest altered structural/functional asymmetry in primary but not secondary auditory cortex in bipolar disorder. *Bipolar Disorders, 11*(4), 371–81. doi:10.1111/j.1399-5618.2009.00701.x

Renvall, H., & Hari, R. (2003). Diminished auditory mismatch fields in dyslexic adults. *Annals of Neurology, 53*(5), 551–7. doi:10.1002/ana.10504

Restuccia, D., Della Marca, G., Marra, C., Rubino, M., & Valeriani, M. (2005). Attentional load of the primary task influences the frontal but not the temporal generators of mismatch negativity. *Cognitive Brain Research, 25*(3), 891–9. doi:10.1016/j.cogbrainres.2005.09.023

Restuccia, D., Marca, G. D., Valeriani, M., Leggio, M. G., & Molinari, M. (2007). Cerebellar damage impairs detection of somatosensory input changes. A somatosensory mismatch-negativity study. *Brain, 130*(1), 276–87. doi:10.1093/brain/awl236

Restuccia, D., Zanini, S., Cazzagon, M., Del Piero, I., Martucci, L., & Della Marca, G. (2009). Somatosensory mismatch negativity in healthy children. *Developmental Medicine & Child Neurology, 51*(12), 991–8. doi:10.1111/j.1469-8749.2009.03367.x

Richman, L. C. (1980). Cognitive patterns and learning disabilities in cleft palate children with verbal deficits. *Journal of Speech Language and Hearing Research, 23*(2), 447–56. doi:10.1044/jshr.2302.447

Richman, L. C., & Eliason, M. (1984). Type of reading disability related to cleft type and neuropsychological patterns. *Cleft Palate Journal, 21*(1), 1–6.

Richman, L. C., Eliason, M. J., & Lindgren, S. D. (1988). Reading disability in children with clefts. *Cleft Palate Journal, 25*(1), 21–25.

Richter, N., Schröger, E., & Rübsamen, R. (2009). Hemispheric specialization during discrimination of sound sources reflected by MMN. *Neuropsychologia, 47*(12), 2652–9. doi:10.1016/j.neuropsychologia.2009.05.017

Rimland, B., & Fein, D. (1988). Special talents of autistic savants. In L. K. Obler & D. Fein (Eds), *The Exceptional Brain: Neuropsychology of talent and special abilities* (pp. 474–92). New York: Guilfor Press.

Rimmele, J., Sussman, E., Keitel, C., Jacobsen, T., & Schröger, E. (2012). Electrophysiological evidence for age effects on sensory memory processing of tonal patterns. *Psychology and Aging, 27*(2), 384–98. doi:10.1037/a0024866

Rinker, T., Kohls, G., Richter, C., Maas, V., Schulz, E., & Schecker, M. (2007). Abnormal frequency discrimination in children with SLI as indexed by mismatch negativity (MMN). *Neuroscience Letters, 413*(2), 99–104. doi:10.1016/j.neulet.2006.11.033

Rinne, T., Alho, K., Alku, P., Holi, M., Sinkkonen, J., Virtanen, J., et al. (1999). Analysis of speech sounds is left-hemisphere predominant at 100–150 ms after sound onset. *NeuroReport, 10*(5), 1113–7.

Rinne, T., Alho, K., Ilmoniemi, R. J., Virtanen, J., & Näätänen, R. (2000). Separate time behaviors of the temporal and frontal mismatch negativity sources. *NeuroImage, 12*(1), 14–19. doi:10.1006/nimg.2000.0591

Rinne, T., Degerman, A., & Alho, K. (2005). Superior temporal and inferior frontal cortices are activated by infrequent sound duration decrements: an fMRI study. *NeuroImage, 26*(1), 66–72. doi:10.1016/j.neuroimage.2005.01.017

Rinne, T., Gratton, G., Fabiani, M., Cowan, N., Maclin, E., Stinard, A., et al. (1999). Scalp-recorded optical signals make sound processing in the auditory cortex visible? *NeuroImage, 10*(5), 620–4.

Rinne, T., Särkkä, A., Degerman, A., Schröger, E., & Alho, K. (2006). Two separate mechanisms underlie auditory change detection and involuntary control of attention. *Brain Research, 1077*(1), 135–43. doi:10.1016/j.brainres.2006.01.043

Rissling, A. J., Braff, D. L., Swerdlow, N. R., Hellemann, G., Rassovsky, Y., Sprock, J., et al. (2012). Disentangling early sensory information processing deficits in schizophrenia. *Clinical Neurophysiology, 123*(10), 1942–9. https://doi.org/10.1016/j.clinph.2012.02.079

Rissling, A. J., Miyakoshi, M., Sugar, C. A., Braff, D. L., Makeig, S., & Light, G. A. (2014). Cortical substrates and functional correlates of auditory deviance processing deficits in schizophrenia. *NeuroImage: Clinical, 6*, 424–37. doi:https://doi.org/10.1016/j.nicl.2014.09.006

Rissling, A. J., Park, S. H., Young, J. W., Rissling, M. B., Sugar, C. A., Sprock, J., et al. (2013). Demand and modality of directed attention modulate 'pre-attentive' sensory processes in schizophrenia patients and nonpsychiatric controls. *Schizophrenia Research, 146*(1–3), 326–35. doi:10.1016/j.schres.2013.01.035

Ritter, W., Deacon, D., Gomes, H., Javitt, D. C., & Vaughan, H. G. (1995). The mismatch negativity of event-related potentials as a probe of transient auditory memory: a review. *Ear and Hearing, 16*(1), 52–67.

Ritter, W., Paavilainen, P., Lavikainen, J., Reinikainen, K., Alho, K., Sams, M., & Näätänen, R. (1992). Event-related potentials to repetition and change of auditory stimuli. *Electroencephalography and Clinical Neurophysiology, 83*(5), 306–21. doi:10.1016/0013-4694(92)90090-5

Ritter, W., Sussman, E., & Molholm, S. (2000). Evidence that the mismatch negativity system works on the basis of objects. *NeuroReport, 11*(1), 61–3.

Roberts, K. L., & Allen, H. A. (2016). Perception and cognition in the ageing brain: A brief review of the short- and long-term links between perceptual and cognitive decline. *Frontiers in Aging Neuroscience, 8*, 38. doi:10.3389/fnagi.2016.00039

Roberts, T. P. L., Cannon, K. M., Tavabi, K., Blaskey, L., Khan, S. Y., Monroe, J. F., et al. (2011). Auditory magnetic mismatch field latency: a biomarker for language impairment in autism. *Biological Psychiatry, 70*(3), 263–9. doi:10.1016/j.biopsych.2011.01.015

Roberts, T. P. L., Heiken, K., Kahn, S. Y., Qasmieh, S., Blaskey, L., Solot, C., et al. (2012). Delayed magnetic mismatch negativity field, but not auditory M100 response, in specific language impairment. *NeuroReport, 23*(8), 463–8. doi:10.1097/WNR.0b013e32835202b6

Robinson, L. J., Thompson, J. M., Gallagher, P., Goswami, U., Young, A. H., Ferrier, I. N., & Moore, P. B. (2006). A meta-analysis of cognitive deficits in euthymic patients with bipolar disorder. *Journal of Affective Disorders, 93*(1–3), 105–15. doi:10.1016/j.jad.2006.02.016

Roeber, U., Berti, S., & Schröger, E. (2003a). Auditory distraction with different presentation rates: an event-related potential and behavioral study. *Clinical Neurophysiology, 114*(2), 341–9. doi:10.1016/S1388-2457(02)00377-2

Roeber, U., Widmann, A., & Schröger, E. (2003b). Auditory distraction by duration and location deviants: a behavioral and event-related potential study. *Cognitive Brain Research, 17*(2), 347–57. doi:10.1016/S0926-6410(03)00136-8

Roeske, D., Ludwig, K., Neuhoff, N., Becker, J., Bartling, J., Bruder, J., et al. (2011). First genome-wide association scan on neurophysiological endophenotypes points to trans-regulation effects on *SLC2A3* in dyslexic children. *Molecular Psychiatry, 16*(1), 97–107.

Roger, C., Hasbroucq, T., Rabat, A., Vidal, F., & Burle, B. (2009). Neurophysics of temporal discrimination in the rat: A mismatch negativity study. *Psychophysiology, 46*(5), 1028–32. doi:10.1111/j.1469-8986.2009.00840.x

Rojas, D. C., Bawn, S. D., Benkers, T. L., Reite, M. L., & Rogers, S. J. (2002). Smaller left hemisphere planum temporale in adults with autistic disorder. *Neuroscience Letters, 328*(3), 237–40. doi:10.1016/S0304-3940(02)00521-9

Roman, S., Canévet, G., Marquis, P., Triglia, J.-M., & Liégeois-Chauvel, C. (2005). Relationship between auditory perception skills and mismatch negativity recorded in free field in cochlear-implant users. *Hearing Research, 201*(1), 10–20. doi:10.1016/j.heares.2004.08.021

Rongve, A., & Aarsland, D. (2006). Management of Parkinson's disease dementia. *Drugs & aging, 23*(10), 807–22.

Rosburg, T. (2003). Left hemispheric dipole locations of the neuromagnetic mismatch negativity to frequency, intensity and duration deviants. *Cognitive Brain Research, 16*(1), 83–90. doi:10.1016/S0926-6410(02)00222-7

Rosburg, T., Haueisen, J., & Kreitschmann-Andermahr, I. (2004). The dipole location shift within the auditory evoked neuromagnetic field components N100m and mismatch negativity (MMNm). *Clinical Neurophysiology, 115*(4), 906–13. doi:10.1016/j.clinph.2003.11.039

Rosburg, T., Trautner, P., Dietl, T., Elger, C. E., Kurthen, M., Schaller, C., et al. (2005). Subdural recordings of the mismatch negativity (MMN) in patients with focal epilepsy. *Brain, 128*(4), 819–28. doi:10.1093/brain/awh442

Rosburg, T., Trautner, P., Ludowig, E., Schaller, C., Kurthen, M., Elger, C. E., & Boutros, N. N. (2007). Hippocampal event-related potentials to tone duration deviance in a passive oddball paradigm in humans. *NeuroImage, 37*(1), 274–81. doi:10.1016/j.neuroimage.2007.05.002

Rowland, L. P., & Shneider, N. A. (2001). Amyotrophic lateral sclerosis. *New England Journal of Medicine, 344*(22), 1688–700.

Roye, A., Jacobsen, T., & Schröger, E. (2007). Personal significance is encoded automatically by the human brain: an event-related potential study with ringtones. *European Journal of Neuroscience, 26*(3), 784–90. doi:10.1111/j.1460-9568.2007.05685.x

Ruusuvirta, T., Astikainen, P., Wikgren, J., & Nokia, M. (2010). Hippocampus responds to auditory change in rabbits. *Neuroscience, 170*(1), 232–37. doi:10.1016/j.neuroscience.2010.06.062

Ruusuvirta, T., Huotilainen, M., Fellman, V., & Näätänen, R. (2003). The newborn human brain binds sound features together. *NeuroReport, 14*(16), 2117–9.

Ruusuvirta, T., Huotilainen, M., Fellman, V., & Näätänen, R. (2004). Newborn human brain identifies repeated auditory feature conjunctions of low sequential probability. *European Journal of Neuroscience, 20*(10), 2819–21. doi:10.1111/j.1460-9568.2004.03734.x

Ruusuvirta, T., Koivisto, K., Wikgren, J., & Astikainen, P. (2007). Processing of melodic contours in urethane-anaesthetized rats. *European Journal of Neuroscience, 26*(3), 701–3. doi:10.1111/j.1460-9568.2007.05687.x

Ruusuvirta, T., Lipponen, A., Pellinen, E., Penttonen, M., Astikainen, P., & Malmierca, M. S. (2013). Auditory cortical and hippocampal-system mismatch responses to duration deviants in urethane-anesthetized rats. *PLoS ONE, 8*(1). doi:10.1371/journal.pone.0054624

Ruusuvirta, T., Penttonen, M., & Korhonen, T. (1998). Auditory cortical event-related potentials to pitch deviances in rats. *Neuroscience Letters, 248*(1), 45–8. doi:10.1016/S0304-3940(98)00330-9

Ruzzoli, M., Pirulli, C., Brignani, D., Maioli, C., & Miniussi, C. (2012). Sensory memory during physiological aging indexed by mismatch negativity (MMN). *Neurobiology of Aging, 33*(3), 625. e621–625.e630. doi:10.1016/j.neurobiolaging.2011.03.021

Ryan, A. K., Goodship, J. A., Wilson, D. I., Philip, N., Levy, A., Seidel, H., et al. (1997). Spectrum of clinical features associated with interstitial chromosome 22q11 deletions: a European collaborative study. *Journal of Medical Genetics, 34*(10), 798–804. doi:10.1136/jmg.34.10.798

Saarinen, J., Paavilainen, P., Schöger, E., Tervaniemi, M., & Näätänen, R. (1992). Representation of abstract attributes of auditory stimuli in the human brain. *NeuroReport, 3*(12), 1149–51.

Sable, J. J., Low, K. A., Whalen, C. J., Maclin, E. L., Fabiani, M., & Gratton, G. (2007). Optical imaging of temporal integration in human auditory cortex. *European Journal of Neuroscience, 25*(1), 298–306. doi:10.1111/j.1460-9568.2006.05255.x

Sabri, M., & Campbell, K. B. (2001). Effects of sequential and temporal probability of deviant occurrence on mismatch negativity. *Cognitive Brain Research, 12*(1), 171–80. doi:10.1016/S0926-6410(01)00026-X

Sabri, M., Kareken, D. A., Dzemidzic, M., Lowe, M. J., & Melara, R. D. (2004). Neural correlates of auditory sensory memory and automatic change detection. *NeuroImage, 21*(1), 69–74. doi:10.1016/j.neuroimage.2003.08.033

Sakata, Y., Tokunaga, K., Yonehara, Y., Bannai, M., Tsuchiya, N., Susami, T., & Takato, T. (1999). Significant association of HLA-B and HLA-DRB1 alleles with cleft lip with or without cleft palate. *Tissue Antigens, 53*(2), 147–52. doi:10.1034/j.1399-0039.1999.530204.x

Salisbury, D. F. (2012). Finding the missing stimulus mismatch negativity (MMN): Emitted MMN to violations of an auditory gestalt. *Psychophysiology, 49*(4), 544–8. doi:10.1111/j.1469-8986.2011.01336.x

Salisbury, D. F., Kuroki, N., Kasai, K., Shenton, M. E., & McCarley, R. W. (2007). Progressive and interrelated functional and structural evidence of post-onset brain reduction in schizophrenia. *Archives of General Psychiatry, 64*(5), 521–9. doi:10.1001/archpsyc.64.5.521

Salisbury, D. F., & McCathern, A. G. (2016). Abnormal complex auditory pattern analysis in schizophrenia reflected in an absent missing stimulus mismatch negativity. *Brain Topography, 29*(6), 867–74. doi:10.1007/s10548-016-0514-2

Salisbury, D. F., McCathern, A. G., Coffman, B. A., Murphy, T. K., & Haigh, S. M. (2018). Complex mismatch negativity to tone pair deviants in long-term schizophrenia and in the first-episode schizophrenia spectrum. *Schizophrenia Research, 191*, 18–24. doi:10.1016/j.schres.2017.04.044

Salisbury, D. F., Polizzotto, N. R., Nestor, P. G., Haigh, S. M., Koehler, J., & McCarley, R. W. (2017). Pitch and duration mismatch negativity and premorbid intellect in the first hospitalized schizophrenia spectrum. *Schizophrenia Bulletin, 43*(2), 407–16. doi:10.1093/schbul/sbw074

Salisbury, D. F., Shenton, M. E., Griggs, C. B., Bonner-Jackson, A., & McCarley, R. W. (2002). Mismatch negativity in chronic schizophrenia and first-episode schizophrenia. *Archives of General Psychiatry, 59*(8), 686–94.

Sallinen, M., Kaartinen, J., & Lyytinen, H. (1994). Is the appearance of mismatch negativity during stage 2 sleep related to the elicitation of K-complex? *Electroencephalography and Clinical Neurophysiology, 91*(2), 140–8. doi:10.1016/0013-4694(94)90035-3

Sallinen, M., Kaartinen, J., & Lyytinen, H. (1996). Processing of auditory stimuli during tonic and phasic periods of REM sleep as revealed by event-related brain potentials. *Journal of Sleep Research, 5*(4), 220–8. doi:10.1111/j.1365-2869.1996.00220.x

Salmelin, R., Helenius, P., & Service, E. (2000a). Neurophysiology of fluent and impaired reading: a magnetoencephalographic approach. *Journal of Clinical Neurophysiology, 17*(2), 163–74.

Salmelin, R., Schnitzler, A., Schmitz, F., & Freund, H. (2000b). Single word reading in developmental stutterers and fluent speakers. *Brain, 123*, 1184–202.

Salmelin, W. R., Schnitzler, W. A., Schmitz, W. F., Jäncke, W. L., Witte, W. O., & Freund, W. H. J. (1998). Functional organization of the auditory cortex is different in stutterers and fluent speakers. *NeuroReport, 9*(10), 2225–9.

Salo, S., Peltola, M. S., Aaltonen, O., Johansson, R., Lang, A. H., & Laurikainen, E. (2002). Stability of memory traces for speech sounds in cochlear implant patients. *Logopedics Phonatrics Vocology, 27*(3), 132–8. doi:10.1080/140154302760834868

Salthouse, T. A. (1991). *Theoretical Perspectives on Cognitive Aging.* Hillsdale, NJ: Erlbaum Associates.

Sambeth, A., Pakarinen, S., Ruohio, K., Fellman, V., van Zuijen, T. L., & Huotilainen, M. (2009). Change detection in newborns using a multiple deviant paradigm: A study using magnetoencephalography. *Clinical Neurophysiology, 120*(3), 530–8. doi:10.1016/j.clinph.2008.12.033

Sams, M., Alho, K., & Näätänen, R. (1983). Sequential effects on the ERP in discriminating two stimuli. *Biological Psychology, 17*(1), 41–58. doi:10.1016/0301-0511(83)90065-0

Sams, M., Alho, K., & Näätänen, R. (1984). Short-term habituation and dishabituation of the mismatch negativity of the ERP. *Psychophysiology, 21*(4), 434–41.

Sams, M., & Hari, R. (1991). Magnetoencephalography in the study of human auditory information processing. *Annals of the New York Academy of Sciences, 620*, 102–17.

Sams, M., Hari, R., Rif, J., & Knuutila, J. (1993). The human auditory sensory memory trace persists about 10 sec: neuromagnetic evidence. *Journal of Cognitive Neuroscience, 5*(3), 363–70.

Sams, M., Hämäläinen, M., Antervo, A., Kaukoranta, E., Reinikainen, K., & Hari, R. (1985). Cerebral neuromagnetic responses evoked by short auditory stimuli. *Electroencephalography and Clinical Neurophysiology, 61*(4), 254–66. doi:10.1016/0013-4694(85)91092-2

Sams, M., Kaukoranta, E., Hämäläinen, M., & Näätänen, R. (1991). Cortical activity elicited by changes in auditory stimuli: different sources for the magnetic N100m and mismatch responses. *Psychophysiology, 28*(1), 21–9.

Sams, M., Paavilainen, P., Alho, K., & Näätänen, R. (1985). Auditory frequency discrimination and event-related potentials. *Electroencephalography and Clinical Neurophysiology/ Evoked Potentials Section, 62*(6), 437–48. doi:10.1016/0168-5597(85)90054-1

Sandmann, P., Kegel, A., Eichele, T., Dillier, N., Lai, W., Bendixen, A., et al. (2010). Neurophysiological evidence of impaired musical sound perception in cochlear-implant users. *Clinical Neurophysiology, 121*(12), 2070–82. doi:10.1016/j.clinph.2010.04.032

Santos, M. A., Munhoz, M. S., Peixoto, M. A., Haase, V. G., Rodrigues, J. L., & Resende, L. M. (2006). Mismatch negativity contribution in multiple sclerosis patients. *Brazilian Journal of Otorhinolaryngology, 72*(6), 800–7.

Sapin, L. R., Berrettini, W. H., Nurnberger Jr, J. I., & Rothblat, L. A. (1987). Mediational factors underlying cognitive changes and laterality in affective illness. *Biological Psychiatry, 22*(8), 979–86. doi:10.1016/0006-3223(87)90007-2

Särkämö, T., Pihko, E., Laitinen, S., Forsblom, A., Soinila, S., Mikkonen, M., et al. (2010a). Music and speech listening enhance the recovery of early sensory processing after stroke. *Journal of Cognitive Neuroscience, 22*(12), 2716–27. doi:10.1162/jocn.2009.21376

Särkämö, T., Tervaniemi, M., & Huotilainen, M. (2013). Music perception and cognition: Development, neural basis, and rehabilitative use of music. *Wiley Interdisciplinary Reviews: Cognitive Science*, 4(4), 441–51. doi:10.1002/wcs.1237

Särkämö, T., Tervaniemi, M., Soinila, S., Autti, T., Silvennoinen, H. M., Laine, M., & Hietanen, M. (2009a). Cognitive deficits associated with acquired amusia after stroke: A neuropsychological follow-up study. *Neuropsychologia*, 47(12), 2642–51. doi:10.1016/j.neuropsychologia.2009.05.015

Särkämö, T., Tervaniemi, M., Soinila, S., Autti, T., Silvennoinen, H. M., Laine, M., & Hietanen, M. (2009b). Amusia and cognitive deficits after stroke: Is there a relationship? *Annals of the New York Academy of Sciences*, 1169(1), 441–5. doi:10.1111/j.1749-6632.2009.04765.x

Särkämö, T., Tervaniemi, M., Soinila, S., Autti, T., Silvennoinen, H. M., Laine, M., et al. (2010b). Auditory and cognitive deficits associated with acquired amusia after stroke: A magnetoencephalography and neuropsychological follow-up study. *PLoS ONE*, 5(12). doi:10.1371/journal.pone.0015157

Sasaki, T., Campbell, K. B., Gordon Bazana, P., & Stelmack, R. M. (2000). Individual differences in mismatch negativity measures of involuntary attention shift. *Clinical Neurophysiology*, 111(9), 1553–60. doi:10.1016/S1388-2457(00)00376-X

Sato, Y., Yabe, H., Hiruma, T., Sutoh, T., Shinozaki, N., Nashida, T., & Kaneko, S. (2000). The effect of deviant stimulus probability on the human mismatch process. *NeuroReport*, 11(17), 3703–8.

Sato, Y., Yabe, H., Todd, J., Michie, P., Shinozaki, N., Sutoh, T., et al. (2003). Impairment in activation of a frontal attention-switch mechanism in schizophrenic patients. *Biological Psychology*, 62(1), 49–63. doi:10.1016/S0301-0511(02)00113-8

Savard, R. J., Rey, A. C., & Post, R. M. (1980). Halstead-reitan category test in bipolar and unipolar affective disorders relationship to age and phase of illness. *Journal of Nervous and Mental Disease*, 168(5), 297–304.

Schachter, S. C. (2004). Epilepsy: major advances in treatment. *Lancet Neurology*, 3(1), 11. doi:10.1016/S1474-4422(03)00611-2

Schall, U. (2016). Is it time to move mismatch negativity into the clinic? *Biological Psychology*, 116, 41–6. doi:10.1016/j.biopsycho.2015.09.001

Schall, U., Johnston, P., Todd, J., Ward, P. B., & Michie, P. T. (2003). Functional neuroanatomy of auditory mismatch processing: an event-related fMRI study of duration-deviant oddballs. *NeuroImage*, 20(2), 729–36. doi:10.1016/S1053-8119(03)00398-7

Schall, U., Müller, B. W., Kärgel, C., & Güntürkün, O. (2015). Electrophysiological mismatch response recorded in awake pigeons from the avian functional equivalent of the primary auditory cortex. *NeuroReport*, 26(5), 239–44.

Scharf, B., & Houtsma, A. J. (1986). Loudness, pitch, localization, aural distortion, pathology. In K. B. Boff, L. Kaufman & J. P. Thomas (Eds), *Handbook of Perception and Human Performance, Vol. 1: Sensory Processes and Perception*. New York: Wiley-Interscience.

Scherer, N. J., & D'Antonio, L. (1997). Language and play development in toddlers with cleft lip and/or palate. *American Journal of Speech-Language Pathology*, 6(4), 48–54. doi:10.1044/1058-0360.0604.48

Scherg, M. (1992). Functional imaging and localization of electromagnetic brain activity. *Brain Topography*, 5(2), 103–11. doi:10.1007/BF01129037

Scherg, M., & Cramon, D. (1986). Psychoacoustic and electrophysiologic correlates of central hearing disorders in man. *European Archives of Psychiatry and Neurological Sciences*, 236(1), 56–60. doi:10.1007/BF00641060

Scherg, M., Vajsar, J., & Picton, T. W. (1989). A source analysis of the late human auditory evoked potentials. *Journal of Cognitive Neuroscience*, 1(4), 336–55. doi:10.1162/jocn.1989.1.4.336

Schiff, S., Valenti, P., Andrea, P., Lot, M., Bisiacchi, P., Gatta, A., & Amodio, P. (2008). The effect of aging on auditory components of event-related brain potentials. *Clinical Neurophysiology*, 119(8), 1795–802. doi:10.1016/j.clinph.2008.04.007

Schmidt, A., Bachmann, R., Kometer, M., Csomor, P. A., Stephan, K. E., Seifritz, E., & Vollenweider, F. X. (2012). Mismatch negativity encoding of prediction errors predicts S-ketamine-induced cognitive impairments. *Neuropsychopharmacology*, *37*(4), 865–75. doi:10.1038/npp.2011.261

Schneider, W., & Shiffrin, R. M. (1977). Controlled and automatic human information processing: I. Detection, search, and attention. *Psychological Review*, *84*(1), 1–66. doi:10.1037/0033-295X.84.1.1

Schreiber, H., Stolz-Born, G., Kornhuber, H. H., & Born, J. (1992). Event-related potential correlates of impaired selective attention in children at high risk for schizophrenia. *Biological Psychiatry*, *32*(8), 634–51. doi:10.1016/0006-3223(92)90294-A

Schroeder, M. M., Ritter, W., & Vaughan, H. (1995). The mismatch negativity to novel stimuli reflects cognitive decline. *Structure And Functions Of The Human Prefrontal Cortex*, *769*, 399–401.

Schroger, E. (1994). An event-related potential study of sensory representations of unfamiliar tonal patterns. *Psychophysiology*, *31*(2), 175–81.

Schroger, E. (1995). Processing of auditory deviants with changes in one versus two stimulus dimensions. *Psychophysiology*, *32*(1), 55–65.

Schröger, E. (1996). A neural mechanism for involuntary attention shifts to changes in auditory stimulation. *Journal of Cognitive Neuroscience*, *8*(6), 527–39. doi:10.1162/jocn.1996.8.6.527

Schröger, E. (1997). On the detection of auditory deviations: A pre-attentive activation model. *Psychophysiology*, *34*(3), 245–57. doi:10.1111/j.1469-8986.1997.tb02395.x

Schröger, E., Bendixen, A., Trujillo-Barreto, N. J., & Roeber, U. (2007). Processing of Abstract Rule Violations in Audition (Abstract Auditory Rules). *PLoS ONE*, *2*(11), e1131. doi:10.1371/journal.pone.0001131

Schröger, E., Giard, M. H., & Wolff, C. (2000). Auditory distraction: event-related potential and behavioral indices. *Clinical Neurophysiology*, *111*(8), 1450–60. doi:10.1016/S1388-2457(00)00337-0

Schröger, E., Paavilainen, P., & Näätänen, R. (1994). Mismatch negativity to changes in a continuous tone with regularly varying frequencies. *Electroencephalography and Clinical Neurophysiology*, *92*(2), 140–7.

Schröger, E., & Winkler, I. (1995). Presentation rate and magnitude of stimulus deviance effects on human pre-attentive change detection. *Neuroscience Letters*, *193*(3), 185–8. doi:10.1016/0304-3940(95)11696-T

Schröger, E., & Wolff, C. (1996). Mismatch response of the human brain to changes in sound location. *NeuroReport*, *7*(18), 3005–8.

Schröger, E., & Wolff, C. (1998a). Attentional orienting and reorienting is indicated by human event-related brain potentials. *NeuroReport*, *9*(15), 3355–8.

Schröger, E., & Wolff, C. (1998b). Behavioral and electrophysiological effects of task-irrelevant sound change: a new distraction paradigm. *Brain Research. Cognitive Brain Research*, *7*(1), 71–87.

Schulte-Körne, G., Deimel, W., Bartling, J., & Remschmidt, H. (1998). Auditory processing and dyslexia: evidence for a specific speech processing deficit. *NeuroReport*, *9*(2), 337–40.

Schönwiesner, M., Novitski, N., Pakarinen, S., Carlson, S., Tervaniemi, M., & Näätänen, R. (2007). Heschl's gyrus, posterior superior temporal gyrus, and mid-ventrolateral prefrontal cortex have different roles in the detection of acoustic changes. *Journal of Neurophysiology*, *97*(3), 2075.

Sculthorpe, L. D., Collin, C. A., & Campbell, K. B. (2008). The influence of strongly focused visual attention on the detection of change in an auditory pattern. *Brain Research*, *1234*, 78–86. doi:10.1016/j.brainres.2008.07.031

Sculthorpe, L. D., Ouellet, D. R., & Campbell, K. B. (2009). MMN elicitation during natural sleep to violations of an auditory pattern. *Brain Research*, *1290*, 52–62. doi:10.1016/j.brainres.2009.06.013

Sculthorpe, L. D., Stelmack, R. M., & Campbell, K. B. (2009). Mental Ability and the Effect of Pattern Violation Discrimination on P300 and Mismatch Negativity. *Intelligence*, *37*(4), 405–11. doi:10.1016/j.intell.2009.03.006

Sculthorpe-Petley, L., Liu, C., Ghosh Hajra, S., Parvar, H., Satel, J., Trappenberg, T. P., et al. (2015). A rapid event-related potential (ERP) method for point-of-care evaluation of brain function: Development of the Halifax Consciousness Scanner. *Journal of Neuroscience Methods, 245*, 64–72. doi:10.1016/j.jneumeth.2015.02.008

Seidl, S. E., & Potashkin, J. A. (2011). The promise of neuroprotective agents in Parkinson's disease. *Frontiers in Neurology, 2*, 68. doi:10.3389/fneur.2011.00068

Serra, J., Escera, C., Sánchez-Turet, M., Sánchez-Sastre, J., & Grau, C. (1996). The H1-receptor antagonist chlorpheniramine decreases the ending phase of the mismatch negativity of the human auditory event-related potentials. *Neuroscience Letters, 203*(2), 77–80. doi:10.1016/0304-3940(95)12265-6

Shafer, V. L., Morr, M. L., Datta, H., Kurtzberg, D., & Schwartz, R. G. (2005). Neurophysiological indexes of speech processing deficits in children with specific language impairment. *Journal of Cognitive Neuroscience, 17*(7), 1168–80. doi:10.1162/0898929054475217

Shafer, V. L., Morr, M. L., Kreuzer, J. A., & Kurtzberg, D. (2000). Maturation of mismatch negativity in school-age children. *Ear and Hearing, 21*(3), 242–51. doi:10.1097/00003446-200006000-00008

Shafer, V. L., Yu, Y. H., & Datta, H. (2010). Maturation of speech discrimination in 4- to 7-yr-old children as indexed by event-related potential mismatch responses. *Ear and Hearing, 31*(6), 735–45. doi:10.1097/AUD.0b013e3181e5d1a7

Shaikh, M., Valmaggia, L., Broome, M. R., Dutt, A., Lappin, J., Day, F., et al. (2012). Reduced mismatch negativity predates the onset of psychosis. *Schizophrenia Research, 134*(1), 42–8. doi:10.1016/j.schres.2011.09.022

Shalgi, S., & Deouell, L. Y. (2007). Direct evidence for differential roles of temporal and frontal components of auditory change detection. *Neuropsychologia, 45*(8), 1878–88. doi:10.1016/j.neuropsychologia.2006.11.023

Sharma, A., & Dorman, M. F. (2006). Central auditory development in children with cochlear implants: Clinical implications. *Advances in Oto-Rhino-Laryngology, 64*, 66–88.

Sharma, M., Purdy, S. C., Newall, P., Wheldall, K., Beaman, R., & Dillon, H. (2006). Electrophysiological and behavioral evidence of auditory processing deficits in children with reading disorder. *Clinical Neurophysiology, 117*(5), 1130–44. doi:10.1016/j.clinph.2006.02.001

Shaywitz, S. E., Shaywitz, B. A., Fletcher, J. M., & Escobar, M. D. (1990). Prevalence of reading disability in boys and girls. Results of the Connecticut Longitudinal Study. *Journal of the American Medical Association, 264*(8), 998–1002.

Shelley, A. M., Silipo, G., & Javitt, D. C. (1999). Diminished responsiveness of ERPs in schizophrenic subjects to changes in auditory stimulation parameters: Implications for theories of cortical dysfunction. *Schizophrenia Research, 37*(1), 65–79. doi:10.1016/S0920-9964(98)00138-8

Shelley, A. M., Ward, P. B., Catts, S. V., Michie, P. T., Andrews, S., & McConaghy, N. (1991). Mismatch negativity: An index of a preattentive processing deficit in schizophrenia. *Biological Psychiatry, 30*(10), 1059–62. doi:10.1016/0006-3223(91)90126-7

Shestakova, J. A., Brattico, J. E., Huotilainen, J. M., Galunov, J. V., Soloviev, J. A., Sams, J. M., et al. (2002). Abstract phoneme representations in the left temporal cortex: magnetic mismatch negativity study. *NeuroReport, 13*(14), 1813–16.

Shestakova, A., Brattico, E., Soloviev, A., Klucharev, V., & Huotilainen, M. (2004). Orderly cortical representation of vowel categories presented by multiple exemplars. *Cognitive Brain Research, 21*(3), 342–50. doi:10.1016/j.cogbrainres.2004.06.011

Shiffrin, R. D., & Schneider, W. (1977). Controlled and automatic human information processing, II: perceptual learning, automatic attending, and a general theory. *Psychological Review, 84*, 127–90.

Shinozaki, N., Yabe, H., Sato, Y., Hiruma, T., Sutoh, T., Matsuoka, T., & Kaneko, S. (2003). Spectrotemporal window of integration of auditory information in the human brain. *Cognitive Brain Research, 17*(3), 563–71. doi:10.1016/S0926-6410(03)00170-8

Shinozaki, N., Yabe, H., Sato, Y., Hiruma, T., Sutoh, T., Nashida, T., et al. (2002). The difference in mismatch negativity between the acute and post-acute phase of schizophrenia. *Biological Psychology*, *59*(2), 105–19. doi:10.1016/S0301-0511(01)00129-6

Shinozaki, N., Yabe, H., Sato, Y., Sutoh, T., Hiruma, T., Nashida, T., & Kaneko, S. (2000). Mismatch negativity (MMN) reveals sound grouping in the human brain. *NeuroReport*, *11*(8), 1597–601.

Shinozaki, N., Yabe, H., Sutoh, T., Hiruma, T., & Kaneko, S. (1998). Somatosensory automatic responses to deviant stimuli. *Cognitive Brain Research*, *7*(2), 165–71. doi:10.1016/S0926-6410(98)00020-2

Shprintzen, R. J. (1995). A new perspective on clefting. In R. J. Shprintzen & J. Bardach (Eds), *Cleft Palate Speech Management. A Multidisciplinary Approac* (pp. 1–15). St. Louis: Mosby Year Book.

Shriberg, L. D., Paul, R., McSweeny, J. L., Klin, A., Cohen, D. J., & Volkmar, F. R. (2001). Speech and prosody characteristics of adolescents and adults with high-functioning autism and Asperger syndrome. *Journal of Speech, Language, and Hearing Research*, *44*(5), 1097–115.

Shtyrov, Y., & Pulvermüller, F. (2007). Early MEG activation dynamics in the left temporal and inferior frontal cortex reflect semantic context integration. *Journal of Cognitive Neuroscience*, *19*(10), 1633–42. doi:10.1162/jocn.2007.19.10.1633

Siegel, L. S., & Faux, D. (1989). Acquisition of certain grapheme-phoneme correspondences in normally achieving and disabled readers. *Reading and Writing*, *1*(1), 37–52. doi:10.1007/BF00178836

Simpson, T. P., Manara, A. R., Kane, N. M., Barton, R. L., Rowlands, C. A., & Butler, S. R. (2002). Effect of propofol anaesthesia on the event-related potential mismatch negativity and the auditory-evoked potential N1. *British Journal of Anaesthesia*, *89*(3), 382–8. doi:10.1093/bja/aef175

Simson, R., Vaughan, H. G., & Ritter, W. (1976). The scalp topography of potentials associated with missing visual or auditory stimuli. *Electroencephalography and Clinical Neurophysiology*, *40*(1), 33–42. doi:10.1016/0013-4694(76)90177-2

Simson, R., Vaughan, H. G., & Ritter, W. (1977). The scalp topography of potentials in auditory and visual discrimination tasks. *Electroencephalography and Clinical Neurophysiology*, *42*(4), 528–35. doi:10.1016/0013-4694(77)90216-4

Singer, W. (1995). Development and plasticity of cortical processing architectures. *Science*, *270*(5237), 758–64.

Singh, S., Liasis, A., Rajput, K., & Luxon, L. (2004a). Short report: methodological considerations in recording mismatch negativity in cochlear implant patients. *Cochlear Implants International*, *5*(2), 76–80. doi:10.1002/cii.128

Singh, S., Liasis, A., Rajput, K., Towell, A., & Luxon, L. (2004b). Event-related potentials in pediatric cochlear implant patients. *Ear and Hearing*, *25*(6), 598–610.

Sinkkonen, J., & Tervaniemi, M. (2000). Towards optimal recording and analysis of the mismatch negativity. *Audiology and Neuro-Otology*, *5*(3–4), 235–46.

Sinkkonen, J., Tiitinen, H., & Näätänen, R. (1995). Gabor filters: an informative way for analysing event-related brain activity. *Journal of Neuroscience Methods*, *56*(1), 99–104. doi:10.1016/0165-0270(94)00111-S

Sivarao, D. V., Chen, P., Yang, Y., Li, Y. W., Pieschl, R., & Ahlijanian K, M. K. (2014). NR2B antagonist CP-101,606 abolishes pitch-mediated deviance detection in awake rats. *Frontiers in Psychiatry*, *5*, 96. doi:10.3389/fpsyt.2014.00096

Smith-Spark, J., & Fisk, J. (2007). Working memory functioning in developmental dyslexia. *Memory*, *15*(1), 34–56. doi:10.1080/09658210601043384

Snowling, M. (2000). *Dyslexia* (2 ed.). Malden, MA: Blackwell Publishing.

Snowling, M. J. (1980). The development of grapheme-phoneme correspondence in normal and dyslexic readers. *Journal of Experimental Child Psychology*, *29*(2), 294–305. doi:10.1016/0022-0965(80)90021-1

Snowling, M. J., & Melby-Lervåg, M. (2016). Oral language deficits in familial dyslexia: A meta-analysis and review. *Psychological Bulletin, 142*(5), 498–545. doi:10.1037/bul0000037

Snyder, E., & Hillyard, S. A. (1976). Long-latency evoked potentials to irrelevant, deviant stimuli. *Behavioral Biology, 16*(3), 319–31. doi:10.1016/S0091-6773(76)91447-4

Sokolov, E. N. (1963). *Perception and the Conditioned Reflex.* New York: Macmillan.

Sokolov, E. N., Spinks, J. A., Näätänen, R., & Lyytinen, H. (2002). *The Orienting Response in Information Processing.* Mahwah, NJ: Lawrence Erlbaum Associates Publishers.

Sonnadara, R. R., Alain, C., & Trainor, L. J. (2006). Effects of spatial separation and stimulus probability on the event-related potentials elicited by occasional changes in sound location. *Brain Research, 1071*(1), 175–85. doi:10.1016/j.brainres.2005.11.088

Spackman, L. A., Boyd, S. G., & Towell, A. (2007). Effects of stimulus frequency and duration on somatosensory discrimination responses. *Experimental Brain Research, 177*(1), 21–30. doi:10.1007/s00221-006-0650-0

Spackman, L. A., Towell, A., & Boyd, S. G. (2010). Somatosensory discrimination: An intracranial event-related potential study of children with refractory epilepsy. *Brain Research, 1310*, 68–76. doi:10.1016/j.brainres.2009.10.072

Squires, K. C., & Donchin, E. (1976). Beyond averaging: The use of discriminant functions to recognize event related potentials elicited by single auditory stimuli. *Electroencephalography and Clinical Neurophysiology, 41*(5), 449–59. doi:10.1016/0013-4694(76)90056-0

Squires, N. K., Squires, K. C., & Hillyard, S. A. (1975). Two varieties of long-latency positive waves evoked by unpredictable auditory stimuli in man. *Electroencephalography and Clinical Neurophysiology, 38*(4), 387–401. doi:10.1016/0013-4694(75)90263-1

Squires, K. C., Wickens, C., Squires, N. K., & Donchin, E. (1976). The effect of stimulus sequence on the waveform of the cortical event-related potential. *Science, 193*(4258), 1142–6. doi:10.1126/science.959831

Stafford, M. R., Jackson, H., Mayo-Wilson, E., Morrison, A. P., & Kendall, T. (2013). Early interventions to prevent psychosis: Systematic review and meta-analysis. *BMJ (Online), 346*(7892). doi:10.1136/bmj.f185

Stagg, C., Hindley, P., Tales, A., & Butler, S. (2004). Visual mismatch negativity: the detection of stimulus change. *NeuroReport, 15*(4), 659–63.

Stefanics, G., Csukly, G., Komlósi, S., Czobor, P., & Czigler, I. (2012). Processing of unattended facial emotions: A visual mismatch negativity study. *NeuroImage, 59*(3), 3042–9. doi:10.1016/j.neuroimage.2011.10.041

Stefanics, G., Kimura, M., & Czigler, I. (2011). Visual mismatch negativity reveals automatic detection of sequential regularity violation. *Frontiers in Human Neuroscience, 5*, 46. doi:10.3389/fnhum.2011.00046

Stein, J. (2001). The magnocellular theory of developmental dyslexia. *Dyslexia, 7*(1), 12–36. doi:10.1002/dys.186

Stoodley, C., & Stein, J. (2013). Cerebellar function in developmental dyslexia. *The Cerebellum, 12*(2), 267–76. doi:10.1007/s12311-012-0407-1

Stothart, G., Kazanina, N., Näätänen, R., Haworth, J., & Tales, A. (2015). Early visual evoked potentials and mismatch negativity in Alzheimer's disease and mild cognitive impairment. *Journal of Alzheimer's Disease, 44*(2), 397–408. doi:10.3233/JAD-140930

Stothart, G., Tales, A., & Kazanina, N. (2013). Evoked potentials reveal age-related compensatory mechanisms in early visual processing. *Neurobiology of Aging, 34*(4), 1302–8. doi:10.1016/j.neurobiolaging.2012.08.012

Stovner, L. J., Hagen, K., Jensen, R., Katsarava, Z., Lipton, R. B., Scher, A. I., et al. (2007). The global burden of headache: A documentation of headache prevalence and disability worldwide. *Cephalalgia, 27*(3), 193–210. doi:10.1111/j.1468-2982.2007.01288.x

Strömmer, J. M., Astikainen, P., & Tarkka, I. M. (2014). Somatosensory mismatch response in young and elderly adults. *Frontiers in Aging Neuroscience*, 6, 293. doi:10.3389/fnagi.2014.00293

Summerfield, C., & Egner, T. (2009). Expectation (and attention) in visual cognition. *Trends in Cognitive Sciences*, *13*(9), 403–9. doi:10.1016/j.tics.2009.06.003

Sun, H. Y., Li, Q., Chen, X. P., & Tao, L. Y. (2015). Mismatch negativity, social cognition, and functional outcomes in patients after traumatic brain injury. *Neural Regeneration Research*, *10*(4), 618–23. doi:10.4103/1673-5374.155437

Sussman, E., Ritter, W., & Vaughan, H. G. (1999). An investigation of the auditory streaming effect using event-related brain potentials. *Psychophysiology*, *36*, 22–34.

Sussman, E., & Winkler, I. (2001). Dynamic sensory updating in the auditory system. *Cognitive Brain Research*, *12*(3), 431–9. doi:10.1016/S0926-6410(01)00067-2

Sutton, S., Braren, M., Zubin, J., & John, E. R. (1965). Evoked-potential correlates of stimulus uncertainty. *Science*, *150*(3700), 1187–8.

Swerdlow, N. R. (2012). Beyond antipsychotics: Pharmacologically-augmented cognitive therapies (PACTs) for schizophrenia. *Neuropsychopharmacology*, *37*(1), 310–11. doi:10.1038/npp.2011.195

Swerdlow, N. R., Bhakta, S., Chou, H.-H., Talledo, J. A., Balvaneda, B., & Light, G. A. (2016). Memantine effects on sensorimotor gating and mismatch negativity in patients with chronic psychosis. *Neuropsychopharmacology*, *41*(2), 419–30.

Swillen, A., Devriendt, K., Legius, E., Prinzie, P., Vogels, A., Ghesquiere, P., & Fryns, J. P. (1999). The behavioural phenotype in velo-cardio-facial syndrome (VCFS): from infancy to adolescence. *Genetic Counseling*, *10*(1), 79–88.

Syka, J., Rybalko, N., Brožek, G., & Jilek, M. (1996). Auditory frequency and intensity discrimination in pigmented rats. *Hearing Research*, *100*(1), 107–13. doi:10.1016/0378-5955(96)00101-3

Takahashi, H., Rissling, A. J., Pascual-Marqui, R., Kirihara, K., Pela, M., Sprock, J., et al. (2013). Neural substrates of normal and impaired preattentive sensory discrimination in large cohorts of nonpsychiatric subjects and schizophrenia patients as indexed by MMN and P3a change detection responses. *NeuroImage*, *66*, 594–603. doi:10.1016/j.neuroimage.2012.09.074

Takegata, R., Brattico, E., Tervaniemi, M., Varyagina, O., Näätänen, R., & Winkler, I. (2005). Preattentive representation of feature conjunctions for concurrent spatially distributed auditory objects. *Cognitive Brain Research*, *25*(1), 169–79. doi:10.1016/j.cogbrainres.2005.05.006

Takegata, R., & Morotomi, T. (1999). Integrated neural representation of sound and temporal features in human auditory sensory memory: an event-related potential study. *Neuroscience Letters*, *274*(3), 207–10. doi:10.1016/S0304-3940(99)00711-9

Takegata, R., Paavilainen, P., Näätänen, R., & Winkler, I. (1999). Independent processing of changes in auditory single features and feature conjunctions in humans as indexed by the mismatch negativity. *Neuroscience Letters*, *266*(2), 109–12. doi:10.1016/S0304-3940(99)00267-0

Takei, Y., Kumano, S., Hattori, S., Uehara, T., Kawakubo, Y., Kasai, K., et al. (2009). Preattentive dysfunction in major depression: A magnetoencephalography study using auditory mismatch negativity. *Psychophysiology*, *46*(1), 52–61. doi:10.1111/j.1469-8986.2008.00748.x

Takei, Y., Kumano, S., Maki, Y., Hattori, S., Kawakubo, Y., Kasai, K., et al. (2010). Preattentive dysfunction in bipolar disorder: A MEG study using auditory mismatch negativity. *Progress in Neuro-Psychopharmacology and Biological Psychiatry*, *34*(6), 903–12. doi:10.1016/j.pnpbp.2010.04.014

Tales, A., Haworth, J., Wilcock, G., Newton, P., & Butler, S. (2008). Visual mismatch negativity highlights abnormal pre-attentive visual processing in mild cognitive impairment and Alzheimer's disease. *Neuropsychologia*, *46*(5), 1224–32. doi:10.1016/j.neuropsychologia.2007.11.017

Tales, A., Newton, P., Troscianko, T., & Butler, S. (1999). Mismatch negativity in the visual modality. *NeuroReport*, *10*(16), 3363–7.

Tales, K. A., Troscianko, R. T., Wilcock, R. G., Newton, R. P., & Butler, R. S. (2002). Age-related changes in the preattentional detection of visual change. *NeuroReport, 13*(7), 969–72.

Tallal, P. (1980). Auditory temporal perception, phonics, and reading disabilities in children. *Brain and Language, 9*(2), 182–98. doi:10.1016/0093-934X(80)90139-X

Tallal, P. (2004). Improving language and literacy is a matter of time. *Nature Reviews Neuroscience, 5*(9), 721–8. doi:1038/nrn1499

Tallal, P., & Gaab, N. (2006). Dynamic auditory processing, musical experience and language development. *Trends in Neurosciences, 29*(7), 382–90. doi:10.1016/j.tins.2006.06.003

Tang, D., Xu, J., Chang, Y., Zheng, Y., Shi, N., Pang, X., & Zhang, B. (2013). Visual mismatch negativity in the detection of facial emotions in patients with panic disorder. *NeuroReport, 24*(5), 207–11. doi:10.1097/WNR.0b013e32835eb63a

Tarasenko, M., Perez, V. B., Pianka, S. T., Vinogradov, S., Braff, D. L., Swerdlow, N. R., & Light, G. A. (2016). Measuring the capacity for auditory system plasticity: An examination of performance gains during initial exposure to auditory-targeted cognitive training in schizophrenia. *Schizophrenia Research, 172*(1–3), 123–30. doi:10.1016/j.schres.2016.01.019

Tarkka, I. M., Luukkainen-Markkula, R., Pitkänen, K., & Hämäläinen, H. (2011). Alterations in visual and auditory processing in hemispatial neglect: An evoked potential follow-up study. *International Journal of Psychophysiology, 79*(2), 272–9. doi:10.1016/j.ijpsycho.2010.11.002

Tata, M. S., & Ward, L. M. (2005). Early phase of spatial mismatch negativity is localized to a posterior "where" auditory pathway. *Experimental Brain Research, 167*(3), 481–6. doi:10.1007/s00221-005-0183-y

Tecchio, F., Benassi, F., Zappasodi, F., Gialloreti, L. E., Palermo, M., Seri, S., & Rossini, P. M. (2003). Auditory sensory processing in autism: a magnetoencephalographic study. *Biological Psychiatry, 54*(6), 647–54. doi:10.1016/S0006-3223(03)00295-6

Tervaniemi, M., Ilvonen, T., Karma, K., Alho, K., & Näätänen, R. (1997). The musical brain: brain waves reveal the neurophysiological basis of musicality in human subjects. *Neuroscience Letters, 226*(1), 1–4. doi:10.1016/S0304-3940(97)00217-6

Tervaniemi, M., Kujala, A., Alho, K., Virtanen, J., Ilmoniemi, R. J., & Näätänen, R. (1999). Functional specialization of the human auditory cortex in processing phonetic and musical sounds: a magnetoencephalographic (MEG) study. *NeuroImage, 9*(3), 330–6. doi:10.1006/nimg.1999.0405

Tervaniemi, M., Maury, S., & Näätänen, R. (1994). Neural representations of abstract stimulus features in the human brain as reflected by the mismatch negativity. *NeuroReport, 5*(7), 844–6.

Tervaniemi, M., Medvedev, S. V., Alho, K., Pakhomov, S. V., Roudas, M. S., Van Zuijen, T. L., & Näätänen, R. (2000). Lateralized automatic auditory processing of phonetic versus musical information: A PET study. *Human Brain Mapping, 10*(2), 74–9. doi:10.1002/(SICI)1097-0193(200006)10:2<74::AID-HBM30>3.0.CO2-2

Tervaniemi, M., Rytkönen, M., Schröger, E., Ilmoniemi, R., & Näätänen, R. (2001). Superior formation of cortical memory traces for melodic patterns in musicians. *Learning & Memory, 8*(5), 295–300.

Tervaniemi, M., Saarinen, J., Paavilainen, P., Danilova, N., & Näätänen, R. (1994). Temporal integration of auditory information in sensory memory as reflected by the mismatch negativity. *Biological Psychology, 38*(2), 157–67. doi:10.1016/0301-0511(94)90036-1

Teter, B., & Ashford, J. W. (2002). Neuroplasticity in Alzheimer's disease. *Journal of Neuroscience Research, 70*(3), 402–37.

Tham, A., Engelbrektson, K., Mathé, A. A., Johnson, L., Olsson, E., & Åberg-Wistedt, A. (1997). Impaired neuropsychological performance in euthymic patients with recurring mood disorders. *Journal of Clinical Psychiatry, 58*(1), 26–9. doi:10.4088/JCP.v58n0105

Thomas, E. J., & Elliott, R. (2009). Brain imaging correlates of cognitive impairment in depression. *Frontiers in Human Neuroscience, 3,* 30. doi:10.3389/neuro.09.030.2009

Thomas, M. L., Green, M. F., Hellemann, G., Sugar, C. A., Tarasenko, M., Calkins, M. E., et al. (2017). Modeling deficits from early auditory information processing to psychosocial functioning in schizophrenia. *JAMA Psychiatry, 74*(1), 37–46. doi:10.1001/jamapsychiatry.2016.2980

Thompson, J. M., Gallagher, P., Hughes, J. H., Watson, S., Gray, J. M., Ferrier, I. N., & Young, A. H. (2005). Neurocognitive impairment in euthymic patients with bipolar affective disorder. *British Journal of Psychiatry, 186,* 32–40. doi:10.1192/bjp.186.1.32

Tiitinen, H., Alho, K., Huotilainen, M., Ilmoniemi, R. J., Simola, J., & Näätänen, R. (1993). Tonotopic auditory cortex and the magnetoencephalographic (MEG) equivalent of the mismatch negativity. *Psychophysiology, 30*(5), 537–40. doi:10.1111/j.1469-8986.1993.tb02078.x

Tiitinen, H., May, P., Reinikainen, K., & Näätänen, R. (1994). Attentive novelty detection in humans is governed by pre-attentive sensory memory. *Nature, 372*(6501), 90–2. doi:10.1038/372090a0

Tikhonravov, D., Neuvonen, T., Pertovaara, A., Savioja, K., Ruusuvirta, T., Näätänen, R., & Carlson, S. (2008). Effects of an NMDA-receptor antagonist MK-801 on an MMN-like response recorded in anesthetized rats. *Brain Research, 1203,* 97–102. doi:10.1016/j.brainres.2008.02.006

Tikhonravov, D., Neuvonen, T., Pertovaara, A., Savioja, K., Ruusuvirta, T., Näätänen, R., & Carlson, S. (2010). Dose-related effects of memantine on a mismatch negativity-like response in anesthetized rats. *Neuroscience, 167*(4), 1175–82. doi:10.1016/j.neuroscience.2010.03.014

Timm, L., Agrawal, D., C. Viola, F., Sandmann, P., Debener, S., Büchner, A., et al. (2012). Temporal Feature Perception in Cochlear Implant Users. *PLoS ONE, 7*(9), e45375. doi:10.1371/journal.pone.0045375

Timm, L., Vuust, P., Brattico, E., Agrawal, D., Debener, S., Buchner, A., et al. (2014). Residual neural processing of musical sound features in adult cochlear implant users. *Frontiers in Human Neuroscience, 8,* 181. doi:10.3389/fnhum.2014.00181

Todd, J., Heathcote, A., Whitson, L. R., Mullens, D., Provost, A., & Winkler, I. (2014). Mismatch negativity (MMN) to pitch change is susceptible to order-dependent bias. *Frontiers in Neuroscience, 8,* 180. doi:10.3389/fnins.2014.00180

Todd, J., Michie, P. T., Budd, T. W., Rock, D., & Jablensky, A. V. (2000). Auditory sensory memory in schizophrenia: inadequate trace formation? *Psychiatry Research, 96*(2), 99–115. doi:10.1016/S0165-1781(00)00205-5

Todd, J., Michie, P. T., & Jablensky, A. V. (2003). Association between reduced duration mismatch negativity (MMN) and raised temporal discrimination thresholds in schizophrenia. *Clinical Neurophysiology, 114*(11), 2061–70. doi:10.1016/S1388-2457(03)00246-3

Todd, J., Michie, P. T., Schall, U., Karayanidis, F., Yabe, H., & Näätänen, R. (2008). Deviant matters: duration, frequency, and intensity deviants reveal different patterns of mismatch negativity reduction in early and late schizophrenia. *Biological Psychiatry, 63*(1), 58–64. doi:10.1016/j.biopsych.2007.02.016

Todd, J., Michie, P. T., Schall, U., Ward, P. B., & Catts, S. V. (2012). Mismatch negativity (MMN) reduction in schizophrenia—impaired prediction-error generation, estimation or salience? *International Journal of Psychophysiology, 83*(2), 222–31.

Todd, J., Myers, R., Pirillo, R., & Drysdale, K. (2010). Neuropsychological correlates of auditory perceptual inference: A mismatch negativity (MMN) study. *Brain Research, 1310,* 113–23. doi:10.1016/j.brainres.2009.11.019

Todd, J., Petherbridge, A., Speirs, B., Provost, A., & Paton, B. (2018). Time as context: The influence of hierarchical patterning on sensory inference. *Schizophrenia Research, 191,* 123–31. doi:10.1016/j.schres.2017.03.033

Toiviainen, P., Tervaniemi, M., Louhivuori, J., Saher, M., Huotilainen, M., & Näätänen, R. (1998). Timbre similarity: Convergence of neural, behavioral, and computational approaches. *Music Perception: An Interdisciplinary Journal, 16*(2), 223–41. doi:10.2307/40285788

Tomblin, J. B., Records, N. L., Buckwalter, P., Zhang, X., Smith, E., & O'Brien, M. (1997). Prevalence of specific language impairment in kindergarten children. *Journal of Speech, Language, and Hearing Research, 40*(6), 1245–60.

Tomé, D., Patricio, B. F., Manchaiah, V., Barbosa, F., & Marques-Teixeira, J. (2015). Mismatch negativity and the n2b component elicited by pure tones and speech sounds in anomic aphasia: a case study. *Journal of Hearing Science, 5*(2), 51–59.

Tomé, D., Sampaio, M., Mendes-Ribeiro, J., Barbosa, F., & Marques-Teixeira, J. (2014). Auditory event-related potentials in children with benign epilepsy with centro-temporal spikes. *Epilepsy Research, 108*(10), 1945–9. doi:10.1016/j.eplepsyres.2014.09.021

Torppa, R., Salo, E., Makkonen, T., Loimo, H., Pykäläinen, J., Lipsanen, J., et al. (2012). Cortical processing of musical sounds in children with cochlear implants. *Clinical Neurophysiology, 123*(10), 1966–79. doi:10.1016/j.clinph.2012.03.008

Trainor, J. L., Samuel, S. S., Desjardins, N. R., & Sonnadara, R. R. (2001). Measuring temporal resolution in infants using mismatch negativity. *NeuroReport, 12*(11), 2443–8.

Trainor, L., McFadden, M., Hodgson, L., Darragh, L., Barlow, J., Matsos, L., & Sonnadara, R. (2003). Changes in auditory cortex and the development of mismatch negativity between 2 and 6 months of age. *International Journal of Psychophysiology, 51*(1), 5–15. doi:10.1016/S0167-8760(03)00148-X

Trautwein, P. G., Ponton, C. W., Kwong, B., & Waring, M. D. (1998). Neurophysiological and psychophysical measures of duration discrimination in normal-hearing adults and adults with cochlear implants. *Journal of the Acoustical Society of America, 103*(5), 2847. doi:10.1121/1.421962

Treisman, A. (1988). Features and objects: The fourteenth Bartlett memorial lecture. *Quarterly Journal of Experimental Psychology Section A, 40*(2), 201–37. doi:10.1080/02724988843000104

Tremblay, K., Kraus, N., Carrell, T. D., & McGee, T. (1997). Central auditory system plasticity: generalization to novel stimuli following listening training. *Journal of the Acoustical Society of America, 102*(6), 3762–73. doi:10.1121/1.420139

Tremblay, K., Kraus, N., & McGee, T. (1998). The time course of auditory perceptual learning: neurophysiological changes during speech-sound training. *NeuroReport, 9*(16), 3556–60.

Troche, S. J., Houlihan, M. E., Stelmack, R. M., & Rammsayer, T. H. (2009). Mental ability, P300, and mismatch negativity: analysis of frequency and duration discrimination. *Intelligence, 37*(4), 365–73. doi:10.1016/j.intell.2009.03.002

Troche, S. J., Houlihan, M. E., Stelmack, R. M., & Rammsayer, T. H. (2010). Mental ability and the discrimination of auditory frequency and duration change without focused attention: An analysis of mismatch negativity. *Personality and Individual Differences, 49*(3), 228–33. doi:10.1016/j.paid.2010.03.040

Tse, C.-Y., & Penney, T. (2007). Preattentive change detection using the event-related optical signal. *Engineering in Medicine and Biology Magazine, IEEE, 26*(4), 52–8. doi:10.1109/MEMB.2007.384096

Tse, C.-Y., & Penney, T. B. (2008). On the functional role of temporal and frontal cortex activation in passive detection of auditory deviance. *NeuroImage, 41*(4), 1462–70. doi:10.1016/j.neuroimage.2008.03.043

Tse, C.-Y., Rinne, T., Ng, K. K., & Penney, T. B. (2013). The functional role of the frontal cortex in pre-attentive auditory change detection. *NeuroImage, 83*, 870–9. doi:10.1016/j.neuroimage.2013.07.037

Tse, C.-Y., Tien, K.-R., & Penney, T. B. (2006). Event-related optical imaging reveals the temporal dynamics of right temporal and frontal cortex activation in pre-attentive change detection. *NeuroImage, 29*(1), 314–20. doi:10.1016/j.neuroimage.2005.07.013

Turetsky, B. I., Calkins, M. E., Light, G. A., Olincy, A., Radant, A. D., & Swerdlow, N. R. (2007). Neurophysiological endophenotypes of schizophrenia: The viability of selected candidate measures. *Schizophrenia Bulletin, 33*(1), 69–94. doi:10.1093/schbul/sbl060

Turetsky, B. I., Dress, E. M., Braff, D. L., Calkins, M. E., Green, M. F., Greenwood, T. A., et al. (2015). The utility of P300 as a schizophrenia endophenotype and predictive biomarker: Clinical and socio-demographic modulators in COGS-2. *Schizophrenia Research, 163*(1–3), 53–62. doi:10.1016/j.schres.2014.09.024

Turgeon, C., Lazzouni, L., Lepore, F., & Ellemberg, D. (2014). An objective auditory measure to assess speech recognition in adult cochlear implant users. *Clinical Neurophysiology, 125*(4), 827–35. doi:10.1016/j.clinph.2013.09.035

Twamley, E. W., Baker, D. G., Norman, S. B., Pittman, J. O. E., Lohr, J. B., & Resnick, S. G. (2013). Veterans health administration vocational services for operation iraqi freedom/operation enduring freedom veterans with mental health conditions. *Journal of Rehabilitation Research and Development, 50*(5), 663–70. doi:10.1682/JRRD.2012.08.0137

Twamley, E. W., Vella, L., Burton, C. Z., Becker, D. R., Bell, M. D., & Jeste, D. V. (2012a). The efficacy of supported employment for middle-aged and older people with schizophrenia. *Schizophrenia Research, 135*(1–3), 100–4. doi:10.1016/j.schres.2011.11.036

Twamley, E. W., Vella, L., Burton, C. Z., Heaton, R. K., & Jeste, D. V. (2012b). Compensatory cognitive training for psychosis: Effects in a randomized controlled trial. *Journal of Clinical Psychiatry, 73*(9), 1212–19. doi:10.4088/JCP.12m07686

Tzovara, A., Rossetti, A. O., Spierer, L., Grivel, J., Murray, M. M., Oddo, M., & De Lucia, M. (2013). Progression of auditory discrimination based on neural decoding predicts awakening from coma. *Brain, 136*(1), 81–9. doi:10.1093/brain/aws264

Umbricht, D., Javitt, D., Novak, G., Bates, J., Pollack, S., Lieberman, J., & Kane, J. (1998). Effects of clozapine on auditory event-related potentials in schizophrenia. *Biological Psychiatry, 44*(8), 716–25. doi:10.1016/S0006-3223(97)00524-6

Umbricht, D., Javitt, D., Novak, G., Bates, J., Pollack, S., Lieberman, J., & Kane, J. (1999). Effects of risperidone on auditory event-related potentials in schizophrenia. *International Journal of Neuropsychopharmacology, 2*(4), 299–304. doi:10.1017/S1461145799001595

Umbricht, D., Koller, R., Schmid, L., Skrabo, A., Grübel, C., Huber, T., & Stassen, H. (2003). How specific are deficits in mismatch negativity generation to schizophrenia? *Biological Psychiatry, 53*(12), 1120–31. doi:10.1016/S0006-3223(02)01642-6

Umbricht, D., Koller, R., Vollenweider, F. X., & Schmid, L. (2002). Mismatch negativity predicts psychotic experiences induced by nmda receptor antagonist in healthy volunteers. *Biological Psychiatry, 51*(5), 400–6. doi:10.1016/S0006-3223(01)01242-2

Umbricht, D., & Krljesb, S. (2005). Mismatch negativity in schizophrenia: A meta-analysis. *Schizophrenia Research, 76*(1), 1–23. doi:10.1016/j.schres.2004.12.002

Umbricht, D., Schmid, L., Koller, R., Vollenweider, F. X., Hell, D., & Javitt, D. C. (2000). Ketamine-induced deficits in auditory and visual context-dependent processing in healthy volunteers: Implications for models of cognitive deficits in schizophrenia. *Archives of General Psychiatry, 57*(12), 1139–47.

Umbricht, D., Vyssotki, D., Latanov, A., Nitsch, R., & Lipp, H. P. (2005). Deviance-related electrophysiological activity in mice: Is there mismatch negativity in mice? *Clinical Neurophysiology, 116*(2), 353–63. doi:10.1016/j.clinph.2004.08.015

Umbricht, D. S. G., Bates, J. A., Lieberman, J. A., Kane, J. M., & Javitt, D. C. (2006). Electrophysiological indices of automatic and controlled auditory information processing in first-episode, recent-onset and chronic schizophrenia. *Biological Psychiatry, 59*(8), 762–72. doi:10.1016/j.biopsych.2005.08.030

Urakawa, T., Inui, K., Yamashiro, K., & Kakigi, R. (2010a). Cortical dynamics of the visual change detection process. *Psychophysiology, 47*(5), 905–12. doi:10.1111/j.1469-8986.2010.00987.x

Urakawa, T., Inui, K., Yamashiro, K., Tanaka, E., & Kakigi, R. (2010b). Cortical dynamics of visual change detection based on sensory memory. *NeuroImage, 52*(1), 302–8. doi:10.1016/j.neuroimage.2010.03.071

Uther, M., Jansen, D. H. J., Huotilainen, M., Ilmoniemi, R. J., & Näätänen, R. (2003). Mismatch negativity indexes auditory temporal resolution: evidence from event-related potential (ERP) and event-related field (ERF) recordings. *Cognitive Brain Research, 17*(3), 685–91. doi:10.1016/S0926-6410(03)00194-0

Uwer, R., Albrecht, R., & Von Suchodoletz, W. (2002). Automatic processing of tones and speech stimuli in children with specific language impairment. *Developmental Medicine and Child Neurology, 44*(8), 527–32. doi:10.1017/S001216220100250X

Vaitulevich, S. F., & Shestopalova, L. B. (2010). Interhemisphere asymmetry of auditory evoked potentials in humans and mismatch negativity during sound source localization. *Neuroscience and Behavioral Physiology, 40*(6), 629–38. doi:10.1007/s11055-010-9305-5

Valenza, E., Simion, F., Cassia, V. M., & Umiltà, C. (1996). Face Preference at Birth. *Journal of Experimental Psychology: Human Perception and Performance, 22*(4), 892–903. doi:10.1037/0096-1523.22.4.892

Van Atteveldt, N., Formisano, E., Goebel, R., & Blomert, L. (2004). Integration of letters and speech sounds in the human brain. *Neuron, 43*(2), 271–82. doi:10.1016/j.neuron.2004.06.025

Van der Lely, H. K. J., & Howard, D. (1993). Children with specific language impairment: Linguistic impairment or short-term memory deficit? *Journal of Speech and Hearing Research, 36*(6), 1193–207.

van Der Stelt, O., & van Boxtel, G. J. M. (2008). Auditory P300 and mismatch negativity in comatose states. *Clinical Neurophysiology, 119*, 2172–4.

Vanhaudenhuyse, A., Laureys, S., & Perrin, F. (2008). Cognitive event-related potentials in comatose and post-comatose states. *Neurocritical Care, 8*(2), 262–70. doi:10.1007/s12028-007-9016-0

van Zuijen, T. L., Plakas, A., Maassen, B. A. M., Been, P., Maurits, N. M., Krikhaar, E., et al. (2012). Temporal auditory processing at 17 months of age is associated with preliterate language comprehension and later word reading fluency: An ERP study. *Neuroscience Letters, 528*(1), 31–5. doi:10.1016/j.neulet.2012.08.058

van Zuijen, T. L., Plakas, A., Maassen, B. A. M., Maurits, N. M., & Leij, A. (2013). Infant ERPs separate children at risk of dyslexia who become good readers from those who become poor readers. *Developmental Science, 16*(4), 554–63. doi:10.1111/desc.12049

van Zuijen, T. L., Simoens, V. L., Paavilainen, P., Näätänen, R., & Tervaniemi, M. (2006). Implicit, intuitive, and explicit knowledge of abstract regularities in a sound sequence: An event-related brain potential study. *Journal of Cognitive Neuroscience, 18*(8), 1292–303. doi:10.1162/jocn.2006.18.8.1292

Vellutino, F. R., Fletcher, J. M., Snowling, M. J., & Scanlon, D. M. (2004). Specific reading disability (dyslexia): what have we learned in the past four decades? *Journal of Child Psychology and Psychiatry, 45*(1), 2–40. doi:10.1046/j.0021-9630.2003.00305.x

Verhaeghen, P., & Salthouse, T. A. (1997). Meta-analyses of age-cognition relations in adulthood: Estimates of linear and nonlinear age effects and structural models. *Psychological Bulletin, 122*, 231–49.

Vinogradov, S., Fisher, M., & De Villers-Sidani, E. (2012). Cognitive training for impaired neural systems in neuropsychiatric illness. *Neuropsychopharmacology, 37*(1), 43–76. doi:10.1038/npp.2011.251

Virtala, P., Berg, V., Kivioja, M., Purhonen, J., Salmenkivi, M., Paavilainen, P., & Tervaniemi, M. (2011). The preattentive processing of major vs. minor chords in the human brain: An event-related potential study. *Neuroscience Letters, 487*(3), 406–10. doi:10.1016/j.neulet.2010.10.066

Virtala, P., Huotilainen, M., Partanen, E., Fellman, V., & Tervaniemi, M. (2013). Newborn infants' auditory system is sensitive to Western music chord categories. *Frontiers in Psychology*, 4, 492. doi:10.3389/fpsyg.2013.00492

Virtala, P., Huotilainen, M., Putkinen, V., Makkonen, T., & Tervaniemi, M. (2012). Musical training facilitates the neural discrimination of major versus minor chords in 13-year-old children. *Psychophysiology*, 49(8), 1125–32. doi:10.1111/j.1469-8986.2012.01386.x

Vuust, P., Brattico, E., Glerean, E., Seppänen, M., Pakarinen, S., Tervaniemi, M., & Näätänen, R. (2011). New fast mismatch negativity paradigm for determining the neural prerequisites for musical ability. *Cortex*, 47(9), 1091–8. doi:10.1016/j.cortex.2011.04.026

Vuust, P., Brattico, E., Seppänen, M., Näätänen, R., & Tervaniemi, M. (2012a). Practiced musical style shapes auditory skills. *Annals of the New York Academy of Sciences*, 12521(1), 139–46. doi:10.1111/j.1749-6632.2011.06409.x

Vuust, P., Brattico, E., Seppänen, M., Näätänen, R., & Tervaniemi, M. (2012b). The sound of music: Differentiating musicians using a fast, musical multi-feature mismatch negativity paradigm. *Neuropsychologia*, 50(7), 1432–43. doi:10.1016/j.neuropsychologia.2012.02.028

Waberski, T. D., Kreitschmann-Andermahr, I., Kawohl, W., Darvas, F., Ryang, Y., Gobbelé, R., & Buchner, H. (2001). Spatio-temporal source imaging reveals subcomponents of the human auditory mismatch negativity in the cingulum and right inferior temporal gyrus. *Neuroscience Letters*, 308(2), 107–10. doi:10.1016/S0304-3940(01)01988-7

Wable, J., van Den Abbeele, T., Gallégo, S., & Frachet, B. (2000). Mismatch negativity: a tool for the assessment of stimuli discrimination in cochlear implant subjects. *Clinical Neurophysiology*, 111(4), 743–51. doi:10.1016/S1388-2457(99)00298-9

Walter, W. G. (1964). The convergence and interaction of visual, auditory, and tactile responses in human nonspecific cortex. *Annals of the New York Academy of Sciences*, 112(1), 320–61. doi:10.1111/j.1749-6632.1964.tb26760.x

Wang, L., Lin, X., Zhou, B., Pöppel, E., & Bao, Y. (2015). Subjective present: a window of temporal integration indexed by mismatch negativity. *Cognitive Processing*, 16, 131–5. doi:10.1007/s10339-015-0687-8

Wang, W., Datta, H., & Sussman, E. (2005). The development of the length of the temporal window of integration for rapidly presented auditory information as indexed by MMN. *Clinical Neurophysiology*, 116(7), 1695–706. doi:10.1016/j.clinph.2005.03.008

Wang, W., Zhu, S. Z., Pan, L. C., Hu, A. H., & Wang, Y. H. (2001). Mismatch negativity and personality traits in chronic primary insomniacs. *Functional Neurology*, 16(1), 3–10.

Wang, X.-D., Gu, F., He, K., Chen, L.-H., & Chen, L. (2012). Preattentive extraction of abstract auditory rules in speech sound stream: a mismatch negativity study using lexical tones (preattentive extraction of abstract auditory rules). *PLoS ONE*, 7(1), e30027. doi:10.1371/journal.pone.0030027

Warren, R. M., & Obusek, C. J. (1972). Identification of temporal order within auditory sequences. *Perception & Psychophysics*, 12(1), 86–90. doi:10.3758/BF03212848

Weber, C., Hahne, A., Friedrich, M., & Friederici, A. D. (2005). Reduced stress pattern discrimination in 5-month-olds as a marker of risk for later language impairment: Neurophysiological evidence. *Cognitive Brain Research*, 25(1), 180–7. doi:10.1016/j.cogbrainres.2005.05.007

Wei, J.-H., Chan, T.-C., & Luo, Y.-J. (2002). A modified oddball paradigm "cross-modal delayed response" and the research on mismatch negativity. *Brain Research Bulletin*, 57(2), 221–30. doi:10.1016/S0361-9230(01)00742-0

Weisz, N., Voss, S., Berg, P., & Elbert, T. (2004). Abnormal auditory mismatch response in tinnitus sufferers with high-frequency hearing loss is associated with subjective distress level. *BMC Neuroscience*, 5, 8.

Wertz, R., Auther, L., Burch-Sims, G. P., Abou-Khalil, R., Kirshner, H., & Duncan, G. (1998). A comparison of the mismatch negativity (MMN) event-related potential to tone and speech stimuli in normal and aphasic adults. *Aphasiology*, *12*(7–8), 499–507. doi:10.1080/02687039808249553

Whitehouse, A. J. O., & Bishop, D. V. M. (2008). Do children with autism 'switch off' to speech sounds? An investigation using event-related potentials. *Developmental Science*, *11*(4), 516–24. doi:10.1111/j.1467-7687.2008.00697.x

Widmann, A., Kujala, T., Tervaniemi, M., Kujala, A., & Schröger, E. (2004). From symbols to sounds: Visual symbolic information activates sound representations. *Psychophysiology*, *41*(5), 709–15. doi:10.1111/j.1469-8986.2004.00208.x

Widmann, A., Schröger, E., Tervaniemi, M., Pakarinen, S., & Kujala, T. (2012). Mapping symbols to sounds: electrophysiological correlates of the impaired reading process in dyslexia. *Frontiers in Psychology*, *3*, 60. doi:10.3389/fpsyg.2012.00060

Wijnen, V. J. M., van Boxtel, G. J. M., Eilander, H. J., & de Gelder, B. (2007). Mismatch negativity predicts recovery from the vegetative state. *Clinical Neurophysiology*, *118*(3), 597–605. doi:10.1016/j.clinph.2006.11.020

Willcutt, E. G., & Pennington, B. F. (2000). Psychiatric Comorbidity in Children and Adolescents with Reading Disability. *Journal of Child Psychology and Psychiatry*, *41*(8), 1039–48.

Winblad, B., Palmer, K., Kivipelto, M., Jelic, V., Fratiglioni, L., Wahlund, L. O., et al. (2004). Mild cognitive impairment – beyond controversies, towards a consensus: report of the International Working Group on Mild Cognitive Impairment. *Journal of Internal Medicine*, *256*(3), 240–6. doi:10.1111/j.1365-2796.2004.01380.x

Wing, L. (1988). The continuum of autistic characteristics. In E. Schopler & G. Mesibov (Eds), *Diagnosis and Assessment in Autism* (pp. 91–110). Boston, MA: Springer.

Winkler, A. I., Teder-Sälejärvi, A. W., Horváth, A. J., Näätänen, A. R., & Sussman, A. E. (2003). Human auditory cortex tracks task-irrelevant sound sources. *NeuroReport*, *14*(16), 2053–6.

Winkler, I. (2007). Interpreting the mismatch negativity. *Journal of Psychophysiology*, *21*(3–4), 147–63. doi:10.1027/0269-8803.21.34.147

Winkler, I., Cowan, N., Csépe, V., Czigler, I., & Näätänen, R. (1996a). Interactions between transient and long-term auditory memory as reflected by the mismatch negativity. *Journal of Cognitive Neuroscience*, *8*(5), 403–15. doi:10.1162/jocn.1996.8.5.403

Winkler, I., Czigler, I., Sussman, E., Horváth, J., & Balázs, L. (2005). Preattentive binding of auditory and visual stimulus features. *Journal of Cognitive Neuroscience*, *17*(2), 320–39. doi:10.1162/0898929053124866

Winkler, I., Karmos, G., & Näätänen, R. (1996b). Adaptive modeling of the unattended acoustic environment reflected in the mismatch negativity event-related potential. *Brain Research*, *742*(1), 239–52. doi:10.1016/S0006-8993(96)01008-6

Winkler, I., Kujala, T., Tiitinen, H., Sivonen, P., Alku, P., Lehtokoski, A., et al. (1999). Brain responses reveal the learning of foreign language phonemes. *Psychophysiology*, *36*, 638–42.

Winkler, I., Kushnerenko, E., Horvath, J., Ceponiene, R., Fellman, V., Huotilainen, M., et al. (2003). Newborn infants can organize the auditory world. *Proceedings of the National Academy of Sciences of the United States*, *100*(20), 11812–15.

Winkler, I., Reinikainen, K., & Näätänen, R. (1993). Event-related brain potentials reflect traces of echoic memory in humans. *Perception & Psychophysics*, *53*(4), 443–9. doi:10.3758/BF03206788

Woldorff, M. G., & Hillyard, S. A. (1991). Modulation of early auditory processing during selective listening to rapidly presented tones. *Electroencephalography and Clinical Neurophysiology*, *79*(3), 170–91. doi:10.1016/0013-4694(91)90136-R

Woldorff, M. G., Hillyard, S. A., Gallen, C. C., Hampson, S. R., & Bloom, F. E. (1998). Magnetoencephalographic recordings demonstrate attentional modulation of mismatch-related neural activity in human auditory cortex. *Psychophysiology, 35*, 283–92.

Wolff, C., & Schröger, E. (2001a). Activation of the auditory pre-attentive change detection system by tone repetitions with fast stimulation rate. *Cognitive Brain Research, 10*(3), 323–7. doi:10.1016/S0926-6410(00)00043-4

Wolff, C., & Schröger, E. (2001b). Human pre-attentive auditory change-detection with single, double, and triple deviations as revealed by mismatch negativity additivity. *Neuroscience Letters, 311*(1), 37–40. doi:10.1016/S0304-3940(01)02135-8

World Health Organization (1993). *The ICD-10 Classification of Mental and Behavioural Disorders: Diagnostic Criteria for Research.* Geneva: World Health Organization.

Wright, B. A., Bowen, R. W., & Zecker, S. G. (2000). Nonlinguistic perceptual deficits associated with reading and language disorders. *Current Opinion in Neurobiology, 10*(4), 482–6. doi:10.1016/S0959-4388(00)00119-7

Wright, B. A., Lombardino, L. J., King, W. M., Puranik, C. S., Leonard, C. M., & Merzenich, M. M. (1997). Deficits in auditory temporal and spectral resolution in language-impaired children. *Nature, 387*(6629), 176–8.

Wunderlich, J. L., & Cone-Wesson, B. K. (2006). Maturation of CAEP in infants and children: A review. *Hearing Research, 212*(1), 212–23. doi:10.1016/j.heares.2005.11.008

Wykes, T., Huddy, V., Cellard, C., McGurk, Sr., & Czobor, P. (2011). A meta-analysis of cognitive remediation for schizophrenia: methodology and effect sizes. *American Journal of Psychiatry, 168*, 472–85.

Wynn, J. K., Sugar, C., Horan, W. P., Kern, R., & Green, M. F. (2010). Mismatch negativity, social cognition, and functioning in schizophrenia patients. *Biological Psychiatry, 67*(10), 940–7. doi:10.1016/j.biopsych.2009.11.024

Yabe, H., Koyama, S., Kakigi, R., Gunji, A., Tervaniemi, M., Sato, Y., & Kaneko, S. (2001a). Automatic discriminative sensitivity inside temporal window of sensory memory as a function of time. *Cognitive Brain Research, 12*(1), 39–48. doi:10.1016/S0926-6410(01)00027-1

Yabe, H., Sato, Y., Sutoh, T., Hiruma, T., Shinozaki, N., Nashida, T., et al. (1999). The duration of the integrating window in auditory sensory memory. *Electroencephalography and Clinical Neurophysiology. Supplement, 49*, 166–9.

Yabe, H., Sutoh, T., Matsuoka, T., Asai, R., Hiruma, T., Sato, Y., et al. (2005). Transient gamma-band response is dissociated from sensory memory as reflected by MMN. *Neuroscience Letters, 380*(1), 80–2. doi:10.1016/j.neulet.2005.01.019

Yabe, H., Tervaniemi, M., Reinikainen, K., & Näätänen, R. (1997). Temporal window of integration revealed by MMN to sound omission. *NeuroReport, 8*(8), 1971–4.

Yabe, H., Tervaniemi, M., Sinkkonen, J., Huotilainen, M., Ilmoniemi, R. J., & Ntnen, R. (1998). Temporal window of integration of auditory information in the human brain. *Psychophysiology, 35*(5), 615–19.

Yabe, H., Winkler, I., Czigler, I., Koyama, S., Kakigi, R., Sutoh, T., et al. (2001b). Organizing sound sequences in the human brain: the interplay of auditory streaming and temporal integration. *Brain Research, 897*(1), 222–7. doi:10.1016/S0006-8993(01)02224-7

Yago, E., Escera, C., Alho, K., & Giard, M.-H. (2001a). Cerebral mechanisms underlying orienting of attention towards auditory frequency changes. *NeuroReport, 12*(11), 2583–7.

Yago, J. E., Corral, J. M., & Escera, J. C. (2001b). Activation of brain mechanisms of attention switching as a function of auditory frequency change. *NeuroReport, 12*(18), 4093–7.

Yang, F. F., McPherson, B., Shu, H., & Xiao, Y. (2012). Central auditory nervous system dysfunction in infants with non-syndromic cleft lip and/or palate. *International journal of pediatric otorhinolaryngology, 76*(1), 82–9.

Yang, L. H., Wonpat-Borja, A. J., Opler, M. G., & Corcoran, C. M. (2010). Potential stigma associated with inclusion of the psychosis risk syndrome in the DSM-V: An empirical question. *Schizophrenia Research, 120*(1–3), 42–8. doi:10.1016/j.schres.2010.03.012

Ylinen, S., & Kujala, T. (2015). Neuroscience illuminating the influence of auditory or phonological intervention on language-related deficits. *Frontiers in Psychology, 6,* 137. doi:10.3389/fpsyg.2015.00137

Yppärilä, H., Karhu, J., Westerén-Punnonen, S., Musialowicz, T., & Partanen, J. (2002). Evidence of auditory processing during postoperative propofol sedation. *Clinical Neurophysiology, 113*(8), 1357–64. doi:10.1016/S1388-2457(02)00158-X

Yung, A. R., & McGorry, P. D. (1996). The initial prodrome in psychosis: Descriptive and qualitative aspects. *Australian and New Zealand Journal of Psychiatry, 30*(5), 587–99. doi:10.3109/00048679609062654

Zamrini, E., Maestu, F., Pekkonen, E., Funke, M., Makela, J., Riley, M., et al. (2011). Magnetoencephalography as a putative biomarker for Alzheimer's disease. *International Journal of Alzheimer's Disease, 2011.* doi:10.4061/2011/280289

Zhang, F., Benson, C., & J. Cahn, S. (2013). Cortical encoding of timbre changes in cochlear implant users. *Journal of the American Academy of Audiology, 24*(1), 46–58. doi:10.3766/jaaa.24.1.6

Zhang, F., Hammer, T., Banks, H.-L., Benson, C., Xiang, J., & Fu, Q.-J. (2011). Mismatch negativity and adaptation measures of the late auditory evoked potential in cochlear implant users. *Hearing Research, 275*(1), 17–29. doi:10.1016/j.heares.2010.11.007

Zhang, X. L., Cohen, H. L., Porjesz, B., & Begleiter, H. (2001). Mismatch negativity in subjects at high risk for alcoholism. *Alcoholism: Clinical and Experimental Research, 25*(3), 330–7.

Zhang, Z., Lu, G., Zhong, Y., Tan, Q., Liao, W., Chen, Z., et al. (2009). Impaired perceptual networks in temporal lobe epilepsy revealed by resting fMRI. *Journal of Neurology, 256*(10), 1705–13. doi:10.1007/s00415-009-5187-2

Zilbovicius, M., Boddaert, N., Belin, P., Poline, J. B., Remy, P., Mangin, J. F., et al. (2000). Temporal lobe dysfunction in childhood autism: a PET study. Positron emission tomography. *American Journal of Psychiatry, 157*(12), 1988–93.

Zilbovicius, M., Garreau, B., Samson, Y., Remy, P., Barthelemy, C., Syrota, A., & Lelord, G. (1995). Delayed maturation of the frontal cortex in childhood autism. *American Journal of Psychiatry, 152*(2), 248–52.

Zuckerman, M. (1994). An alternative five-factor model for personality. In C. F. K. Halverson, G. A. & R. P. Martin (Eds), *The Developing Structure of Temperament and Personality from Infancy to Adulthood* (pp. 53–68). New York: Lawrence Erlbaum Associates.

Zuckerman, M., & Kuhlman, D. M. (2000). Personality and risk-taking: common bisocial factors. *Journal of Personality, 68*(6), 999–1029.

Zwislocki, J. (1960). Theory of temporal auditory summation. *Journal of the Acoustical Society of America, 32*(8), 1046–60. doi:10.1121/1.1908276

Zwislocki, J., Pirodda, E., & Rubin, H. (1959). On some poststimulatory effects at the threshold of audibility. *Journal of the Acoustical Society of America, 31*(1), 9–14. doi:10.1121/1.1907619

Zwislocki, J. J. (1969). Temporal summation of loudness: an analysis. *Journal of the Acoustical Society of America, 46*(2), 431–41.

Zwislocki, J. J. (1972). A theory of central auditory masking and its partial validation. *Journal of the Acoustical Society of America, 52*(2B), 644–59. doi:10.1121/1.1913154

Author Index

Subject Index